Absolute Risk

Methods and Applications in Clinical Management and Public Health

MONOGRAPHS ON STATISTICS AND APPLIED PROBABILITY

General Editors

F. Bunea, V. Isham, N. Keiding, T. Louis, R. L. Smith, and H. Tong

1. Stochastic Population Models in Ecology and Epidemiology *M.S. Barlett* (1960)
2. Queues *D.R. Cox and W.L. Smith* (1961)
3. Monte Carlo Methods *J.M. Hammersley and D.C. Handscomb* (1964)
4. The Statistical Analysis of Series of Events *D.R. Cox and P.A.W. Lewis* (1966)
5. Population Genetics *W.J. Ewens* (1969)
6. Probability, Statistics and Time *M.S. Barlett* (1975)
7. Statistical Inference *S.D. Silvey* (1975)
8. The Analysis of Contingency Tables *B.S. Everitt* (1977)
9. Multivariate Analysis in Behavioural Research *A.E. Maxwell* (1977)
10. Stochastic Abundance Models *S. Engen* (1978)
11. Some Basic Theory for Statistical Inference *E.J.G. Pitman* (1979)
12. Point Processes *D.R. Cox and V. Isham* (1980)
13. Identification of Outliers *D.M. Hawkins* (1980)
14. Optimal Design *S.D. Silvey* (1980)
15. Finite Mixture Distributions *B.S. Everitt and D.J. Hand* (1981)
16. Classification *A.D. Gordon* (1981)
17. Distribution-Free Statistical Methods, 2nd edition *J.S. Maritz* (1995)
18. Residuals and Influence in Regression *R.D. Cook and S. Weisberg* (1982)
19. Applications of Queueing Theory, 2nd edition *G.F. Newell* (1982)
20. Risk Theory, 3rd edition *R.E. Beard, T. Pentikäinen and E. Pesonen* (1984)
21. Analysis of Survival Data *D.R. Cox and D. Oakes* (1984)
22. An Introduction to Latent Variable Models *B.S. Everitt* (1984)
23. Bandit Problems *D.A. Berry and B. Fristedt* (1985)
24. Stochastic Modelling and Control *M.H.A. Davis and R. Vinter* (1985)
25. The Statistical Analysis of Composition Data *J. Aitchison* (1986)
26. Density Estimation for Statistics and Data Analysis *B.W. Silverman* (1986)
27. Regression Analysis with Applications *G.B. Wetherill* (1986)
28. Sequential Methods in Statistics, 3rd edition *G.B. Wetherill and K.D. Glazebrook* (1986)
29. Tensor Methods in Statistics *P. McCullagh* (1987)
30. Transformation and Weighting in Regression *R.J. Carroll and D. Ruppert* (1988)
31. Asymptotic Techniques for Use in Statistics *O.E. Bandorff-Nielsen and D.R. Cox* (1989)
32. Analysis of Binary Data, 2nd edition *D.R. Cox and E.J. Snell* (1989)
33. Analysis of Infectious Disease Data *N.G. Becker* (1989)
34. Design and Analysis of Cross-Over Trials *B. Jones and M.G. Kenward* (1989)
35. Empirical Bayes Methods, 2nd edition *J.S. Maritz and T. Lwin* (1989)
36. Symmetric Multivariate and Related Distributions *K.T. Fang, S. Kotz and K.W. Ng* (1990)
37. Generalized Linear Models, 2nd edition *P. McCullagh and J.A. Nelder* (1989)
38. Cyclic and Computer Generated Designs, 2nd edition *J.A. John and E.R. Williams* (1995)
39. Analog Estimation Methods in Econometrics *C.F. Manski* (1988)
40. Subset Selection in Regression *A.J. Miller* (1990)
41. Analysis of Repeated Measures *M.J. Crowder and D.J. Hand* (1990)
42. Statistical Reasoning with Imprecise Probabilities *P. Walley* (1991)
43. Generalized Additive Models *T.J. Hastie and R.J. Tibshirani* (1990)
44. Inspection Errors for Attributes in Quality Control *N.L. Johnson, S. Kotz and X. Wu* (1991)
45. The Analysis of Contingency Tables, 2nd edition *B.S. Everitt* (1992)
46. The Analysis of Quantal Response Data *B.J.T. Morgan* (1992)
47. Longitudinal Data with Serial Correlation—A State-Space Approach *R.H. Jones* (1993)

48. Differential Geometry and Statistics *M.K. Murray and J.W. Rice* (1993)
49. Markov Models and Optimization *M.H.A. Davis* (1993)
50. Networks and Chaos—Statistical and Probabilistic Aspects
O.E. Barndorff-Nielsen, J.L. Jensen and W.S. Kendall (1993)
51. Number-Theoretic Methods in Statistics *K.-T. Fang and Y. Wang* (1994)
52. Inference and Asymptotics *O.E. Barndorff-Nielsen and D.R. Cox* (1994)
53. Practical Risk Theory for Actuaries *C.D. Daykin, T. Pentikäinen and M. Pesonen* (1994)
54. Biplots *J.C. Gower and D.J. Hand* (1996)
55. Predictive Inference—An Introduction *S. Geisser* (1993)
56. Model-Free Curve Estimation *M.E. Tarter and M.D. Lock* (1993)
57. An Introduction to the Bootstrap *B. Efron and R.J. Tibshirani* (1993)
58. Nonparametric Regression and Generalized Linear Models *P.J. Green and B.W. Silverman* (1994)
59. Multidimensional Scaling *T.F. Cox and M.A.A. Cox* (1994)
60. Kernel Smoothing *M.P. Wand and M.C. Jones* (1995)
61. Statistics for Long Memory Processes *J. Beran* (1995)
62. Nonlinear Models for Repeated Measurement Data *M. Davidian and D.M. Giltinan* (1995)
63. Measurement Error in Nonlinear Models *R.J. Carroll, D. Rupert and L.A. Stefanski* (1995)
64. Analyzing and Modeling Rank Data *J.J. Marden* (1995)
65. Time Series Models—In Econometrics, Finance and Other Fields
D.R. Cox, D.V. Hinkley and O.E. Barndorff-Nielsen (1996)
66. Local Polynomial Modeling and its Applications *J. Fan and I. Gijbels* (1996)
67. Multivariate Dependencies—Models, Analysis and Interpretation *D.R. Cox and N. Wermuth* (1996)
68. Statistical Inference—Based on the Likelihood *A. Azzalini* (1996)
69. Bayes and Empirical Bayes Methods for Data Analysis *B.P. Carlin and T.A Louis* (1996)
70. Hidden Markov and Other Models for Discrete-Valued Time Series *I.L. MacDonald and W. Zucchini* (1997)
71. Statistical Evidence—A Likelihood Paradigm *R. Royall* (1997)
72. Analysis of Incomplete Multivariate Data *J.L. Schafer* (1997)
73. Multivariate Models and Dependence Concepts *H. Joe* (1997)
74. Theory of Sample Surveys *M.E. Thompson* (1997)
75. Retrial Queues *G. Falin and J.G.C. Templeton* (1997)
76. Theory of Dispersion Models *B. Jørgensen* (1997)
77. Mixed Poisson Processes *J. Grandell* (1997)
78. Variance Components Estimation—Mixed Models, Methodologies and Applications *P.S.R.S. Rao* (1997)
79. Bayesian Methods for Finite Population Sampling *G. Meeden and M. Ghosh* (1997)
80. Stochastic Geometry—Likelihood and computation
O.E. Barndorff-Nielsen, W.S. Kendall and M.N.M. van Lieshout (1998)
81. Computer-Assisted Analysis of Mixtures and Applications—Meta-Analysis, Disease Mapping and Others
D. Böhning (1999)
82. Classification, 2nd edition *A.D. Gordon* (1999)
83. Semimartingales and their Statistical Inference *B.L.S. Prakasa Rao* (1999)
84. Statistical Aspects of BSE and vCJD—Models for Epidemics *C.A. Donnelly and N.M. Ferguson* (1999)
85. Set-Indexed Martingales *G. Ivanoff and E. Merzbach* (2000)
86. The Theory of the Design of Experiments *D.R. Cox and N. Reid* (2000)
87. Complex Stochastic Systems *O.E. Barndorff-Nielsen, D.R. Cox and C. Klüppelberg* (2001)
88. Multidimensional Scaling, 2nd edition *T.F. Cox and M.A.A. Cox* (2001)
89. Algebraic Statistics—Computational Commutative Algebra in Statistics
G. Pistone, E. Riccomagno and H.P. Wynn (2001)
90. Analysis of Time Series Structure—SSA and Related Techniques
N. Golyandina, V. Nekrutkin and A.A. Zhigljavsky (2001)
91. Subjective Probability Models for Lifetimes *Fabio Spizzichino* (2001)
92. Empirical Likelihood *Art B. Owen* (2001)
93. Statistics in the 21st Century *Adrian E. Raftery, Martin A. Tanner, and Martin T. Wells* (2001)
94. Accelerated Life Models: Modeling and Statistical Analysis
Vilijandas Bagdonavicius and Mikhail Nikulin (2001)

95. Subset Selection in Regression, Second Edition *Alan Miller* (2002)
96. Topics in Modelling of Clustered Data *Marc Aerts, Helena Geys, Geert Molenberghs, and Louise M. Ryan* (2002)
97. Components of Variance *D.R. Cox and P.J. Solomon* (2002)
98. Design and Analysis of Cross-Over Trials, 2nd Edition *Byron Jones and Michael G. Kenward* (2003)
99. Extreme Values in Finance, Telecommunications, and the Environment *Bärbel Finkenstädt and Holger Rootzén* (2003)
100. Statistical Inference and Simulation for Spatial Point Processes *Jesper Møller and Rasmus Plenge Waagepetersen* (2004)
101. Hierarchical Modeling and Analysis for Spatial Data *Sudipto Banerjee, Bradley P. Carlin, and Alan E. Gelfand* (2004)
102. Diagnostic Checks in Time Series *Wai Keung Li* (2004)
103. Stereology for Statisticians *Adrian Baddeley and Eva B. Vedel Jensen* (2004)
104. Gaussian Markov Random Fields: Theory and Applications *Håvard Rue and Leonhard Held* (2005)
105. Measurement Error in Nonlinear Models: A Modern Perspective, Second Edition *Raymond J. Carroll, David Ruppert, Leonard A. Stefanski, and Ciprian M. Crainiceanu* (2006)
106. Generalized Linear Models with Random Effects: Unified Analysis via H-likelihood *Youngjo Lee, John A. Nelder, and Yudi Pawitan* (2006)
107. Statistical Methods for Spatio-Temporal Systems *Bärbel Finkenstädt, Leonhard Held, and Valerie Isham* (2007)
108. Nonlinear Time Series: Semiparametric and Nonparametric Methods *Jiti Gao* (2007)
109. Missing Data in Longitudinal Studies: Strategies for Bayesian Modeling and Sensitivity Analysis *Michael J. Daniels and Joseph W. Hogan* (2008)
110. Hidden Markov Models for Time Series: An Introduction Using R *Walter Zucchini and Iain L. MacDonald* (2009)
111. ROC Curves for Continuous Data *Wojtek J. Krzanowski and David J. Hand* (2009)
112. Antedependence Models for Longitudinal Data *Dale L. Zimmerman and Vicente A. Núñez-Antón* (2009)
113. Mixed Effects Models for Complex Data *Lang Wu* (2010)
114. Intoduction to Time Series Modeling *Genshiro Kitagawa* (2010)
115. Expansions and Asymptotics for Statistics *Christopher G. Small* (2010)
116. Statistical Inference: An Integrated Bayesian/Likelihood Approach *Murray Aitkin* (2010)
117. Circular and Linear Regression: Fitting Circles and Lines by Least Squares *Nikolai Chernov* (2010)
118. Simultaneous Inference in Regression *Wei Liu* (2010)
119. Robust Nonparametric Statistical Methods, Second Edition *Thomas P. Hettmansperger and Joseph W. McKean* (2011)
120. Statistical Inference: The Minimum Distance Approach *Ayanendranath Basu, Hiroyuki Shioya, and Chanseok Park* (2011)
121. Smoothing Splines: Methods and Applications *Yuedong Wang* (2011)
122. Extreme Value Methods with Applications to Finance *Serguei Y. Novak* (2012)
123. Dynamic Prediction in Clinical Survival Analysis *Hans C. van Houwelingen and Hein Putter* (2012)
124. Statistical Methods for Stochastic Differential Equations *Mathieu Kessler, Alexander Lindner, and Michael Sørensen* (2012)
125. Maximum Likelihood Estimation for Sample Surveys *R. L. Chambers, D. G. Steel, Suojin Wang, and A. H. Welsh* (2012)
126. Mean Field Simulation for Monte Carlo Integration *Pierre Del Moral* (2013)
127. Analysis of Variance for Functional Data *Jin-Ting Zhang* (2013)
128. Statistical Analysis of Spatial and Spatio-Temporal Point Patterns, Third Edition *Peter J. Diggle* (2013)
129. Constrained Principal Component Analysis and Related Techniques *Yoshio Takane* (2014)
130. Randomised Response-Adaptive Designs in Clinical Trials *Anthony C. Atkinson and Atanu Biswas* (2014)
131. Theory of Factorial Design: Single- and Multi-Stratum Experiments *Ching-Shui Cheng* (2014)
132. Quasi-Least Squares Regression *Justine Shults and Joseph M. Hilbe* (2014)
133. Data Analysis and Approximate Models: Model Choice, Location-Scale, Analysis of Variance, Nonparametric Regression and Image Analysis *Laurie Davies* (2014)
134. Dependence Modeling with Copulas *Harry Joe* (2014)
135. Hierarchical Modeling and Analysis for Spatial Data, Second Edition *Sudipto Banerjee, Bradley P. Carlin, and Alan E. Gelfand* (2014)

136. Sequential Analysis: Hypothesis Testing and Changepoint Detection *Alexander Tartakovsky, Igor Nikiforov, and Michèle Basseville* (2015)
137. Robust Cluster Analysis and Variable Selection *Gunter Ritter* (2015)
138. Design and Analysis of Cross-Over Trials, Third Edition *Byron Jones and Michael G. Kenward* (2015)
139. Introduction to High-Dimensional Statistics *Christophe Giraud* (2015)
140. Pareto Distributions: Second Edition *Barry C. Arnold* (2015)
141. Bayesian Inference for Partially Identified Models: Exploring the Limits of Limited Data *Paul Gustafson* (2015)
142. Models for Dependent Time Series *Granville Tunnicliffe Wilson, Marco Reale, John Haywood* (2015)
143. Statistical Learning with Sparsity: The Lasso and Generalizations *Trevor Hastie, Robert Tibshirani, and Martin Wainwright* (2015)
144. Measuring Statistical Evidence Using Relative Belief *Michael Evans* (2015)
145. Stochastic Analysis for Gaussian Random Processes and Fields: With Applications *Vidyadhar S. Mandrekar and Leszek Gawarecki* (2015)
146. Semialgebraic Statistics and Latent Tree Models *Piotr Zwiernik* (2015)
147. Inferential Models: Reasoning with Uncertainty *Ryan Martin and Chuanhai Liu* (2016)
148. Perfect Simulation *Mark L. Huber* (2016)
149. State-Space Methods for Time Series Analysis: Theory, Applications and Software
Jose Casals, Alfredo Garcia-Hiernaux, Miguel Jerez, Sonia Sotoca, and A. Alexandre Trindade (2016)
150. Hidden Markov Models for Time Series: An Introduction Using R, Second Edition
Walter Zucchini, Iain L. MacDonald, and Roland Langrock (2016)
151. Joint Modeling of Longitudinal and Time-to-Event Data
Robert M. Elashoff, Gang Li, and Ning Li (2016)
152. Multi-State Survival Models for Interval-Censored Data
Ardo van den Hout (2016)
153. Generalized Linear Models with Random Effects: Unified Analysis via H-likelihood, Second Edition
Youngjo Lee, John A. Nelder, and Yudi Pawitan (2017)
154. Absolute Risk: Methods and Applications in Clinical Management and Public Health
Ruth M. Pfeiffer and Mitchell H. Gail (2017)

Monographs on Statistics and Applied Probability 154

Absolute Risk

Methods and Applications in Clinical Management and Public Health

Ruth M. Pfeiffer
National Cancer Institute
Rockville, Maryland, USA

Mitchell H. Gail
National Cancer Institute
Rockville, Maryland, USA

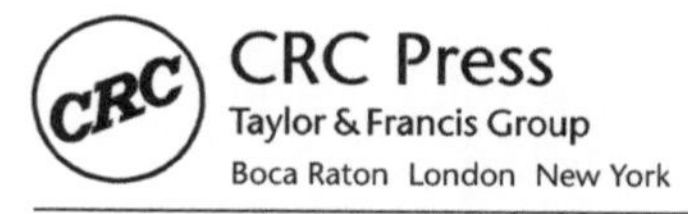
CRC Press
Taylor & Francis Group
Boca Raton London New York

CRC Press is an imprint of the
Taylor & Francis Group, an **informa** business
A CHAPMAN & HALL BOOK

CRC Press
Taylor & Francis Group
6000 Broken Sound Parkway NW, Suite 300
Boca Raton, FL 33487-2742

First issued in paperback 2020

Published in 2018 by Taylor & Francis Group, LLC
CRC Press is an imprint of Taylor & Francis Group, an Informa business

ISBN-13: 978-1-4665-6165-6 (hbk)
ISBN-13: 978-0-367-65781-9 (pbk)

Library of Congress Cataloging-in-Publication Data

Names: Pfeiffer, Ruth M., author. | Gail, Mitchell H., author.
Title: Absolute risk : methods and applications in clinical management and public health / Ruth M. Pfeiffer, Mitchell M. Gail.
Description: Boca Raton : Taylor & Francis, a CRC title, part of the Taylor & Francis imprint, a member of the Taylor & Francis Group, the academic division of T&F Informa plc, 2017. |
Series: Chapman & Hall/CRC monographs on statistics & applied probability | Includes bibliographical references.
Identifiers: LCCN 2017011272| ISBN 9781466561656 (hardback) | ISBN 9781466561687 (pdf).
Subjects: LCSH: Health risk assessment--Popular works. | Public health—Risk assessment.
Classification: LCC RA427.3 .P45 2017 | DDC 362.1--dc23
LC record available at https://lccn.loc.gov/2017011272

Visit the Taylor & Francis Web site at
http://www.taylorandfrancis.com

and the CRC Press Web site at
http://www.crcpress.com

Contents

List of Figures

List of Tables

Symbols

Symbol Description

Symbol	Description
$\alpha_{ij}(t)$	Transition rate from state i to j in a multi-state model
$AR(t)$	Attributable risk for age group t
AUC	Area under the ROC curve or the probability that a randomly selected case has a risk greater than that of a randomly selected non-case
$\boldsymbol{\beta}$	Parameters such as log relative hazards for cause-specific hazard models
C	Censoring time (with distribution 1-G)
C_{FN}	Cost of a false negative outcome
C_{FP}	Cost of a false positive outcome
C_{TN}	Cost of a true negative outcome
C_{TP}	Cost of a true positive outcome
D	Disease indicator is 1 for case, 0 for non-case in case-control data
$\delta(t)$	Event indicator at time t. Absent competing risks, $\delta(t) = 1$ if $T \leq C$. With competing risks, the process $\delta(t)$ indicates which of the competing events occurred at or before t and is 0 if none occurred.
$\Delta_i(\cdot)$	Influence deviate operator for individual i
$\vec{E}(\boldsymbol{\beta}_m, t)$	Expected covariate value in risk set at at time t, $\frac{\sum_{i=1}^{n} Y_i(t)\exp(\boldsymbol{\beta}'_m \mathbf{Z}_i^m)\mathbf{Z}_i^m}{\sum_{i=1}^{n} Y_i(t)\exp(\boldsymbol{\beta}'_m \mathbf{Z}_i^m)}$
$\mathcal{E}(\hat{\boldsymbol{\beta}}_m)$	Observed information from the partial likelihood
$F(\cdot)$	Distribution function either of population absolute risks, or in other contexts, of survival times
$f(t)$	Density of distribution $F(\cdot)$, including survival distributions
FP	False positive probability, $P(R > r^*\vert O = 0)$, i.e., 1-specificity
$g\{r_m(t)\}$	Link function for cumulative incidence regression
$\mathbf{G}$	Joint genotypes in a family
$G(\cdot)$	Distribution of absolute risk in cases, $P(R \leq r\vert O = 1)$; also used as distribution of censoring times
$\boldsymbol{\gamma}$	Parameters such as log relative sub-distrbution hazards for cumulative incidence regression
$h_m(t, \mathbf{Z})$	Hazard of the sub-distribution function for cumulative incidence regression for cause m
$K(\cdot)$	Distribution of absolute risk in non-cases, $P(R \leq r\vert O = 0)$
$\lambda(t)$	Hazard for a survival distribution
$\lambda_m(t)$	Cause-specific hazard for cause m
$\lambda_{0m}(t)$	Cause-specific baseline hazard for cause m
$\lambda_m^*(t)$	Composite hazard for cause m in a population with various combinations of covariates
$\lambda_m^p(t)$	Pure or net hazard for cause m
$\Lambda(t)$	Cumulative hazard for a survival distribution
$\Lambda_m(t)$	Cumulative cause-specific hazard for cause m
$\Lambda_{0m}(t)$	Cumulative cause-specific baseline hazard for cause m
$N_i(t)$	The counting process, $I(X_i \leq t, \delta_i = 1), t \geq 0$ for individual i
$N(t)$	The aggregate counting process, $\sum_{i=1}^{n} N_i(t)$
$NB(t)$	Net benefit function
NPV	Negative predictive value

NRI	Net reclassification improvement
O_i	Indicator of whether the cause of interest occurred in individual i or not
π	Prior probability of of disease
$PCF(p)$	Proportion of cases followed, $1 - G \circ F^{-1}(1-p)$
$iPCF(p^*)$	Weighted integral of $PCF(p)$ from p^* to 1.
PMC	Probability of misclassification
$PNF(q)$	Proportion needed to follow, $1 - F \circ G^{-1}(1-q)$
$iPNF(q^*)$	Weighted integral of $PNF(q)$ from q^* to 1.
PPV	Positive predictive value
$r_m(t_0, t_1)$	Absolute risk of cause m, $P(t_0 < T \leq t_1, \delta(T) = m \mid T \geq t_0)$
$r_m(t_0, t_1; \mathbf{z})$	Absolute risk of cause m given covariates, $P(t_0 < T \leq t_1, \delta = m \mid T \geq t_0, \mathbf{z})$
R_i	Estimated absolute risk for individual i
r^*	Risk threshold
$RCC(t)$	Relative cost curve; analogous to relative utility curve
ROC	Receiver operating characteristic curve, namely plot of TP against FP as the threshold varies
$S(t)$	Survival distribution, $P(T > t) = 1 - F(t)$
$sens(t)$	Sensitivity at threshold t, $P(R > t \mid O = 1)$
S_g	Subgroup of a partition for assessing calibration of the individuals in a population
$spec(t)$	Specificity at threshold t, $P(R \leq t \mid O = 0)$
T	Time to an event
TP	True positive probability or sensitivity, $P(R > r^* \mid O = 1)$
$\vec{U}(\boldsymbol{\beta}_m)$	Score contribution at time t from partial likelihood, $\sum_{i=1}^{n} dN_{mi}(t)\{\mathbf{z}_i^m - \vec{E}(\boldsymbol{\beta}_m, t_i)\}$
X	Time to the earlier of event or censoring
$\mathbf{X}$	Covariates in model to which additional covariates are to be added
$\mathbf{Y}$	Joint phenotypes of family members
$Y_i(t)$	At risk indicator at time t for individual i
$Y(t)$	Number at risk at time t, $\sum_{i=1}^{n} Y_i(t)$
t^*	Risk threshold for decision
$\mathbf{Z}$	Covariates that affect any of the competing causes
$\mathbf{Z}^m$	Covariates that affect cause m

Preface

This book provides a theoretical basis and examples to demonstrate the importance of absolute disease risk in counseling patients, in devising public health strategies, and in clinical management. We wrote this book for epidemiologists, clinicians, and statisticians, with sufficient technical detail to allow others to estimate, test, and use models of absolute risk, and with a range of examples to inspire broader application of the models. The development and proper use of absolute risk models requires a collaborative effort to identify a good application, to gather the required clinical or epidemiologic data, and to build and test the model on sound statistical principles. This book is broad enough to inform the various research participants needed for such a collaboration.

Dr. Mitchell Gail's interest in absolute risk arose during a consultation with Dr. John J. Mulvihill, who was counseling women at elevated risk of breast cancer and observed that many women greatly overestimated their risk. Dr. Mulvihill's desire to obtain realistic estimates grew into a collaboration involving epidemiologists and statisticians at the National Cancer Institute, National Institutes of Health, that led to the "Gail" model, published in 1989, to project breast cancer risk based on an analysis that took competing risks into account. The U.S. National Cancer Institute's Breast Cancer Risk Assessment Tool (BCRAT) incorporates updates to that model. Dr. Gail and Dr. Ruth Pfeiffer have continued to pursue research on methods for estimating and evaluating absolute risk models, taking advantage of many advances made by the statistical community in survival analysis and in understanding how epidemiologic data and analyses fit into a general modeling framework. They have also promoted applications of risk models. For example, the Gail model was useful in designing and interpreting a clinical trial of tamoxifen to prevent breast cancer. The model was used to plan the study and decide who should be eligible. After the trial, the model gave a means to weigh risks and benefits for deciding who might benefit from tamoxifen chemoprevention. Likewise, risk models can be used to stratify the population into those who might most benefit from screening or from high risk interventions. Dr. Pfeiffer led the development of criteria to evaluate the public health impact of such applications.

There are several excellent books on survival methods for modeling pure risk of disease, with most applications concerning prognosis following a disease diagnosis. Four books have recently appeared that account for competing risks and elaborate on theoretical aspects of absolute risk, sometimes called cumulative incidence. Again, most of the applications concern prognosis. The present book adds to this literature on absolute risk in several respects. In addition to presenting the theoretical background for absolute risk, including a treatment of competing risks, this book: (1) discusses various sampling designs for estimating absolute risk and for estimating criteria to evaluate models; (2) provides details on statistical inference, including construction of confidence intervals, for the various sampling designs; (3) discusses criteria for evaluating risk models and for comparing risk models, including both general criteria and problem-specific expected losses in well-defined clinical and public health applications; and (4) describes a wealth of applications, encompassing both disease prevention and prognosis, and ranging from counseling individual patients, to clinical decision making, to assessing the impact of risk-based public health strategies.

Much of the material in this book is based on work with others. While it is not possible to name all who helped shape our ideas, we particularly want to thank the following collaborators who have contributed to several aspects of this work including Jacques Bénichou, David P. Byar, Raymond J. Carroll, Nilanjan Chatterjee, Jinbo Chen, Joseph P. Costantino, Andrew N. Freedman, Laurence S. Freedman, Barry I. Graubard, Sylvan B. Green, Stephanie Kovalchik, Ju-Hyun Park, David Pee, Elisabetta Petracci, and Catherine Schairer. We thank the Intramural Research Program of the Division of Cancer Epidemiology and Genetics, National Cancer Institute, National Institutes of Health, for sustained support for research on absolute risk and for the writing of this book, and David Check for help with figures, tables, and bibliography. We also thank John Kimmel at Chapman and Hall for his advice and help.

We dedicate this book to our parents, Irving and Ada Gail, and Franz and Liselotte Pfeiffer.

Chapter 1

Introduction

A 40-year-old woman visits her doctor and is reassured to learn that her mammogram gave no indication of breast cancer. However, her mother had breast cancer diagnosed at age 60. The woman asks: "What is the chance that I will have a diagnosis of breast cancer by age 60?" The answer to this question is an estimate of her *absolute risk* of breast cancer over a defined age interval. Several features of this question are important. First, her chance of being diagnosed with breast cancer is reduced by the possibility that she will die of some cause unrelated to breast cancer before age 60. Thus, competing causes of mortality need to be taken into account to answer this question. Second, the chance of being diagnosed with breast cancer depends on the duration of the risk projection interval, in this case the 20 years from age 40 to age 60. The longer the projection interval, the higher is the absolute risk. Third, the absolute risk depends on the age of the woman when she came to her doctor for counseling. This is because the incidence rate of breast cancer increases with age, as do mortality rates from competing causes of death. Finally, risk factors present at the time of counseling influence the estimate of absolute risk. In this example, the fact that the woman's mother had had breast cancer increases the estimate of her absolute risk.

The previous example concerned the absolute risk of developing a disease, breast cancer. Absolute risk is also a clinically useful parameter after a disease has been diagnosed. For example, suppose a 70-year-old male is diagnosed with prostate cancer, and the histopathology ("Gleason score") from the biopsy is favorable. The absolute risk that the man will die from prostate cancer may be quite small even with conservative management (Albertsen et al., 2005), in part because many such men will die of other causes before the prostate cancer progresses. Thus, an estimate of absolute risk may be helpful in deciding whether more aggressive treatments, such as surgery or radiation, are warranted.

The literature on competing risks sometimes uses other words for the concept of absolute risk. "Crude risk" (Gail, 1975; Tsiatis, 2005), "marginal probability" (Pepe and Mori, 1993), and "cumulative incidence" (Gray, 1988) are three such terms, although "cumulative incidence" is also sometimes used to denote the cumulative "pure" (Gail, 1975) risk or the integrated cause-specific hazard (Andersen et al., 1993). Absolute risk should not be confused with "pure" risk, which is the hypothetical probability of the event (e.g., breast cancer) if other competing causes of mortality could be eliminated. In contrast to absolute risk, *pure risk* is not estimable without strong assumptions (Gail, 1975; Tsiatis, 1975; Prentice et al., 1978). Pure risk is also less relevant for many clinical decisions, because in fact the patient will be subject to mortality from competing risks. Absolute risk is also different from *relative risk*, which is the ratio of risk for a person with one set of characteristics to the risk for a reference person, who is often chosen to have all risk factors set to their lowest (baseline) levels.

Although relative risks are useful for assessing the strength of risk factors, they are not nearly as useful as absolute risks for making clinical decisions or establishing policies for disease prevention. Such decisions or policies often weigh the favorable effects of an intervention on the health outcomes of interest against the unfavorable effects that the intervention might have on other health outcomes. The common currency for such decisions is the (possibly weighted) absolute risk for each of the health outcomes in the presence and absence of intervention.

The following sections of this introduction give examples of widely used risk models and some of their special features, discuss applications of absolute risk models in disease prevention and prognostication following disease onset, and outline the contents and structure of the book.

1.1 Examples of risk models for disease incidence

1.1.1 Breast cancer incidence

1.1.1.1 A brief survey of models

Several models are available for projecting the risk of breast cancer, as previously reviewed (Amir et al., 2010; Gail and Mai, 2010). Some of these models are based only on age and detailed family history, such as the model of Claus et al. (1994). Two other such models,"BRCAPRO" (Berry et al., 1997; Chen and Parmigiani, 2007) and "BOADICEA" (Antoniou et al., 2008a), also allow one to include information on the status of BRCA1 or BRCA2 mutations that greatly increase cancer risk. Other models, such as the National Cancer Institute's Breast Cancer Risk Assessment Tool (BCRAT)(Gail et al., 1989; Costantino et al., 1999; Gail et al., 2007; Matsuno et al., 2011), which is sometimes called the "Gail model", and "IBIS" (Tyrer et al., 2005), which is sometimes called the "Tyrer–Cuzick model", include factors in addition to family history, such as results of biopsies, and age at first live birth. IBIS also includes information on BRCA1 and BRCA1 mutation carrier status. The invasive breast cancer absolute risk model BC2013 (Pfeiffer et al., 2013), that we discuss later in the book, includes potentially modifiable risk factors, such as hormone replacement therapy, alcohol use, and body mass index, as does the model of age-specific incidence by Colditz and Rosner (2000).

A more detailed summary of the risk factors in some of these models is provided in Table 1.1. The variation in choice of risk factors is noteworthy. Other differences are also depicted. BOADICEA and IBIS are calibrated to breast cancer rates in England and Wales, whereas the Claus model and BCRAT are calibrated to age-specific breast cancer incidence rates from the National Cancer Institute's Surveillance, Epidmiology and End Results (SEER) Program. Rates in England and Wales are 5–25% lower than SEER rates in women over age 55 years. Not all the models account for the effects of competing causes of mortality in projecting breast cancer risk. Although the effects of competing risks are small for short-term projections, such as 5 years, lifetime projections or 20-year projections of absolute risk can be reduced appreciably by competing mortality. Other differences include the detailed approaches to model building and the quality and coherence of the types of data that went into these models.

With the exception of studies on BCRAT, there is a paucity of independent validation data to determine how well these models are calibrated and how effective they are at discriminating women who will eventually develop breast cancer from those who will not. BCRAT is thought to be well calibrated for use in the general U.S. population. Some models that include more information on family history and BRCA1 or BCRA2 mutation status are widely used in high-risk clinics for women with strong family histories of breast cancer. Thus, one needs to think carefully about the intended application before choosing a model (Amir et al., 2010; Gail and Mai, 2010). In addition to the primary publications, helpful information is available at the following web sites: for BRCAPRO, http://bcb.dfci.harvard.edu/bayesmendel/brcapro.php; for BOADICEA, http://ccge.medschl.cam.ac.uk/boadicea/web-application/; for IBIS, http://www.ems-trials.org/riskevaluator/; and for BCRAT, http://www.cancer.gov/bcrisktool/

Table 1.1: Features of several models to project absolute or pure risk of breast cancer in women without a previous breast cancer diagnosis

Model	**Claus**	**BRCAPRO**	**BOADICEA**	**IBIS**	**BCRAT**
Risk Factors*					
Family history of breast cancer in relative	Ages at onset in 1st, 2nd degree	Ages at onset in 1st, 2nd degree; ovarian cancer; bilateral; male breast cancer	Ages at onset in 1st, 2nd, 3rd degree; ovarian cancer; bilateral; male breast cancer	Ages at onset in 1st, 2nd degree; ovarian cancer, bilateral	Number of 1st degree relatives with breast cancer
Previous breast disease				Atypical hyperplasia; LCIS	Number of biopsies; atypical hyperplasia
Hormonal factors				Age at menarche; age at first live birth; age at menopause; oral contraceptive use	Age at menarche; age at first live birth
BRCA1, BRCA2		Included	Included	Included	
Other				Body mass index	
Exclusions*	Absence of affected 1st degree relatives				LCIS; DCIS; BRCA1 or BRCA2 mutation**
Accounts for competing mortality	No	Yes	No	Default is no, but optional	Yes
Calibrated to incidence in	SEER	Meta-analysis for BRCA1 or BRCA2 carriers; SEER for non-carriers	England/ Wales	England/ Wales	SEER

*All models include age; all models exclude patients with previous breast cancer.
**Other methods to project risk are more appropriate for women with previous radiation therapy to the chest for the treatment of Hodgkin lymphoma, for women with certain other mutations, and for women who have recently immigrated to the United States from regions of Asia where breast cancer risk is low. Further, BCRAT may not be appropriate for women living outside the United States. BCRAT risk calculations assume that a woman is screened for breast cancer as in the general U.S. population. A woman who does not have mammograms will have somewhat lower chances of a diagnosis of breast cancer. Abbreviations: LCIS=Lobular carcinoma *in situ* ; DCIS=ductal carcimoma *in situ*; SEER= Surveillance, Epidemiology and End Results Program of the U.S. National Cancer Institute.

gives a description and risk projection for the online user, whereas http://dceg.cancer.gov/bb gives links to SAS programs and other programs to perform BCRAT calcuations more flexibly.

1.1.1.2 The National Cancer Institute's (NCI's) Breast Cancer Risk Assessment Tool, BCRAT

In this section we describe how BCRAT was developed and updated, some of its features, and efforts to test its calibration and discriminatory accuracy. BCRAT was originally derived from data from the Breast Cancer Detection Demonstration Project (BCDDP), which was designed to encourage women to be screened with mammography to detect breast cancer. From 1973 to 1975, over 280,000 women volunteered for the initial screening mammography, and many were followed with annual mammography for 4 subsequent years. Some prevalent cancers were detected at the time of the initial mammographic screen, but incident invasive and *in situ* cancers detected during follow-up formed the basis of a case-control study of white women. Data from 2,852 women with breast cancer (cases) and 3,146 controls yielded estimates of the relative risks of breast cancer that were associated with risk factors such as age at menarche, age at first live birth, numbers of previous biopsies that yielded benign histology, and number of mother or sisters with a previous diagnosis of breast cancer. Table 1.2 describes the coding and estimated relative risks for these risk factors based on analyses in Gail et al. (1989). The combined relative risk, compared to a woman at the lowest risk level of each factor, is given by multiplying factors A,B,C, and D in Table 1.2 that correspond to the various risk factors (see footnote to Table 1.2). For example, a 40-year-old nulliparous white woman who began menstruating at age 14 years (A=1), who has had no biopsies (B=1 and D=1), and whose sister had breast cancer (C=2.76) has an overall relative risk of $1.00 \times 1.00 \times 2.76 \times 1.00 = 2.76$.

To convert relative risks to absolute risks, Gail et al. (1989) combined information on relative risks with age-specific breast cancer incidence rates estimated from 243,211 white women followed in BCDDP and with national mortality rates from non-breast cancer competing causes of mortality. A key step was determining the baseline age-specific incidence rate for a woman with all risk factors at their lowest levels. The baseline incidence rate was estimated by multiplying the age-specific BCDDP breast cancer rates, which represent women with various risk factor combinations, times {1-AR(t)}, where AR(t) is the age-specific attributable risk at age t. The conversion factor {1-AR(t)} estimates the reciprocal of the average relative risk among those age t in the population. Gail et al. (1989) estimated this factor from cases in the case-control study, using a formula of Bruzzi et al. (1985). Chapters 4 and 5 show how the baseline incidence rates and relative risks for breast cancer can be combined with national mortality rates to compute absolute risk.

The resulting absolute risk model is referred to as "Gail Model 1" by Costantino et al. (1999). Statisticians at the National Surgical Adjuvant Breast and Bowel Project (NSABP) modified Gail Model 1 by substituting age-specific invasive breast cancer incidence rates from the National Cancer Institute's Surveillance, Epidemiology and End Results (SEER) Program for BCDDP incidence rates and by modifying the estimate of AR(t) accordingly, but not the relative risks, to produce "Gail Model 2," as described in the Appendix to Costantino et al. (1999). Unless otherwise noted, we refer hereafter only to Gail Model 2, which is incorporated in BCRAT. Estimates of absolute breast cancer risk from Gail Model 2 (i.e., BCRAT) can vary considerably, depending on the woman's age at counseling, her risk factors, and the age interval for the risk projection. For example, the projected 5-year risk for the previously described 40-year-old nulliparous woman is 1%, but her risk to age 90 is 17%. A 60-year-old woman who began menstruating at age 11, had her first child at age 25, has had a breast biopsy with atypical hyperplasia, and whose mother had breast cancer has a 5-year risk of 7%, and a risk to age 90 of 31%. Chapter 5 describes how to estimate

Table 1.2: Relative risk calculations for the Breast Cancer Risk Assessment Tool (BCRAT)

Risk factor		**Relative risk for each factor or combination of factors**
A. Age at menarche (years)		
≥ 14		1.00 (ref)
12-13		1.10
< 12		1.21
B. Number of breast biopsies		
Age at counseling < 50 years		
0		1.00 (ref)
1		1.70
≥ 2		2.88
Age at counseling ≥ 50 years		
0		1.00 (ref)
1		1.27
≥ 2		1.62
C. Age at first live birth (years)	**Number of mother/sisters with breast cancer**	
< 20	0	1.00 (ref)
	1	2.61
	≥ 2	6.80
20-24	0	1.24
	1	2.68
	≥ 2	5.78
25-29 or nulliparous	0	1.55
	1	2.76
	≥ 2	4.91
≥ 30	0	1.93
	1	2.83
	≥ 2	4.17
D. Atypical hyperplasia (AH)		
No biopsies		1.00 (ref)
At least one biopsy and no AH on found on any biopsy		0.93
No AH found and AH status unknown for at least one biopsy		1.00
AH found on at least one biopsy		1.82

To compute the overall relative risk, multiply the four component relative risks from categories A, B, C, and D. For example, a 40-year-old nulliparous woman who began menstruating at 14, who has had no biopsies, and whose sister had breast cancer has an overall relative risk of $1.00 \times 1.00 \times 2.76 \times 1.00 = 2.76$.

absolute risk by combining relative and attributable risks from case-control or cohort data with registry data on incidence rates and mortality rates, as was done to produce BCRAT.

The fact that women with previous breast biopsies with hyperplasia and a strong family history of breast cancer are at much higher risk than women without these factors can influence clinical management and preventive efforts. However, before such actions are taken on the basis of a risk model, one should have evidence that the model yields valid predictions, ideally by evaluating the model in independent data from the data used to develop the model (Harrell, 2001; Steyerberg, 2009; van Houwelingen and Putter, 2012). One of the most important criteria to be satisfied is that the model be well *calibrated.* As described in detail in Chapter 6, a model is said to be well calibrated if the ratio of events observed in the independent validation data to the number of events expected based on the model is near 1.0. This ratio should be near 1.0 not only for the entire validation cohort, but in various subsets defined by combinations of risk factors and by levels of projected risk.

One cause of poor calibration is "over-fitting" that can arise when the data are fitted to many covariates, some of which may have been selected on the basis of preliminary univariate analyses on the same data. Methods to ameliorate this problem have been described (Copas, 1987; van Houwelingen, 2000, 2001; Harrell, 2001; Steyerberg et al., 2004; Steyerberg, 2009; van Houwelingen and Putter, 2012). Systematic errors can also lead to poor calibration. For example, BCRAT is not appropriate for women who have had a previous breast cancer, women who have had a previous diagnosis of certain breast lesions (lobular carcinoma *in situ* or ductal carcinoma *in situ*), women known to have strong genetic predispositions to breast cancer from mutations in the BRCA1 or BRCA2 genes and certain other genes, and women who were treated with radiation to the chest for Hodgkin lymphoma, which increases breast cancer risk (Travis et al., 2005). The model may also lead to miscalibrated risk estimates when applied to populations that differ from those in which the model was developed. For example, BCRAT was developed with data from white women initially; it has subsequently been improved for African-American and Asian-American populations by modifications based on data from those populations. The model was designed for women who were screened with mammography regularly, as in the BCDDP population. A study in the Nurses Health Study population showed that Gail Model 1 overestimated risk during 1976–1988, when women were not being screened regularly (Spiegelman et al., 1994), but a subsequent study of this population during 1992–1997, when screening was widely applied, showed good calibration of Gail Model 2 (BCRAT) (Rockhill et al., 2001). Thus, absolute risks can be influenced by the type of surveillance being applied, and by other factors that might cause secular changes in disease rates (Schonfeld et al., 2010).

Another important feature of a risk model is its *discriminatory accuracy.* A model has good disciminatory accuracy if the distribution of risks in those who develop disease has little overlap with the risk distribution among those who do not develop disease and whose risks tend to be lower. Discriminatory accuracy is often measured as the area under the receiver operating characteristic curve (AUC)(see Chapter 6). The AUC for BCRAT is only about 0.60, and the model has been criticized for lack of discriminatory accuracy (Rockhill et al., 2001). Initial efforts to increase the discriminatory accuracy by including information from single nucleotide polymorphisms (SNPs) only improved the AUC to about 0.62 (Gail, 2009b; Wacholder et al., 2010), and inclusion of information on mammographic density only increased AUC to about 0.65 (Chen et al., 2006a). By adding mammographic density and all the SNPs that have been associated with breast cancer to other standard risk factors, Garcia-Closas et al. (2014) estimated that an AUC of 0.68 was achievable. Nonetheless additional strong risk factors beyond SNPs and mammographic density are needed to improve the discriminatory accuracy of models like BCRAT. Polymorphisms and mammographic density are not currently used in BCRAT.

1.1.2 Other models of cancer incidence

Models to predict the incidence of nine cancers in addition to breast cancer are documented at http://epi.grants.cancer.gov/cancer_risk_prediction/# overview. These include bladder, cervical, colorectal, lung, ovarian, pancreatic, prostate and testicular cancers, and melanoma. We will be using data from a model for breast cancer by (Pfeiffer et al., 2013) to illustrate the development of a risk model (Chapter 4) and its validation in independent data (Chapter 6). This model of absolute risk which we call BC2013, was developed by combining estimates of relative and attributatble risk from large cohorts with SEER invasive breast cancer incidence rates and U.S. non-breast cancer mortality rates. As in BCRAT, age was the time scale used for risk projections.

1.1.3 Framingham Model for incidence of coronary heart disease

The Framingham Model estimates the pure 10-year cumulative risk of coronary heart disease, defined as angina pectoris, coronary insufficiency, myocardial infarction, or death ascribed to coronary heart disease (Wilson et al., 1998). Risk projections from this model are widely used to make recommendations for interventions to prevent heart disease, including the use of statins (Expert Panel on Detection and Evaluation and Treatment of High Blood Cholesterol in Adults, 2001). Gender-specific models were based on follow-up of cohorts of 2489 men and 2856 women aged 30 to 74 years old at recruitment in Framingham, Massachusetts from 1971 to 1974. The Framingham data were analyzed on the time scale of time since recruitment, unlike BCRAT which used age as the primary time scale. The Cox proportional hazards model (Cox, 1972) was used to incorporate the predictors, age, treatment for hypertension, smoking, diabetes, total cholesterol, and high density lipoprotein cholesterol. The Framingham model treated death from other causes as censoring and thus estimated the cumulative pure 10-year risk, not the absolute risk. Over a relatively short interval like 10 years, pure and absolute risk may not differ greatly, but for longer projections the Framingham model was recently adapted by incorporating competing hazard of death from other causes (see Chapters 3 and 4) to compute absolute risk (Lloyd-Jones et al., 2006).

The validity of the Framingham Model has been tested in data from independent cohorts (D'Agostino et al., 2001). Although the model seemed well calibrated for white and black men and women, it overestimated risk in other ethnic and racial groups, such as Japanese-American men, Hispanic men, and Native American men and women. After recalibration, the models were well calibrated in those groups, except for evidence of residual overestimation of risk in the highest decile of predicted risk. The AUC values for white men ranged from 0.63 to 0.79 and those for white women from 0.66 to 0.83 in three independent cohorts. These values are higher than for BCRAT. However, AUC values for BCRAT are often estimated from women in narrow age strata to evaluate BCRAT's disciminatory accuracy from factors other than age. Part of the discriminatory accuracy measured for the Framingham Model derives from the fact that older men and women are at higher risk of coronary heart disease than younger men and women, and age is treated as a covariate in the model.

1.2 Applications of risk models for disease incidence

Risk models have applications in the clinical management of individuals at risk of incident disease and in public health and population studies.

Risk models can provide reliable and useful *perspective* on the level of risk. For example, BCRAT was motivated initially by the need for accurate risk assessments for women who thought they had very high risks of breast cancer and were considering drastic measures to avoid it, such as prophylactic mastectomy. Often such women overestimated their risks and were pleasantly surprised to find that the projections from BCRAT were much lower than they had feared. This perspective is useful background information for making more rational decisions regarding breast cancer prevention. As another example, there has been ongoing debate regarding whether women in their forties should undergo routine screening mammography, whereas it is widely recommended for women age 50 and older. If a 45-year old women has the risk of a 50-year old woman, however, as the result of having adverse risk factors, she may well want to consider screening mammography (Gail and Rimer, 1998;

Gail and Schairer, 2010; Wu et al., 2012). The Framingham model likewise provides useful information on levels of risk that guide clinical management (Expert Panel on Detection and Evaluation and Treatment of High Blood Cholesterol in Adults, 2001).

Models of absolute risk also play a role in the more *formal weighing of the risks and benefits* of an intervention, because the absolute risks of the various health outcomes affected by the intervention are central to this calculus. For example, preventive use of tamoxifen reduces the risk of invasive breast cancer by nearly half, but it increases the risks of stroke and endometrial cancer (Fisher et al., 1998). In order for a woman to have a net benefit from this intervention, her risk of breast cancer must be high enough that the absolute reduction in breast cancer risk outweighs the increases in absolute risks of adverse outcomes caused by tamoxifen. Tables have been developed to guide the decision to take interventions such as tamoxifen (Gail et al., 1999a; Freedman et al., 2011) or raloxifene (Freedman et al., 2011) based on level of breast cancer risk. There is no single level of breast cancer risk that determines whether a woman should take these interventions, because that level depends on the absolute risks of the other outcomes in the presence and absence of the intervention. Screening for persons at high risk of disease or with prevalent disease is another type of intervention with risks and benefits, because false positive and false negative screens each have adverse consequences. Risk models usually need to have high discriminatory accuracy to be useful in deciding who should be screened and who not (Chapter 6).

Some public health applications of models of absolute risk do not require high discriminatory accuracy. For example, statisticians at NSABP used Gail Model 2 (BCRAT) to calculate the *required sample sizes* for the Breast Cancer Prevention Trial (or "P-1" Trial) of tamoxifen to prevent invasive breast cancer (Fisher et al., 1998). The required sample size for this trial depended on the number of incident breast cancers arising during the trial, which reflects the average absolute risk of the trial participants. BCRAT predicted the observed number of events well (Costantino et al., 1999). The concept of absolute risk was also used to define eligibility for the trial because the investigators only wanted to give tamoxifen to women with high enough breast cancer risk that they might benefit. Thus women over age 59 were eligible, as were younger women with at least the average 5-year risk of a 60-year old woman, namely 1.66%.

Absolute risk models can also be used to assess the *burden of disease in populations* with known distributions of risk factors, because the risk in the population represents the average over the joint risk factor distribution of the conditional absolute risk given the risk factors. A special application of these ideas arises if the risk model includes modifiable risk factors. For example, Petracci et al. (2011) included alcohol consumption, leisure physical activity, and body mass index as risk factors in an absolute risk model for breast cancer in Italian women that also included factors such as those in BCRAT. By varying the levels of these modifiable risk factors, they estimated the reductions in absolute risk in the entire population and in high-risk subgroups of the population. These reductions in absolute risk, though potentially meaningful, were much smaller than one would imagine based on quantities such as population attributable risk. Thus, absolute risk models can give added perspective on the potential effects of interventions to reduce modifiable exposures. We present a similar analysis for U.S. women based on BC2013 (Pfeiffer et al., 2013) in Chapter 10. One should be aware, however, that several assumptions must hold in order that these estimates of intervention effect be valid. In particular, one must assume that the hypothesized intervention will actually achieve the desired modification in risk factor levels, and that the effect on disease incidence from these changes in risk factors is reliably predicted from observational data on the associations between the risk factors and disease.

1.3 Prognosis after disease diagnosis

The concept of absolute risk is also clinically useful for patients who have developed a disease. In particular, one may be interested in the absolute risk of a cancer recurrence in a defined time interval following initial cancer treatment, or in the chance of dying from that cancer in a defined time interval following initial cancer treatment. Both these events are observed in the presence of the risk of dying from other causes. Thus, we are concerned with the absolute risks of these events. If the risks are low, no further treatments may be needed. If the risks are high, further possibly toxic treatments may be justified. Indeed, much of the literature on risk modeling has focussed on disease prognosis following initial diagnosis and treatment (Harrell, 2001; Steyerberg, 2009; van Houwelingen and Putter, 2012; Geskus, 2016). Often cumulative pure risk is used instead of absolute risk, but when the time interval is long and the risks of mortality from competing causes are appreciable, as in elderly men with prostate cancer, absolute risks, which are smaller than pure risks, add an essential perspective (Albertsen et al., 2005).

Stratification of patients based on risk of recurrence or risk of death from the initial disease following disease diagnosis is one aspect of "personalized medicine", because it allows doctors and patients to guage the extent to which further treatment may be necessary. Another aspect, not to be confused with stratification on absolute risk, is the use of molecular and other data to identify subsets of patients who might respond particularly well to a given treatment. The terms "prognostic marker" and "predictive marker" are sometimes used to distinguish these two very different concepts (Simon et al., 2009). The methods in this book are useful for prognostic risk stratification. Other methods to search for interactions between treatment and patient characteristics are needed to discover predictive markers.

1.4 Contents of book

Chapter 2 defines basic concepts and notation for survival analysis of a single endpoint. Chapter 3 extends these ideas for multiple competing outcomes to formally define the absolute risk of a particular outcome of interest. The concepts of pure and absolute risk are distinguished and non-parametric estimates are given. Chapter 4 discusses the analysis of cohort data with covariates and shows how various risk factors (or covariates) can be introduced into models for competing risks so that absolute risk projections are individualized to take covariates into account. One formulation introduces covariates into cause-specific hazard functions (Prentice et al., 1978; Gail et al., 1989), while another uses covariates to modulate the absolute risk directly, for example (Fine and Gray, 1999). Designs based on sampling covariate data from a cohort, such as the case-cohort design (Prentice, 1986) and the nested case-control design (Liddell et al., 1977) also lead to individualized estimates of absolute risk via cause-specific models, provided the times of all events arising in the cohort are known(Chapter 4). The strategy of estimating absolute risk by combining information on relative risks and attributable risk from case-control studies with registry data, such as SEER data on cancer incidence, is described in detail in Chapter 5. Chapter 6 gives criteria to evaluate risk models, including calibration, discriminatory accuracy, other general criteria, and more specific criteria applicable when the losses from classification errors can be specified. Chapter 7 describes methods of inference to compare two risk models. Chapter 8 discusses model-building, variable selection and strategies for updating risk models to incorporate new covariates. Chapter 9 describes estimation of risk from family-based designs and the role of SNPs in risk modeling. Chapter 10 touches on four topics related to absolute risk: use of absolute risk in disease prognosis; analyses that allow for missing information on the type of health outcome that has occurred; absolute risk predictions with time-varying covariates; and a review of applications of risk models in individual counseling and public health.

Chapter 2

Definitions and basic concepts for survival data in a cohort without covariates

2.1 Basic survival concepts

In this section we describe survival concepts for a single outcome or event type. Later we discuss absolute risk in the presence of competing risks. Among the many excellent books covering these topics, we recommend Kalbfleisch and Prentice (2002) and Chapter 2 of Andersen et al. (1993). A more specialized introduction to multistate models and competing risk analysis can be found, for example, in Beyersmann et al. (2012) and Geskus (2016).

Classic survival analysis focuses on the time from a given starting point to a subsequent event; the time to that event is called the *survival* or *event time*, T, and has range $[0, \infty)$. The primary interest lies in the survival function, conventionally denoted by S, and defined as

$$S(t) = P(T > t). \tag{2.1}$$

The *survival function* S(t) is a non-increasing function of time and for many applications one assumes $S(0) = 1$. A related quantity is the *lifetime distribution function*, defined as

$$F(t) = P(T \leq t) = 1 - S(t).$$

If F is absolutely continuous, one can compute the density function of the lifetime distribution,

$$f(t) = F'(t) = \frac{d}{dt}F(t) = -\frac{d}{dt}S(t) = -S'(t).$$

A widely used quantity in biomedical research is the *hazard function*, also called *hazard rate*, of S, defined as the event rate at time t conditional on survival until time t or later,

$$\lambda(t) = \lim_{\epsilon \to 0^+} P(t \leq T < t + \epsilon \,|\, T \geq t)/\epsilon. \tag{2.2}$$

If F is absolutely continuous, this definition implies that

$$\lambda(t) = \frac{f(t)}{S(t)} = -\frac{S'(t)}{S(t)} = -\frac{d \log\{S(t)\}}{dt}.$$

Integrating both sides and using that $S(0) = 1$ yields the *cumulative hazard function*,

$$\Lambda(t) = \int_0^t \lambda(u)\, du = -\log S(t),$$

and

$$S(t) = \exp\{-\Lambda(t)\} = \exp\left\{-\int_0^t \lambda(u) du\right\}.$$

Example: An example of an absolutely continuous distribution is the Weibull distribution, with survival function $S(t) = \exp(-\gamma t^{\alpha})$, where $\alpha > 0$ is the shape parameter and $\gamma > 0$ is the scale parameter of the distribution. From the previous formulas, its hazard is $\lambda(t) = \gamma\alpha t^{\alpha-1}$, which is increasing for $\alpha > 1$ and decreasing for $\alpha < 1$. For $\alpha = 1$, the hazard is constant over time, and $\lambda(t) = \gamma$ corresponds to the exponential distribution.

When T is a discrete random variable taking values $t_1 < t_2 < \ldots$ with probabilities

$$f(t_i) = P(T = t_i), \quad i = 1, 2, \ldots,$$

the hazard function at t_i is given by

$$\lambda_i = \lambda(t_i) = P(T = t_i | T \geq t_i) = \frac{f(t_i)}{S(t_i-)}, \tag{2.3}$$

where $S(t) = \sum_{j:t_j > t} f(t_j)$ is the survival function and $S(t-) = \lim_{\epsilon \to 0+} S(t - \epsilon)$.

The cumulative hazard function of a survival time T whose distribution has both continuous and discrete components is given by $\Lambda(t) = \int_0^t \lambda_c(u)du + \sum_{i:t_i \leq t} \lambda_i$, where λ_c is the continuous hazard function and λ_i are the hazards corresponding to the discrete event times t_i. The overall survival function of T is thus given by

$$S(t) = \exp\left\{-\int_0^t \lambda(u)du\right\} \prod_{j:t_j \leq t} (1 - \lambda_j).$$

The general definition of the cumulative hazard function of an arbitrary distribution function F is given by the Lebesgue–Stieltjes integral,

$$\Lambda(t) = \int_0^t \frac{1}{S(u-)} dF(u), t \geq 0, \tag{2.4}$$

or equivalently,

$$F(t) = 1 - S(t) = \int_0^t S(u-)d\Lambda(u). \tag{2.5}$$

2.2 Choice of time scale: age, time since diagnosis, time since accrual or counseling

An important issue in survival analysis is the choice of time scale. It is often useful to choose the time scale that is most strongly associated with the risk of experiencing the event of interest. In clinical studies a natural choice may be *time-on-study*, namely the time since a particular event that marks the beginning of study observation. For example, one may be interested in the time from diagnosis and treatment of breast cancer to a subsequent event, such as breast cancer recurrence or death from breast cancer. The left panel of Figure 2.1 shows the experience of four women on the scale of time-on-study. The follow-up starts at the same time origin for each woman, namely when each woman is diagnosed with breast cancer, after which she starts being at risk for breast cancer recurrence or breast cancer death. During follow-up, women 1 and 3 experience a recurrence (solid circles) and women 2 and 4 are censored (open circles). Censoring occurs if follow-up ends before the patient has the event of interest (e.g., breast cancer recurrence). When woman 1 fails (i.e., has a breast cancer recurrence), three of the four woman are at risk for failure. The sets of women at risk at the failure times (called "risk sets") thus decrease monotonically.

In cohort studies of disease etiology or incidence, subjects without a given disease are followed up to detect the time of occurrence of that disease. However, in contrast to many clinical studies, the time when a subject first comes under observation, typically the time of

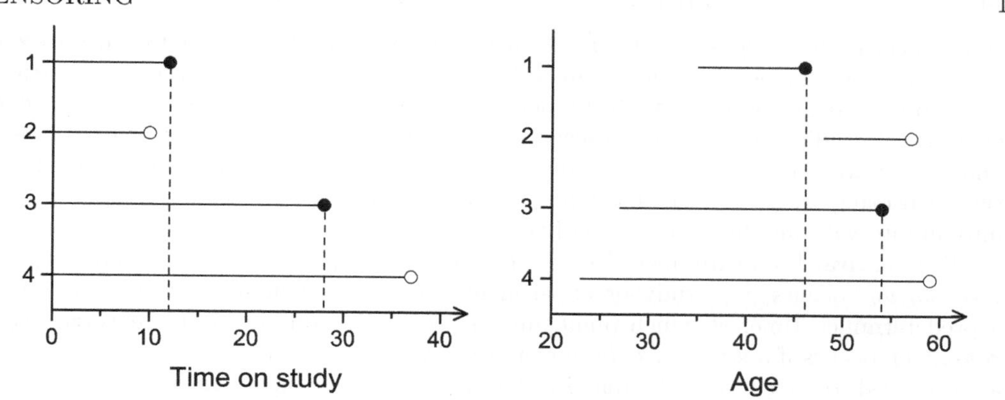

Figure 2.1: Time scales for survival analysis: time on study scale (left panel) and age scale (right panel).

administration of a questionnaire or an interview, usually does not coincide with the time when the subject first becomes at risk for the disease of interest. In addition, the effect of age usually needs to be tightly controlled in epidemiologic cohort studies because the incidence of most diseases, especially chronic diseases, is strongly influenced by age. Because the time variable is tightly modeled in survival analyses, age is a natural time-scale. When using age as the time scale, the hazard function (2.2) can be directly interpreted as the age-specific incidence function. Survival methods can model this hazard flexibly, giving tighter control for age than models that include age as a covariate. However, analyzing survival data on the age scale is more complex than analyzing survival data on the time-on-study scale, because follow-up begins at different ages for different subjects. Using age as the time scale therefore implies staggered or delayed entry into the study, and at any given age, some subjects are not yet under observation whereas others are no longer under follow-up. The right panel of Figure 2.1 shows the same four follow-up times as the left panel, but now on the age scale. The start of follow-up is the age at which each woman was diagnosed with breast cancer, which ranges from 21 to 48 years. This starting age is indicated by the left end of each horizontal follow-up line. When woman 1 fails, woman 2 has not yet entered the study, and thus not yet under observation. Therefore only three women are at risk at the age when the first failure occurs. Thus, the number of subjects at risk does not decrease monotonically with age and risk sets are not nested, unlike the risk sets on the time-on-study scale. Another feature that may arise when using the age scale is left truncation, that occurs when there are study restrictions on the age at inclusion. In the right panel of Figure 2.1, the minimal age of inclusion is 20 years, and individuals who failed at younger ages are not part of the study. This feature of the data is not apparent on the time-on-study scale plot. Left truncation is discussed more formally in the Section 2.4.

2.3 Censoring

Survival data are subject to a special missing data problem, namely censoring. In medical studies one often finds that the event of interest has occurred in some but not all study subjects when the observation period ends. For example, in a study of breast cancer recurrence after breast cancer diagnosis and treatment, some women will have died of non-breast cancer causes before breast cancer recurrence. In addition, some women will have dropped out of the study or be lost to follow-up before breast cancer recurrence, and some women will remain alive and without breast cancer recurrence at the end of follow-up. These partially observed times to breast cancer recurrence are called *censored* survival times. Several types of censoring are possible. Data are *right censored* when they are not observed exactly, but only known to be above a certain value. *Left censoring* occurs when an observation is not observed but only known to be below a certain value. Left censoring may occur for example in studies of infectious diseases, where the time of infection of a person is only known to have occurred before the time of a positive test for the infection. Both left and right censoring are special cases of *interval censoring*, where an observation is known to fall into an interval, but the exact value of the survival time is not observed.

The survival literature also distinguishes between type 1 and type 2 censoring. *Type I censoring* occurs if a study or experiment with a given number of subjects stops at a predetermined time, at which point any subjects remaining are right-censored. *Type II censoring* occurs if a study or experiment stops when a predetermined number of subjects are observed to have failed; the remaining subjects are then right-censored.

A common assumption is that censoring is not-informative, that is, each subject has a censoring time that is statistically independent of his or her failure time.

2.3.1 Right censoring

We define notation for right censoring, which is the most common type of censoring in observational and clinical studies. Reasons for right censoring include cessation of follow-up at the end of the study, sometimes called *administrative censoring*, and other loss to follow-up (e.g., individuals move away or do not respond to study inquiries). Right censoring also occurs when a person dies from a cause unrelated to the outcome of interest. The assumption that the censoring time is independent of the survival time of interest is plausible for administrative censoring and for some types of loss to follow-up, but may be questionable for certain types of loss to follow-up or deaths from other causes.

Let C be a nonnegative random variable that is independent of T. Under right censoring one only observes the minimum of the censoring time and the survival time, $X = \min(C,T)$ and the indicator for the event, $\delta(t) = I(T = t, C \geq t)$, where $I(.)$, the indicator function, is 1 if the argument is true and 0 otherwise. Thus T is completely observable only if $T \leq C$, i.e., when $\delta(t) = 1$. The data for an individual at time t are $(X, \delta(t))$. If T and C are independent, the survival function of $X = \min(C,T)$ is the product

$$S_X(t) = S(t)S_C(t),$$

where S_C denotes the survival function for the censoring variable C. Here $S(.)$ and $\Lambda(.)$ are the survival function and the cumulative hazard function of T. Using that $dF(t) = S(t-)d\Lambda(t)$ from expression (2.5), it follows that

$$P(X \leq t, \delta = 1) = P(T \leq t, C > t) = \int_0^t S_C(u-)dF(u) = \int_0^t S_X(u-)d\Lambda(u),$$

and solving for Λ yields

$$\Lambda(t) = \int_0^t S_X^{-1}(u-)dP(X \leq u, \delta(u) = 1). \tag{2.6}$$

Thus, under the assumption of independent censoring, $P(X \leq t, \delta = 1)$ and $S_X(t)$ uniquely determine the cumulative hazard function $\Lambda(t)$ of T, and Λ is estimable from the observed censored survival data on $0 \leq t \leq t^*$, where t^* is the smaller of the two values $\max(T)$ and $\max(C)$. The assumption of independence of C and T cannot be tested, however, but has to be justified based on the nature of the censoring process.

2.4 Truncation

Another form of missing data that is often encountered in survival analysis is *truncation.* A truncated sample contains information only on subjects who satisfy a truncation condition, such as women at least fifty years old at study entry. A truncated sample provides no information on those not satisfying the truncation condition, not even how many there were. In contrast, censored observations are part of the study sample, and the censoring times or intervals are used in the analysis.

Left truncation occurs when the study is restricted to individuals who are a certain age or older at recruitment. For example a study of breast cancer incidence might include only women aged fifty or older. Women whose event time occurs before that age are not observed, and no information is available for them. *Right truncation* occurs when the study is restricted to individuals who have experienced the event at or before a given date. For example, a study population might only include persons who developed clinical acquired immune deficiency syndrome (AIDS) before 1990.

In the presence of truncation, the non-truncated observations have a survival distribution that is conditional on not being truncated.

2.5 Life-table estimator

One of the oldest estimators of the survival function is based on life tables (see, e.g., (Chiang, 1968)). A life table is a summary of survival data grouped into intervals. It is often applied in situations when actual failure and censoring times are not available, and only total numbers of failures and individuals at risk are given for particular intervals. An example of a life table for women who died from breast cancer between ages 60 and 75 is given in Table 2.1. Let d_i denote the number of failures (or events) in the ith time interval $I_i = [t_{i-1}, t_i)$, c_i the

Table 2.1: Life-table estimate of breast cancer mortality in 1000 60-year-old women diagnosed with breast cancer

Age Interval	i	n_i	d_i	c_i	q_i	$\hat{S}_i = \prod_{j \leq i}(1 - q_j)$
$[60, 65)$	1	1000	17	44	0.017	0.983
$[65, 70)$	2	939	20	63	0.022	0.961
$[70, 75)$	3	856	22	89	0.027	0.935

number of censored observations and n_i the number of individuals at risk at the beginning of the time interval, which is equal to the number of individuals who neither experienced the event nor were censored up to time t_{i-1}. The censoring can be assumed to occur at the beginning, the end or on average halfway through each interval. The last assumption is appropriate if censoring occurs uniformly throughout the intervals and yields the standard life-table estimate of the conditional probability of failure in I_i, $\hat{q}_i = 0$ if $n_i = 0$ and

$$\hat{q}_i = \frac{d_i}{n_i - c_i/2}$$

otherwise. The corresponding estimate of the survival function at the end of the ith interval is

$$LT(t_i) = \hat{S}(t_i) = \prod_{l \leq i}(1 - \hat{q}_l). \tag{2.7}$$

The variance of this estimate can be obtained by the following heuristic derivation (see Greenwood (1926)) that relies on the fact that outcomes in various intervals are uncorrelated, as follows from the conditional independence of events in subsequent intervals given outcomes in previous intervals. Thus $\text{cov}(\hat{q}_i, \hat{q}_j) = 0$ for $i < j$, and $\hat{p}_i = 1 - \hat{q}_i$ has the binomial variance $\widehat{\text{var}}(\hat{p}_i) = \hat{p}_i\hat{q}_i/(n_i - c_i/2)$. Applying the delta method (Cramer, 1947, p. 353) to $\log \hat{S}(t) = \sum_i \log(1 - \hat{q}_i) = \sum_i \log(\hat{p}_i)$ yields $\text{var}(\log \hat{p}_i) \approx \hat{q}_i/\{\hat{p}_i(n_i - c_i/2)\}$ and thus

$$\text{var}\{\log \hat{S}(t)\} \approx \sum_i \frac{\hat{q}_i}{\hat{p}_i(n_i - c_i/2)} = \sum_i \frac{d_i}{(n_i - c_i/2)(n_i - d_i - c_i/2)}.$$

Using $S(t) = \exp\{\log S(t)\}$, and applying the delta method leads to the Greenwood-type formula for variance,

$$\widehat{\text{var}}\{\hat{S}(t)\} = \{\hat{S}(t)\}^2 \sum_i \frac{d_i}{(n_i - c_i/2)(n_i - d_i - c_i/2)}. \tag{2.8}$$

2.5.1 Kaplan–Meier survival estimate

The Kaplan–Meier or product limit estimator is the limit of the life-table estimator when intervals are so small that at most one distinct failure time occurs within an interval. There may be more than one failure at that time, however. This estimator is the non-parametric maximum likelihood estimate of the survival function under right-censoring (Kaplan and Meier, 1958). By convention, it is a right continuous step function which takes jumps only at the event times.

Let $d(t)$ denote the number of events at time t. Typically $d(t)$ is either zero or one, but we also allow tied event times, in which case $d(t)$ can be greater than one. Let $n(t)$ denote the number of individuals at risk just prior to time t. Then the Kaplan–Meier estimate is defined as

$$KM(t) = \hat{S}(t) = \prod_{u \le t} \left\{1 - \frac{d(u)}{n(u)}\right\}. \tag{2.9}$$

The above product changes only at times t where $d(t) > 0$, that is at times when events occur. Due to its form and its limit relationship to the life-table estimate, Kaplan and Meier (1958) called the estimator (2.9) the *product limit* estimator. Note that in the absence of censoring, KM is identical to $1 - F_n$, where F_n is the usual empirical distribution function of the observed event times, $F_n(t) = (1/n)\sum_{i=1}^n I(T_i \le t)$.

Because $\exp(-x) \approx 1 - x$ for values of x that are close to zero, the Kaplan-Meier estimate can also be approximated by

$$KM(t) = \hat{S}(t) \approx \prod_{u \le t} \exp\left\{-\frac{d(u)}{n(u)}\right\} = \exp\left\{-\sum_{u \le t} \frac{d(u)}{n(u)}\right\}.$$

Several variance estimators are available, including Greenwood's formula,

$$\widehat{\text{var}}\{\widehat{S}(t)\} = \{\hat{S}(t)\}^2 \sum_{t_i \le t} \frac{d_i}{n_i(n_i - d_i)}.$$

Rigorous derivations of the variance, that confirm the validity of Greenwood's formula, can be found in the counting process literature for survival analysis (e.g., (Andersen et al., 1993)).

A non-parametric estimate of the cumulative hazard rate function, the Nelson–Aalen estimator (Nelson, 1969; Aalen, 1976), is given by

$$\hat{\Lambda}(t) = \sum_{t_i \le t} \frac{d_i}{n_i}.$$

Its variance estimate is $\widehat{\text{var}}\{\hat{\Lambda}(t)\} = \sum_{t_i \le t} d_i/[n_i(n_i - d_i)]$. Applying the delta method to the relationship $\log S(t) = -\Lambda(t)$, one again obtains the Greenwood formula.

2.6 Counting processes and Markov methods

Aalen (1978) introduced multivariate counting processes into the study of lifetime data, under a variety of censoring mechanisms, including right censoring. We briefly outline this very useful approach and notation that we later use to derive distributional properties of various estimates.

We assume that for each of n individuals in a cohort we observe the random vector $(X_i, \delta_i), i = 1, \ldots, n$, where the observed event time $X_i = \min(C_i, T_i)$ is the minimum of the censoring time C_i and the survival time T_i, and $\delta_i(t) = I(T_i = t, C_i \geq t)$ is the event indicator for the ith individual. For individual i the *counting process* $N_i(t)$ is defined as $N_i(t) = I(X_i \leq t, \delta_i = 1), t \geq 0$. The process jumps when the individual experiences the event. Typically $N_i(0) = 0$. The "at risk process" for the ith individual is $Y_i(t) = I(X_i \geq t)$ for $t \geq 0$. Under the assumption of independent censoring and given the past up to and including time t, represented by σ-fields $\{\mathcal{F}_t\}$, $N_i(t)$ has the *intensity process* $\lambda_i(t)$, given by

$$\lambda_i(t)Y_i(t)dt = P(dN_i(t) = 1|\mathcal{F}_t),$$

where $dN_i(t) = N_i(t) - N_i(t-)$ is the increment of N_i at time t. We let $N_i(t-) = \lim_{\epsilon \to 0+} N(t - \epsilon)$. As N_i is a binary process, we can reformulate the above relationship as

$$E(dN_i(t) - \lambda_i(t)Y_i(t)|\mathcal{F}_t) = 0.$$

Thus the process $M_i(t) = N_i(t) - \int_0^t \lambda_i(s)Y_i(s)ds \equiv N_i(t) - \int_0^t Y_i(s)d\Lambda_i(s)$ has expectation zero. The expression $\Lambda_i(t) = \int_0^t \lambda_i(s)ds$ is called the *cumulative intensity* of N_i.

For the whole cohort, the aggregated processes

$$N(t) = \sum_{j=1}^{n} N_j(t)$$

and

$$Y(t) = \sum_{j=1}^{n} Y_j(t), t \geq 0$$

count the number of events through time t and the number of individuals still at risk of failure just before time t, respectively. The sample paths of N jump whenever events occur, and are thus non-decreasing step functions, i.e., for $s \leq t$, $N(s) \leq N(t)$. The step size at time t, $dN(t) = N(t) - N(t-)$, is the number of events occurring exactly at t. In the absence of ties, $dN(t) = 1$ when an event occurs at time t or 0 otherwise. The number of individuals censored at time t is $w(t) = [Y(t) - Y(t-)] - dN(t)$.

In the counting process notation, the sample counterparts of the survival function $S_X(t)$ and the probability $P(T \leq t, \delta = 1)$ are

$$\hat{S}_X(t-) = Y(t)/n \text{ and } \hat{P}(T \leq t, \delta = 1) = N(t)/n.$$

Substituting these two expression into Equation (2.6) yields an estimate of the cumulative hazard process, the Nelson–Aalen estimator

$$\hat{\Lambda}(t) = \int_0^t \frac{dN(u)}{Y(u)} = \sum_{t_i \leq t} \frac{dN(t_i)}{Y(t_i)}, \tag{2.10}$$

which is an increasing right-continuous step function with increments $dN(t_i)/Y(t_i)$ at the observed event times t_i. In the absence of ties the estimate further simplifies to $\hat{\Lambda}(t) = \sum_{t_i \leq t} \frac{1}{Y(t_i)}$.

Aalen (1978) showed that the process

$$M(t) = \frac{1}{\sqrt{n}} \left\{ N(t) - \int_0^t Y(u) d\Lambda(u) \right\}$$

is a square integrable martingale with respect to the past up to and including time t, represented by σ-fields $\{\mathcal{F}_t\}$. The martingale can be regarded as a centered error process. Martingales are fundamental stochastic processes for which a large body of theory has been developed. Given the past, i.e., $\{\mathcal{F}_t\}$, $Y(t)$ is fixed, and not random. In brief, a martingale $\{M(t), t \geq 0\}$ is a stochastic process whose increments over an interval $(t_0, t_1]$ given $\{\mathcal{F}_{t_0}\}$, have expectation zero, $E(M(t_1) - M(t_0)|\mathcal{F}_{t_0}) = 0$. Given $\mathcal{F}_t$, $M(t)$ is fixed. Central limit theorems for martingales allow the derivation of asymptotic properties of estimators and test statistics based on $N(t)$. For example, the process $\sqrt{n}\{\hat{\Lambda}(t) - \Lambda(t)\}$ also is a martingale with respect to $\{\mathcal{F}_t\}$. From the martingale central limit theorem (Rebolledo, 1980), this process converges weakly to a Gaussian process for each t. The unbiasedness and asymptotic normality of $\hat{\Lambda}(t)$ allow us to compute asymptotic normal pointwise confidence intervals for $\Lambda(t)$ at time t, given by $[\hat{\Lambda}(t) - z_{1-\alpha/2} se\{\hat{\Lambda}(t)\}, \hat{\Lambda}(t) + z_{1-\alpha/2} se\{\hat{\Lambda}(t)\}]$, where z_α denotes the α quantile of the standard normal distribution and se stands for the standard error. Simultaneous confidence bands for $\hat{\Lambda}(t)$ are also available, and are discussed in detail in Chapter IV.1.3 of Andersen et al. (1993). As $\hat{S}(t) = \exp\{-\hat{\Lambda}(t)\}$, this result can also be used to construct 95% confidence intervals for the survival function $S(t)$, given by $\exp[-\hat{\Lambda}(t) \pm z_{1-\alpha/2} se\{\hat{\Lambda}(t)\}]$.

The Kaplan–Meier estimator in (2.9) and the life-table estimator in (2.7) can be written in counting-process notation as

$$KM(t) = \hat{S}(t) = \lim_{\epsilon \to 0+} \prod_{u: u+\epsilon \leq t} \left\{ 1 - \frac{dN(u)}{Y(u)} \right\} \tag{2.11}$$

$$LT(t) = \lim_{\epsilon \to 0+} \prod_{u: u+\epsilon \leq t} \left\{ 1 - \frac{dN(u)}{Y(u) - w(u)/2} \right\},$$

respectively. In Equation (2.9), $n(u)$ was used instead of $Y(u)$ and $d(u)$ was used instead of $dN(u)$, to be consistent with the earlier literature. As the Kaplan–Meier estimate (2.11) is asymptotically equivalent to $\exp\{-\hat{\Lambda}(t)\}$, it's properties can be obtained from those of $\hat{\Lambda}(t)$.

Chapter 3

Competing risks

3.1 Concepts and definitions

In Chapter 2 we assumed that only one event, such as breast cancer recurrence, could occur, apart from independent censoring. If deaths from other causes occurred, they were treated as independent censoring. Now we consider the possibility that any of M events can occur, apart from censoring. If the occurrence of one of these events precludes any subsequent event, the M events are called *competing risks.* Often the focus is on a particular risk, or a subset of risks. For example, in a long term study of a new treatment for women diagnosed with breast cancer, the main outcome of interest might be death from breast cancer. However, some women will die of causes other than breast cancer, and either of these two types of death precludes the other. One therefore needs to account for the competing effects of death from other causes to appropriately assess the impact of treatment on breast cancer mortality (Figure 3.1). The chance of dying from breast cancer may be reduced either because treatment forestalls breast cancer death or, possibly, because it increases risk of mortality from other causes.

We now formalize these ideas for $M \geq 2$ competing risks (Figure 3.2). These ideas are discussed in several textbooks for survival methods (Andersen et al., 1993; Kalbfleisch and Prentice, 2002; Pintilie, 2006; Beyersmann et al., 2012; Geskus, 2016). A person is in state $\delta = 0$ until one of M competing events (say event m) occurs, at which time the person is in the absorbing state m (Figure 3.2). In particular, we observe the state process $\delta(t)$ that takes values in $\{0, 1, \ldots, M\}$ with $\delta(0) = 0$ and describes the state a person is in at time t. We also observe the time T to the first of $M \geq 2$ event types. Thus $T = \inf\{t > 0 : \delta(t) \neq 0\}$ is the first time when the process δ is no longer in the initial state and $\delta(T)$ corresponds to the type of event and extends the event indicator in Section 2.6 to multiple event types. For practical applications it is also necessary to account for right censoring. As in Section 2.3.1, we let C denote the censoring process, that is assumed to be independent of T. The observed event time is the minimum of the censoring time and the survival time, $X = \min(C, T)$. The state indicator δ also captures censoring; if a person is censored at a particular time s, then no event of types 1 through M has occurred, and thus the person remains in the initial state, i.e., $\delta(s) = 0$. Although we assume that censoring is independent from T, we make no assumptions regarding the dependence of the M times to competing events.

The transition rate from state 0 to state m is described by the cause-specific hazard function,

$$\lambda_m(t) = \lim_{\epsilon \to 0+} \frac{P\left(t \leq T < t + \epsilon, \delta(T) = m | T \geq t\right)}{\epsilon}. \tag{3.1}$$

λ_m gives the instantaneous failure rate from cause m at time t in the presence of all other failure types. For example, suppose one is primarily interested in mortality from breast cancer as in Figure 3.1. Letting $m = 1$ denote death from breast cancer and $m = 2$ death from other causes, we define $\lambda_1(t)$ as the mortality rate from breast cancer death among women alive at age t, and $\lambda_2(t)$ as the mortality rate from all other causes among women alive at age t.

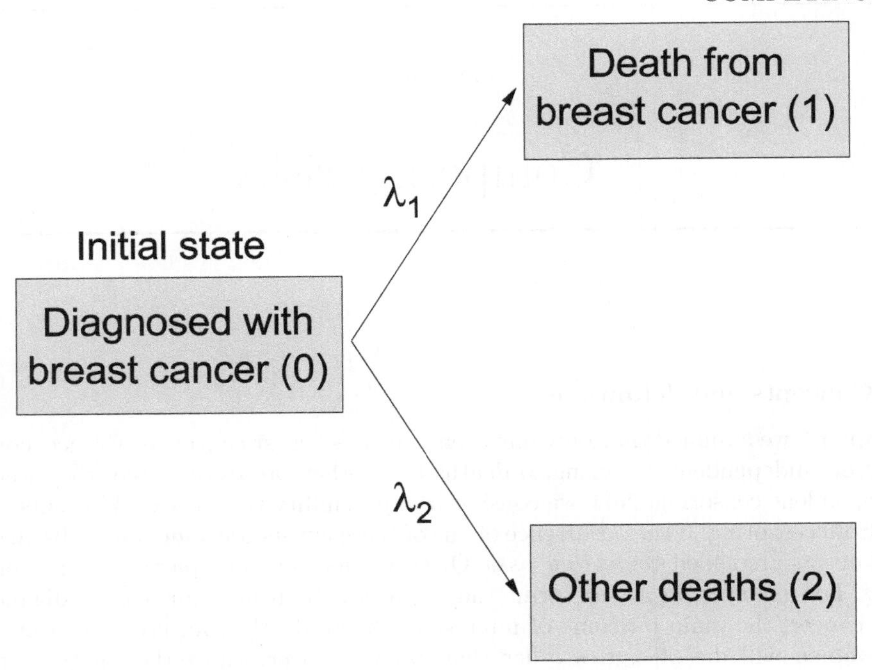

Figure 3.1: Competing risks of death from breast cancer or death from other causes following breast cancer diagnosis and treatment. Corresponding cause-specific hazards are λ_1 and λ_2, respectively.

The cause-specific hazard functions for M competing events are depicted in Figure 3.2. Assuming that only one failure type can occur at a given time t, the overall hazard of T is

$$\lambda(t) = \sum_{m=1}^{M} \lambda_m(t),$$

and the probability of having no event at or before t is

$$S(t) = P(T > t) = \exp\left\{-\int_0^t \lambda(u)du\right\} = \exp\left\{-\int_0^t \sum_{m=1}^{M} \lambda_m(u)du\right\}. \tag{3.2}$$

We also define, by analogy with $S(t)$, the function $S_m(t) = \exp\left\{-\int_0^t \lambda_m(u)du\right\}$, where $\Lambda_m(t) = \int_0^t \lambda_m(u)du$ is the integrated or cumulative cause-specific hazard for cause m. Note however that $S_m(t)$ does not have a survival function interpretation (see Kalbfleisch and Prentice (2002), p. 252, and Prentice et al. (1978)) without further assumptions that are discussed in Section 3.2.

Example: When the cause-specific hazard functions $\lambda_m(t) = \gamma_m \alpha_m t^{\alpha_m - 1}, m = 1, \ldots, M$ arise from Weibull distributions, the overall hazard $\lambda(t) = \sum_m \lambda_m(t) = \sum_m \gamma_m \alpha_m t^{\alpha_m - 1}$. The overall survival function $S(t) = \prod_m \exp(-\gamma_m t_m^{\alpha})$.

A key quantity is $r_m = P(T \leq t, \delta(T) = m)$, the *cumulative incidence function* or *absolute risk*, for a failure of type m, namely the probability of experiencing an event from cause m by time t in the presence of $M-1$ competing events. The absolute risk is also known as the *crude risk* in the literature. In order to define r_m we first define the *sub-density function* for the time to a failure of type m,

$$f_m(t) = \lim_{\epsilon \to 0+} \frac{P(t \leq T < t + \epsilon, \delta(T) = m)}{\epsilon} = \lambda_m(t)S(t), m = 1, \ldots, M. \tag{3.3}$$

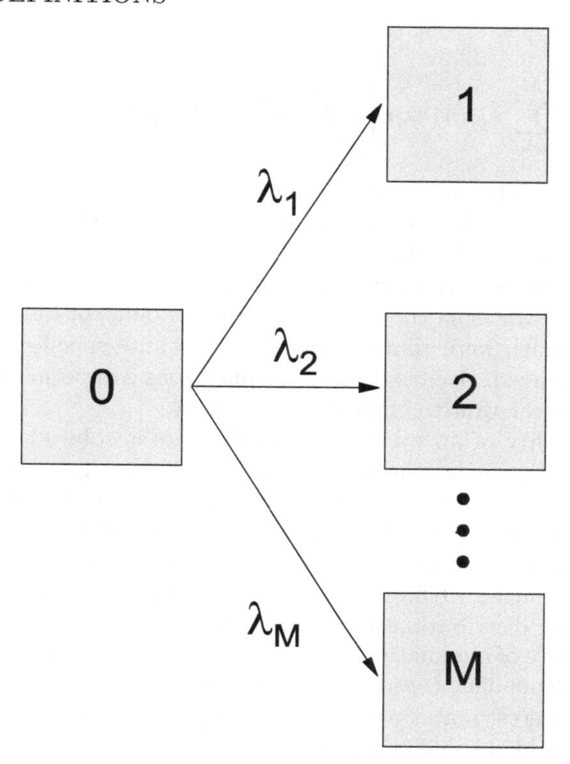

Figure 3.2: Competing risk model with M competing events and with cause-specific hazard functions $\lambda_m(t)$.

Then the absolute risk of event type m in the interval $(0, t]$ is

$$r_m(t) = P(T \leq t, \delta(T) = m) = \int_0^t f_m(u)du = \int_0^t \lambda_m(u)S(u-)du = \int_0^t \lambda_m(u) \prod_{i=1}^{M} S_i(u-)du. \tag{3.4}$$

The probability of ever having an event of type m is given by $p_m = \lim_{t\to\infty} r_m(t)$, and $\sum_{m=1}^{M} p_m = 1$. As typically $p_m < 1$, r_m is not a proper distribution but a *sub-distribution.* Note that $r_m(t)$ is a functional of $\{\lambda_k\}_{k=1}^{M}$ and hence is identifiable from observable data (Section 3.2).

In practical applications a conditional version of r_m is often used, namely the conditional probability of experiencing an event from cause m within the time interval $(t_0, t_1]$ in the presence of $M - 1$ competing events, given survival up to t_0,

$$\begin{aligned} r_m(t_0, t_1) = P(t_0 < T \leq t_1, \delta(T) = m | T \geq t_0) &= \frac{\int_{t_0}^{t_1} \lambda_m(u)S(u-)du}{S(t_0-)} \\ &= \frac{\int_{t_0}^{t_1} \lambda_m(u) \prod_{k=1}^{M} S_k(u-)du}{\prod_{k=1}^{M} S_k(t_0-)} \\ &= \int_{t_0}^{t_1} \lambda_m(u) \exp\left\{ - \int_{t_0}^{u} \sum_{k=1}^{M} \lambda_k(s)ds \right\} du. \end{aligned} \tag{3.5}$$

Notice also that

$$\sum_{m=1}^{M} r_m(t_0,t_1) = \int_{t_0}^{t_1} \sum_{m=1}^{M} \lambda_m(u) \exp\left\{-\int_{t_0}^{u} \sum_{k=1}^{M} \lambda_k(s)ds\right\} du = 1 - \exp\left\{-\int_{t_0}^{t_1} \sum_{k=1}^{M} \lambda_k(s)ds\right\}$$

is one minus the probability of event-free survival in the interval $(t_0, t_1]$.

In contrast to the absolute risk, which refers to the probability of a particular event in the presence of all competing risks, the *net or pure probability* is the hypothetical probability of that event if it were the only risk acting on a population. For example, the pure probability of death from breast cancer is the hypothetical probability of dying from breast cancer if all other causes of death were eliminated and if the cause-specific hazard of breast cancer mortality were unchanged. Because in most applications competing risks are inevitable, the absolute risk is more relevant to clinical management.

The pure probability of an event is larger than its absolute risk, which is reduced by the action of competing risks. The pure probability is usually estimated as one minus the Kaplan-Meier survival curve estimate for the event of interest, with all competing events treated as independent censoring. Calculations of pure risk depend on non-identifiable assumptions regarding the joint distribution of latent failure times for the several competing events (Cox, 1959; Tsiatis, 1975; Gail, 1975). Assuming independence of the failure times defines one such joint distribution and is consistent with the observable data (see Section 3.2). Thus the estimate of cumulative risk based on the Kaplan-Meier curve that treats competing events as independent censoring is an estimate of the pure probability of the event of interest, and it overestimates absolute risk, especially over long time intervals $(t_0, t_1]$. Special software is needed to estimate absolute risk.

Competing risk models are a special case of multistate models, that may also describe events that occur after a primary event of interest. For example, in a multistate model one could have the states "well", "cancer" and "death". The transition to the absorbing state "death" can happen from either the "cancer" or the "well" state. States from which no further transition is possible are typically termed "absorbing" states. The competing risk setting can be thought of as a multistate model where all M states are absorbing. Excellent overviews of multistate models and related software in *R* are given in Beyersmann et al. (2012) and Geskus (2016). We discuss multistate models further in Section 10.4.2.

3.2 Pure versus cause-specific hazard functions

We contrast the cause-specific hazard λ_m for the m-th cause defined in (3.1) with the *net or pure hazard function* for cause m,

$$\lambda_m^p(t) = \lim_{\epsilon \to 0+} \frac{P\left(t \le T < t + \epsilon | T \ge t, \text{ no other causes acting}\right)}{\epsilon}. \tag{3.6}$$

To illustrate the difference it is helpful to introduce the notion of latent failure times. Letting the variable T_m denote the time of failure for an event of cause m, the observed time until the first of M event types can be written as $T = \min(T_1, \ldots, T_M)$. Given the joint survival function of the M causes,

$$S(t_1, \ldots, t_M) = P(T_1 > t_1, \ldots, T_M > t_M),$$

one interpretation of "no other causes acting" is that T_m has the marginal survival function $P(T_m > t_m) = S(0, \ldots, 0, t_m, 0, \ldots, 0)$. The pure hazard function for T_m is then obtained from the marginal survival function as

$$\lambda_m^p(t) = -\frac{\partial}{\partial t_m} \log\{S(t_1, \ldots, t_M)\}|_{t_m = t, t_k = 0, k \ne m}.$$

The cause-specific hazard function, however, is based on the relationship

$$\lambda_m(t) = -\frac{\partial}{\partial t_m} \log\{S(t_1, \ldots, t_M)\}|_{t_1=\ldots=t_M=t}.$$

Note that $S(t, \ldots, t) = P(T_1 > t, \ldots, T_M > t) = \exp\left\{-\int_0^t \sum_{m=1}^M \lambda_m(u)du\right\}$ is equal to the overall survival probability $S(t)$ given in (3.2), which is estimable from the observed data. The cause-specific hazards are estimable because we can observe the instantaneous risk of event m among those at risk at t. In fact, assuming T is independent of censoring, the observed data for a subject contribute the factor $S(t)\prod_{m=1}^M \{\lambda_m(t)\}^{I\{\delta_m(t)=1\}}$ to the likelihood. This factor is a function only of the cause-specific hazards, showing they are estimable (Prentice et al., 1978). Because λ_m is estimable from observed data, any function that depends only on the cause-specific hazards is also estimable. In contrast, the joint survival function $S(t_1, \ldots, t_M)$ is only identifiable from observed data under parametric models or under the assumption that the failure times T_m are independent (Tsiatis, 1975; Gail, 1975). Neither of these modeling assumptions can be tested with available data. Under independence of the T_m, the cause-specific hazard for cause m, λ_m, is equal to the pure hazard function, λ_m^p, and hence $S_m(t)$ is a survival function. However, the independence assumption is especially dubious in medical applications, because a person at high risk of one such event may also be at elevated risk of other causes. Moreover, medical interventions designed to reduce risk for or eliminate one event may also effect the hazard functions of other types of events. Although no independence assumptions are required to estimate cause-specific hazards $\lambda_m(t)$ or any functionals of them (Prentice et al., 1978), the censoring time C is assumed to be independent of the event time T and the distribution of C is assumed to be functionally independent of $\{\lambda_m(t)\}$.

Before we discuss covariate modeling for absolute risk in Chapter 4, we present non-parametric estimates of absolute risk based on observations from a cohort in Section 3.3.

3.3 Non-parametric estimation of absolute risk

We consider a cohort of n individuals who are followed prospectively. Recall that we observe the time $X = \min(T, C)$, which is the minimum of the time T to the first of M event types or censoring, C. The state process is $\delta(t)$, where $\delta(t) = m$ if an event of type m occurs at or before time t, $m = 1, 2, ..., M$. If no events have occurred, $\delta(t) = 0$. Extending the notation in Section 2.6, we define the cause-specific counting process $N_{im}(t) = I(X_i \leq t, \delta(t) = m)$ for individual i, and let $N_m(t) = \sum_{i=1}^n N_{im}(t), t \geq 0, m = 1, \ldots, M$ denote the number of events of type m that have occurred in the interval $(0, t]$ and $dN_m(t)$ denote the number of events of type m occurring exactly at time t. The total number of events in $(0, t]$ is given by $N(t) = \sum_{m=1}^M N_m(t)$. The number of individuals at risk just prior to time t is $Y(t)$. Truncation can also be accommodated in this setup, but for ease of exposition we only consider right censoring. We let $t_i, i = 1, \ldots, N(\infty)$ denote the observed event times of any of the M events types, but not censoring.

A non-parametric estimate of the probability of overall survival up to time t is obtained from the Kaplan-Meier estimate as

$$\hat{P}(T \leq t) = 1 - \hat{S}(t) = 1 - \prod_{t_i \leq t}\left\{1 - \frac{dN(t_i)}{Y(t_i)}\right\} = \sum_{t_i \leq t}\left\{\frac{dN(t_i)}{Y(t_i)}\hat{S}(t_i-)\right\}. \quad (3.7)$$

Because $P(T \leq t) = \sum_{m=1}^M P(T \leq t, \delta(T) = m)$ and $dN(t_i) = \sum_{m=1}^M dN_m(t_i)$, an estimate of $r_m(t)$ can be derived from the above expression as

$$\hat{r}_m(t) = \sum_{t_i \leq t}\left\{\frac{dN_m(t_i)}{Y(t_i)}\hat{S}(t_i-)\right\} \equiv \sum_{t_i \leq t}\hat{\lambda}_m(t_i)\hat{S}(t_i-). \quad (3.8)$$

The right-hand side of Equation (3.8) is a non-parametric estimator of (3.4). The overall survival estimate $\hat{S(t)}$ depends on all M events and is obtained without any assumption of independence. As mentioned previously, an estimate of the "pure risk" of event type m is obtained by treating all other events as independent censoring and applying life-table or Kaplan-Meier procedures. This estimate of the hypothetical probability of event type m in the absence of other causes of failure is only valid if the intervention to eliminate other causes of failure does not alter $\lambda_m(t)$ and if the unverifiable independence assumption holds.

Gaynor et al. (1993) derived the variance of $\hat{r}_m(t)$ in (3.8), using a first order Taylor approximation, as

$$\widehat{\text{var}}\{\hat{r}_m(t)\} = \sum_{j:t_j \le t} \widehat{\text{var}}\left\{\hat{\lambda}_m(t_j)\hat{S}(t_j-)\right\} + 2 \sum_{\{j:t_j<t\}} \sum_{\{k:t_j<t_k \le t\}} \widehat{\text{cov}}\left\{\hat{\lambda}_m(t_j)\hat{S}(t_j-), \hat{\lambda}_m(t_k)\hat{S}(t_k-)\right\}.$$

The terms in the previous equation are

$$\widehat{\text{var}}\left\{\hat{\lambda}_m(t_j)\hat{S}(t_j-)\right\} = \left\{\hat{\lambda}_m(t_j)\hat{S}(t_j-)\right\}^2 \left\{\frac{Y(t_j) - dN_m(t_j)}{dN_m(t_j)Y(t_j)} + \sum_{k=1}^{j-1} \frac{dN_m(t_k)}{Y(t_k)\{Y(t_k) - dN_m(t_k)\}}\right\}$$

and

$$\widehat{\text{cov}}\left\{\hat{\lambda}_m(t_j)\hat{S}(t_j-), \hat{\lambda}_m(t_k)\hat{S}(t_{k-1})\right\} = \hat{\lambda}_m(t_j)\hat{S}(t_j-)\hat{\lambda}_m(t_k)\hat{S}(t_k-) \times \left\{-\frac{1}{Y(t_j)} + \sum_{l=1}^{j-1} \frac{dN_m(t_l)}{Y(t_l)\{Y(t_l) - dN_m(t_l)\}}\right\}.$$

Andersen et al. (1993) (Section IV.4) presented a Greenwood-type estimate for the variance of $\hat{r}_m(t)$ in Equation (3.8).

Example: We now illustrate the non-parametric estimate of r_m and contrast it with the Kaplan–Meier estimate of "pure risk". We assume that $M = 2$, that the primary outcome $m = 1$ denotes deaths due to breast cancer, and that the second outcome corresponds to deaths from causes other than breast cancer (Figure 3.1). We also assume no censoring in this example, which simplifies the computations. The numbers in Table 3.1 are the same as

Table 3.1: Life-table of breast cancer mortality and other-cause mortality in 1000 women diagnosed with breast cancer at age 60

Age Interval	n_i	d_{1i}	d_{2i}
[60, 65)	1000	17	44
[65, 70)	939	20	63
[70, 75)	856	22	89

The number at risk at the beginning of the interval is n_i, and the numbers dying of breast cancer and of other causes are, respectively, d_{1i} and d_{2i}.

in Table 2.1, but the censoring column in Table 2.1 becomes deaths from causes other than breast cancer (d_{2i}) in Table 3.1. Applying formula (3.8) to the numbers in Table 3.1, we see that the absolute risk of dying from breast cancer by age 75 is

$$\hat{r}_1(75) = \frac{17}{1000} + \frac{20}{939}\frac{939}{1000} + \frac{22}{856}\frac{856}{1000} = \frac{17 + 20 + 22}{1000} = 0.059.$$

In contrast, the Kaplan–Meier estimate of the pure probability of dying from breast cancer by treating other causes of death as censoring is

$$1 - KM(75) = 1 - \hat{S}(75) = 1 - \left(1 - \frac{17}{1000}\right)\left(1 - \frac{20}{939}\right)\left(1 - \frac{22}{856}\right) = 0.063.$$

The estimate $\hat{r}_1(75) = 0.059$ is smaller than the Kaplan–Meier estimate of "pure risk", 0.063, because a woman who may die of non-breast cancer causes has a reduced chance of dying of breast cancer, compared to a hypothetical woman who is not at risk from non-breast cancer mortality. Although the difference between the absolute and pure risk is small in this example, risk projections over long time periods can be quite different.

Chapters 4 and 5 describe methods for estimating absolute risk $r_m(t)$ from cohort data and other types of data, with the inclusion of covariates.

Chapter 4

Regression models for absolute risk estimated from cohort data

In Chapter 3 we discussed how to estimate absolute risk non-parametrically for a single homogeneous cohort. Interest often centers on estimating absolute risk for persons with specific characteristics measured by covariates. If there are only a few combinations of categorical risk factors, one might be able to use the methods of the previous chapter separately for strata defined by these combinations. Usually, however, the data are too sparse for the stratification approach and one uses modeling to incorporate covariate information and to obtain covariate-specific estimates of absolute risk. There are two basic approaches to incorporate information on covariates $\mathbf{Z} = (Z_1, \ldots, Z_p)$. In the first approach, r_m depends on $\mathbf{Z}$ through the cause-specific hazard functions $\lambda_m, m = 1, \ldots, M$, any or all of which may depend on $\mathbf{Z}$. Some components of $\mathbf{Z}$ may affect some cause-specific hazards and not others. In the second approach, often referred to as *cumulative incidence regression*, see e.g., Fine and Gray (1999), one directly models $r_m(t)$ as a function of $\mathbf{Z}$. We discuss estimating absolute risk for both approaches. For the cause-specific hazard models, we also discuss estimation from sub-samples of a cohort, including nested case-control and case-cohort studies, and from cohorts obtained by complex sampling from a general population. In Chapter 5, under the cause-specific hazards model, we show how to combine estimates of relative and attributable risk from observational studies with overall population incidence rates of the primary and competing events to estimate absolute risk. We present methods for estimating absolute risks, with examples, in Sections 4.1, 4.2, 4.3, 4.4, and 4.5. Variance calculations and confidence interval construction are discussed in a concluding Section 4.6.

4.1 Cause-specific hazard regression

Cause-specific hazard regression incorporates covariates as in panel a of Figure 4.1 to calculate the absolute risk r_m of experiencing the mth event type within the time interval $(t_0, t_1]$ in the presence of $M - 1$ competing events. Given that one is alive and failure-free at t_0, the absolute risk is

$$r_m(t_0, t_1; \mathbf{Z} = \mathbf{z}) = P(t_0 < T \leq t_1, \delta = m | T > t_0, \mathbf{z}) = \int_{t_0}^{t_1} \lambda_m(u, \mathbf{z}^m) S(u-) du =$$

$$\int_{t_0}^{t_1} \lambda_m(u; \mathbf{z}^m) \exp\{-\int_{t_0}^{u} \sum_{k=1}^{M} \lambda_k(s; \mathbf{z}^k) ds\} du, \quad (4.1)$$

where T is the time to the first event, $\mathbf{z}$ is the vector of all covariates that affect any of the M cause-specific hazards, $\mathbf{z}^m$ denotes the subset of covariates in $\mathbf{z}$ that affect $\lambda_m, m = 1, \ldots, M$ and δ denotes the event type. $\mathbf{Z}$ denotes a random covariate vector, whereas $\mathbf{z}$ denotes a particular realization of $\mathbf{Z}$.

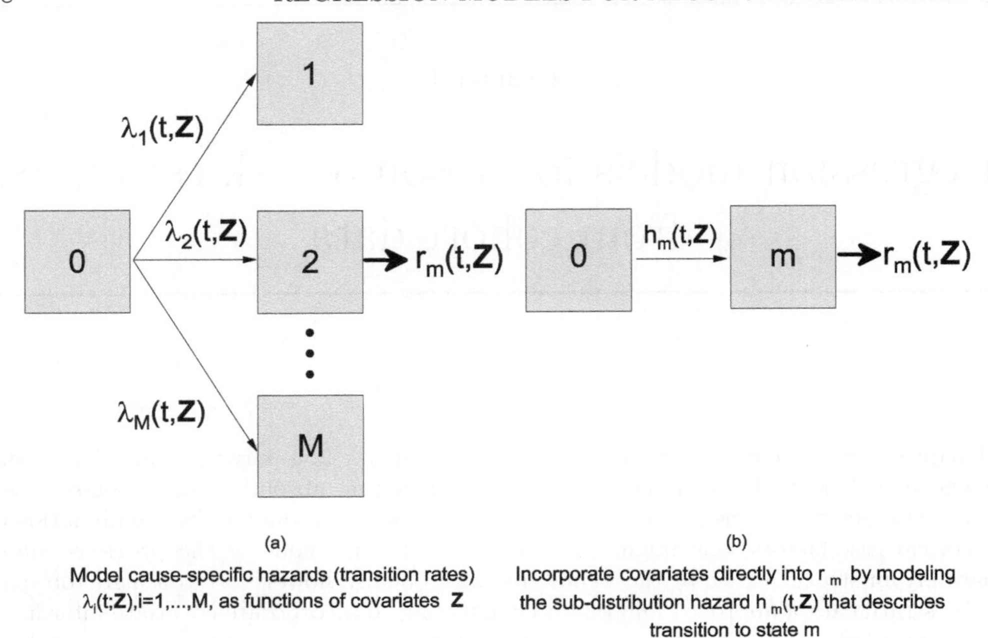

Figure 4.1: Incorporating covariates **Z** into estimates of absolute risk r_m via the cause-specific hazard functions (transition rates) $\lambda_k, k = 1, \ldots, M$ or directly, via cumulative incidence regression.

We assume that covariates in (4.1) remain fixed at their values at the beginning of the projection interval, t_0. However, expression (4.1) is valid if $\mathbf{z}$ or some components of it vary with time, provided that the cause-specific hazard functions are correctly specified, and provided the covariates are "external" (Kalbfleisch and Prentice, 2002). We defer discussion of time-dependent covariates to Section 10.4.1. The risk time scale could be age or time since diagnosis of a particular disease.

To estimate r_m, one plugs estimates $\hat{\lambda}_k, k = 1, \ldots, M$ of the cause-specific hazard functions into Equation (4.1), i.e.,

$$\hat{r}_m(t_0, t_1; \mathbf{z}) = \int_{t_0}^{t_1} \hat{\lambda}_m(u; \mathbf{z}^m) \exp\{-\int_{t_0}^{u} \sum_{k=1}^{M} \hat{\lambda}_k(s; \mathbf{z}^k) ds\} du. \tag{4.2}$$

The most common models for cause-specific hazard functions are relative risk models, that assume that the vector of covariates **Z** influences the hazard function through

$$\lambda_m(t; \mathbf{z}^m) = \lambda_{0m}(t) rr(\boldsymbol{\beta}_m' \mathbf{z}^m), m = 1, \ldots, M, \tag{4.3}$$

where rr denotes the relative hazard, a non-negative scalar function of $\boldsymbol{\beta}_m' \mathbf{z}^m$, and $\lambda_{0m}(t) = \lambda_m(t; \mathbf{z}_0)$ stands for the baseline hazard function for cause m at time t at the referent or baseline covariate level $\mathbf{z}_0$. When rr is the exponential function, one obtains the enormously popular Cox regression model (Cox, 1972),

$$\lambda_m(t; \mathbf{z}^m) = \lambda_{0m}(t) \exp(\boldsymbol{\beta}_m \mathbf{z}^m), m = 1, \ldots, M. \tag{4.4}$$

If individuals 1 and 2 have the same values for all components of $\mathbf{z}_m$ except component k, and values $z_k + 1$ and z_k for that component, respectively, their relative hazard from (4.4) is

$$\frac{\lambda_m(t; \mathbf{z}_1^m)}{\lambda_m(t; \mathbf{z}_2^m)} = \exp\{\boldsymbol{\beta}_m'(\mathbf{z}_1^m - \mathbf{z}_2^m)\} = \exp(\beta_{mk}),$$

where β_{mk} is the log relative hazard for component k. Thus the effect of a unit increase in z_k with all other components of $\mathbf{Z}$ fixed is to multiply the hazard function by $\exp(\beta_{mk})$, which is also referred to as the *relative risk* associated with z_k. If covariates are fixed in Equation (4.4), the relative risk for two individuals with different covariates are constant over time, but not if the covariates vary.

In the next section we outline inference for absolute risk in Equation (4.2) from cohort data when the cause-specific hazard functions are modeled by (4.4), as was first discussed by Benichou and Gail (1990a) for a piecewise constant baseline hazard function and for a non-parametric baseline hazard function. We present point estimates for r_m for non-parametric and for piecewise constant baseline hazard functions. Variance estimates are in Section 4.6.

4.1.1 Estimation of the hazard ratio parameters

We now show how to estimate the regression parameters for the cause-specific hazard functions under a Cox proportional hazards assumption, following (Cheng et al., 1998). We allow for right censoring that may depend on covariates in the model. Left truncation can be accommodated by proper definition of the "at risk" indicator $Y_i(t)$. The observations for individual i in the cohort are $X_i = \min(C_i, T_i)$, the covariates $\mathbf{Z}_i$, and $\delta_i(t)$, that takes values in $\{0, 1, \ldots, M\}$ and denotes the state individual i is in at time t. The "at risk" indicator $Y_i(t) = 1$, if $t \geq$ the entry time for possibly left truncated data and if $t \leq X_i$; otherwise $Y_i(t) = 0$. Thus left truncation as well as right censoring are accommodated by adjusting the risk set. The quantity $\{N_{mi}(t) = I[X_i \leq t, \delta_i = m], t \geq 0\}$ denotes a process that jumps when individual i experiences an event of type m. Extending the notation of Section 2.6, we set $N_m(t) = \sum_{i=1}^{n} N_{mi}(t)$ and $Y(t) = \sum_{i=i}^{n} Y_i(t), t \geq 0$, which count the number of events of type m and the number of individuals still at risk at time t, respectively. Note that in Figure 4.1, Panel a, $Y_i(t) = 0$ following any event or censoring.

Due to the semi-parametric form of (4.4), standard likelihood methods cannot be applied to estimate the regression coefficients $\boldsymbol{\beta}$. Instead, Cox (1972, 1975) estimated $\boldsymbol{\beta}$ based on a *partial likelihood.* The conditional probability that individual i had an event of type m at time t, given that there was exactly one event of type m at that time and given all those at risk at time t, is

$$\frac{\lambda_m(t, \mathbf{Z}_i^m)}{\sum_{j=1}^{n} \lambda_m(t, \mathbf{Z}_j^m) Y_j(t)} = \frac{\exp(\boldsymbol{\beta}_m' \mathbf{Z}_i^m)}{\sum_{j=1}^{n} \exp(\boldsymbol{\beta}_m' \mathbf{Z}_j^m) Y_j(t)}, \tag{4.5}$$

where the factor λ_{0m} has canceled out of the numerator and denominator. In the competing risk setting, the partial likelihood for $\boldsymbol{\beta}$ is the product over all failures times t_l of the conditional probabilities for all m event types, and thus independent of the baseline hazard functions; the partial likelihood is

$$PL(\boldsymbol{\beta}) = \prod_{m=1}^{M} \prod_{i=1}^{n} \prod_{t \geq 0} \left(\frac{Y_i(t) \exp(\boldsymbol{\beta}_m' \mathbf{Z}_i^m)}{\sum_{j=1}^{n} Y_j(t) \exp(\boldsymbol{\beta}_m' \mathbf{Z}_j^m)} \right)^{dN_{mi}(t)}. \tag{4.6}$$

Hereafter we assume that the components of $\boldsymbol{\beta}$ that correspond to each of the outcomes $m = 1, \ldots, M$ are distinct, and functionally independent. In particular, there is no assumption of any common effects of any of the covariates on the M outcomes. Then the partial likelihood (4.6) factors into separate partial likelihoods,

$$PL(\boldsymbol{\beta}) = \prod_{m=1}^{M} PL(\boldsymbol{\beta}_m). \tag{4.7}$$

In this usual case, estimates for the cause-specific regression coefficients $\hat{\boldsymbol{\beta}}_m$ can be obtained by maximizing M partial likelihood functions for each event type separately, i.e., by solving separate vector equations

$$\vec{U}(\boldsymbol{\beta}_m) = \sum_{i=1}^{n} dN_{mi}(t_i)\{\mathbf{z}_i^m - \vec{E}(\boldsymbol{\beta}_m, t_i)\}, m = 1, \ldots, M, \tag{4.8}$$

where

$$\vec{E}(\boldsymbol{\beta}_m, t) = \frac{\sum_{i=1}^{n} Y_i(t) \exp(\boldsymbol{\beta}_m' \mathbf{Z}_i^m) \mathbf{Z}_i^m}{\sum_{i=1}^{n} Y_i(t) \exp(\boldsymbol{\beta}_m' \mathbf{Z}_i^m)}. \tag{4.9}$$

Standard statistical software such as *PROC PHREG* in SAS (SAS Institute Inc., 2011) or the package *survival* written in R can be utilized to obtain $\hat{\boldsymbol{\beta}}_m$, by treating all event types $k \neq m$ as censoring events. In addition to point estimates, this approach also provides valid estimates of the variance of $\hat{\boldsymbol{\beta}}_m$. Alternatively, standard optimization algorithms can be used to obtain the maximum partial likelihood estimator $\hat{\boldsymbol{\beta}}_m$ such that $\vec{U}(\hat{\boldsymbol{\beta}}_m) = 0$.

Prentice et al. (1978) pointed out that the full likelihood factored, analogous to Equation (4.7), and indicated that the cause-specific hazards were therefore estimable and that event types $k \neq m$ could be regarded as censoring for estimating λ_m.

4.1.2 Non-parametric estimation of the baseline hazard

When no distributional assumption is made for the cause-specific baseline hazard function $\lambda_{0m}(t)$, an estimator (Aalen, 1978) is

$$\hat{\lambda}_{0m}(t) = \frac{\sum_{i=1}^{n} dN_{mi}(t)}{\sum_{i=1}^{n} Y_i(t) \exp(\hat{\boldsymbol{\beta}}_m' \mathbf{Z}_i^m)}, \tag{4.10}$$

where $\hat{\boldsymbol{\beta}}_m$ maximizes the corresponding factor in (4.7). The non-parametric Nelson–Aalen estimate of the cumulative cause-specific baseline hazard at time t is

$$\hat{\Lambda}_{0m}(t) = \int_0^t \hat{\lambda}_{0m}(s) ds = \sum_{u_j^m \leq t} \hat{\lambda}_{0m}(u_j^m), \tag{4.11}$$

with $u_1^m < u_2^m < \ldots < u_{N_m}^m$ denoting the N_m observed event times for the mth event type. The estimators $\hat{\boldsymbol{\beta}}_m$ and $\hat{\Lambda}_{0m}$ are consistent, asymptotically normal, and asymptotically efficient among semi-parametric Cox models (Andersen et al., 1993, Sect VIII 4.3). Specifically, $n^{1/2}(\hat{\boldsymbol{\beta}}_m - \boldsymbol{\beta}_m)$ converges to a normal distribution with mean zero and a covariance matrix that can be estimated by $n\mathcal{E}_m^{-1}$ where $\mathcal{E}_m = -\partial^2 \log PL(\boldsymbol{\beta})/\partial \boldsymbol{\beta}_m^2$ is evaluated at $\hat{\boldsymbol{\beta}}_m$. We also define the estimated cumulative hazard for event type m,

$$\hat{\Lambda}_m(t; \mathbf{z}_m) = \sum_{u_j^m \leq t} \hat{\lambda}_{0m}(u_j^m) \exp(\hat{\boldsymbol{\beta}}_m' \mathbf{z}_m) = \hat{\Lambda}_{0m}(t) \exp(\hat{\boldsymbol{\beta}}_m' \mathbf{z}_m). \tag{4.12}$$

4.1.3 Semi-parametric estimation of absolute risk r_m

The semi-parametric estimate of absolute risk of event type m within the interval $(t_0, t_1]$, given $\mathbf{z}$ and given no events until time t_0 is

$$\hat{r}_m(t_0, t_1; \mathbf{z}) = \exp(\hat{\boldsymbol{\beta}}_m' \mathbf{z}^m) \sum_{t_0 < u_j \leq t_1} \hat{\lambda}_{0m}(u_j) \exp\left[-\sum_{k=1}^{M} \{\hat{\Lambda}_k(u_j; \mathbf{z}^k) - \hat{\Lambda}_k(t_0; \mathbf{z}^k)\}\right], \tag{4.13}$$

where u_j are the observed event times of type m occurring in $(t_0, t_1]$. Gerds et al. (2017) developed the R package *riskRegression* to perform these calculations when $t_0 = 0$.

4.1.4 *Estimation of a piecewise exponential baseline hazard model*

While a non-parametric baseline hazard function allows the most flexibility, we also consider the piecewise constant baseline hazard model here for two reasons. First, data are sometimes reduced for Poisson regression into numbers of events of various types and person-years exposure within cells defined by time categories, such as ages $30-34, 35-39, \ldots$ years, and by cross-classifications on covariate levels. Such data are sufficient for estimation of the piecewise constant baseline hazard model. A second motivation is that a parametric model can greatly increase efficiency in comparison to semi-parametric methods when it is a reasonable approximation to the true baseline. The piecewise exponential model is a flexible choice among parametric models. In simulation studies for cohort data, Benichou and Gail (1990a) reported up to fourfold efficiency gains for estimating absolute risk for the piecewise exponential model compared to a non-parametric baseline hazard. Other flexible parametric hazard functions such as splines could also be fit to the data.

We define a set of ordered possibly unequally spaced time intervals $\mathcal{I}_1, \mathcal{I}_2, \ldots$, with $\mathcal{I}_q = [\tau_{0q}, \tau_{1q})$ and $\tau_{1q} = \tau_{0(q+1)}$. Denote the constant cause-specific baseline hazard during the qth time interval by $\lambda_{0m}(\mathcal{I}_q)$. The baseline hazard function for cause m under the piecewise exponential model is

$$\lambda_{0m}(t) = \sum_q \lambda_{0m}(\mathcal{I}_q) I(t \in \mathcal{I}_q).$$

As in Benichou and Gail (1990a), the estimated absolute risk of event type m in $(\tau_{0k}, \tau_{1l}]$ given no events before τ_{0k} is

$$\hat{r}_m(\tau_{0k}, \tau_{1l}; \mathbf{z}) = \sum_{q=k}^{l} \hat{S}(\mathcal{I}_q) \hat{P}_m(\mathcal{I}_q) \left[1 - \exp\{-\sum_{v=1}^{M} \hat{\lambda}_{0v}(\mathcal{I}_q) \exp(\hat{\boldsymbol{\beta}}_v' \mathbf{z}^v)(\tau_{1q} - \tau_{0q})\} \right], \quad (4.14)$$

where $\hat{P}_m(\mathcal{I}_q) = \hat{\lambda}_{0m}(\mathcal{I}_q) \exp(\hat{\boldsymbol{\beta}}_m' \mathbf{z}^m) / \sum_v \hat{\lambda}_{0v}(\mathcal{I}_q) \exp(\hat{\boldsymbol{\beta}}_v' \mathbf{z}^v)$ and

$$\hat{S}(\mathcal{I}_q) = \begin{cases} 1 & q = k \\ \prod_{j=k}^{q-1} \exp\{-\sum_i \hat{\lambda}_{0i}(\mathcal{I}_j) \exp(\hat{\boldsymbol{\beta}}_i \mathbf{z}^i)(\tau_{1j} - \tau_{0j})\} & q > k \end{cases}. \quad (4.15)$$

Let t_{0i} be the time that the ith individual in the cohort is first at-risk and t_i the time last at risk. In the competing risk setting, t_i occurs at the earlier of the time of any event or censoring. Then the at-risk time for this individual during the qth interval is

$$\mathcal{A}_i(\tau_q) = I(t_{0i} < \tau_{1q} \cap t_i > \tau_{0q}) \{\min\{t_i, \tau_{1q}\} - \max\{t_{0i}, \tau_{0q}\}\}. \quad (4.16)$$

Note that the definition of $\mathcal{A}_i$ allows for left truncation. Set $D^m(\mathcal{I}_q)$ equal to the total weighted person-time during the qth interval,

$$D^m(\mathcal{I}_q) = \sum_{i=1}^{n} \mathcal{A}_i(\tau_q) \exp(\hat{\boldsymbol{\beta}}_m' \mathbf{z}_i^m).$$

Then given $d^m(\mathcal{I}_q) = \sum_{i=1}^n I(\delta_i(t_i) = m, \tau_{0q} \le t_i < \tau_{1q})$ observed events of type m in $[\tau_{0q}, \tau_{1q})$, the estimate for $\lambda_{0m}(\mathcal{I}_q)$ is

$$\hat{\lambda}_{0m}(\mathcal{I}_q) = \frac{d^m(\mathcal{I}_q)}{D^m(\mathcal{I}_q)}.$$

This estimator is equivalent to (4.10) when the event times fall at the endpoints $\tau_{iq}, i = 0, 1$ of the intervals on which λ_{0m} is constant.

Under the piecewise exponential model, the baseline cumulative hazard from τ_{0k} to time $t \ge \tau_{0k}$ is

$$\hat{\Lambda}_{0m}(t) = \sum_{q:\tau_{0q} < t} \hat{\lambda}_{0m}(\mathcal{I}_q) (\min\{t, \tau_{1q}\} - \tau_{0q}).$$

4.1.5 Alternative hazard models

The methodology can be applied to a broader set of hazard models by generalizing Equation (4.4), so that

$$\lambda_m(t; \mathbf{z}^m) = \lambda_{0m}(t) rr(\boldsymbol{\beta}_m; \mathbf{z}^m), \tag{4.17}$$

where $rr(\boldsymbol{\beta}_m; \mathbf{z}^m)$ is a known non-negative scalar function of $\boldsymbol{\beta}_m$ and covariates $\mathbf{z}^m$. If the $\mathbf{z}^m$ include a continuous exposure variable, z_1^m (e.g., cumulative pack-years smoked or absorbed radiation), one might consider an excess relative risk (ERR) model for z_1^m (Preston et al., 1993), such as

$$rr(\boldsymbol{\beta}_m; \mathbf{z}^m) = (1 + \beta_{m1} z_1^m) \exp(\boldsymbol{\beta}'_{m2} \mathbf{z}_2^m). \tag{4.18}$$

To obtain the absolute risk estimates and variances for any model of the form of Equation (4.17), one derives estimating equations for β_m from a partial likelihood by replacing all instances of $\exp(\boldsymbol{\beta}'_m \mathbf{z}^m)$ in Equation (4.4) and its first and second derivatives with $rr(\boldsymbol{\beta}_m; \mathbf{z}^m)$, $\partial rr(\boldsymbol{\beta}_m; \mathbf{z}^m)/\partial \boldsymbol{\beta}_m$, and $\partial^2 rr(\boldsymbol{\beta}_m; \mathbf{z}^m)/\partial \boldsymbol{\beta}_m \partial \boldsymbol{\beta}'_m$, respectively. Given the estimator $\hat{\boldsymbol{\beta}}_m$, one would substitute $rr(\hat{\boldsymbol{\beta}}_m; \mathbf{z}^m)$ and its first derivative for their corresponding quantities in the formulas of Sections 4.1.1 and 4.1.2 to derive point estimates and in the formulas in Section 4.6.1 to estimate variances for absolute risk. Note that the estimate of β_{m1} in (4.18) is constrained so that $(1 + \beta_{m1} z_1^m) > 0$ for all feasible z_1^m.

As an alternative to the proportional hazards model, Aalen (1989) proposed the additive hazard model

$$\lambda(t, \mathbf{Z}) = \alpha_0(t) + \boldsymbol{\alpha}(t)' \mathbf{Z}. \tag{4.19}$$

Shen and Cheng (1999) studied estimates of absolute risk (4.1) based on a special case of the additive model in (4.19), namely

$$\lambda_m(t, \mathbf{Z}) = \alpha_{0m}(t) + \boldsymbol{\beta}'_m \mathbf{Z}^m. \tag{4.20}$$

This model was first proposed by Lin and Ying (1994) who showed that estimates of $\boldsymbol{\beta}$ in Equation (4.20) can be obtained in a closed form. Shen and Cheng (1999) discussed estimation and prediction of the absolute risk r_m when Equation (4.20) is used for the cause-specific hazard functions and also constructed simultaneous confidence intervals for r_m. If Equation (4.20) holds for all M competing events, then the impact of the covariates $\mathbf{Z}$ on the total hazard is given by the sum of their effects on the cause-specific hazard functions, $\sum_m \lambda_m(t) = \sum_m \alpha_{m0}(t) + \sum_m \boldsymbol{\beta}'_m \mathbf{Z}$. Schaubel and Wei (2007) established connections between the model of Lin and Ying (1994) and both Cox and least squares regression and showed how standard statistical software may be used to fit the additive hazards model.

Scheike and Zhang (2002, 2003) proposed a flexible additive-multiplicative hazard model, the Cox–Aalen model, that combines the Cox proportional hazards model with the additive model of Aalen,

$$\lambda_m(t, \mathbf{Z}) = \{\boldsymbol{\alpha}_m(t)' \mathbf{Z}_1^m\} \exp(\boldsymbol{\beta}'_m \mathbf{Z}_2^m), \tag{4.21}$$

where the first entry of the vector $\mathbf{Z}_1^m$ is equal to one. This model reduces to the Cox model when $\mathbf{Z}_1^m = 1$ and to Aalen's additive model when all components of $\mathbf{Z}_2^m$ are zero. Scheike and Zhang (2002) studied estimates $\hat{r}_m(t)$ based on the Cox–Aalen hazard model and also provided variance estimates.

Although these alternative approaches to modeling cause-specific hazards are potentially useful, we rely on the Cox model (4.4) in our examples and in Section 4.6 on variance estimation.

4.2 Cumulative incidence regression

In the cause-specific hazards model, the absolute risk $r_m(t) = P(T \leq t, \delta = m|\mathbf{Z})$ depends on the cause-specific hazards $\lambda_k, k = 1, \ldots, M$, of the main cause of interest, m, and of the

$M-1$ competing causes through a complex nonlinear relationship given in Equation (4.1). It is therefore difficult to understand the effects of covariates on r_m by simply examining $\hat{\boldsymbol{\beta}}_m$. A related issue is that standard methods for model assessment and covariate selection for the cause-specific hazard model may apply to the individual estimated cause-specific hazards, but not to modeling absolute risk itself. It is possible that a covariate influences the absolute risk r_m, but may not be strongly associated with any of the cause-specific hazards, and therefore not be chosen for cause-specific modeling of absolute risk.

Cumulative incidence regression avoids these problems by incorporating covariates directly into $r_m(t, \mathbf{Z})$ via a link function,

$$g\{r_m(t)\} = \psi_0(t) + \boldsymbol{\gamma}'\mathbf{Z}, \tag{4.22}$$

where ψ_0 is an unspecified invertible and monotone increasing function that captures the baseline failure probability, see, e.g., (Fine, 1999). In this framework $\boldsymbol{\gamma}$ measures the distance from the baseline probability $g^{-1}\{\psi_0(t)\}$ on the scale of g. There is no subindex m for $\boldsymbol{\gamma}$, because $\boldsymbol{\gamma}$ is the only vector of regression coefficients that is estimated. Cumulative incidence regression thus directly estimates this transformation model for r_m without estimating models for the other competing causes $k = 1, \ldots, M, k \neq m$. Recall from Section 3.1 that not all individuals will experience an event of type m because $\lim_{t\to\infty} r_m(t) < 1$. Thus r_m is referred to as a sub-distribution function, and some authors refer to regression models for r_m as sub-distribution regression models.

Before discussing cumulative incidence models in more detail, we describe a process (Beyersmann and Schumacher, 2008) that helps formalize this approach to modeling r_m. Beyersmann and Schumacher (2008) defined the sub-distribution process $\delta^*(t)$ in terms of the original competing risk process $\delta(t)$ as

$$\delta^*(t) = I(\delta(t) = m)\delta(t) + I(\delta(t) = k, k \neq m)\delta(T-),$$

where $T = \inf\{t : \delta(t) > 0\}$. From this definition, the process δ^* has only two states, 0 and m, and remains in the initial state 0 if an individual experiences one of the $M-1$ competing events. Thus the two processes δ and δ^* have to be interpreted differently. If $\delta^*(t) = 0$, then an individual has not experienced an event of type m, while $\delta(t) = 0$ is interpreted as "no event by time t". The corresponding time to the occurrence of an event of type m is then $T^* := \inf\{t > 0 | \delta^*(t) \neq 0\}$. Thus $T^* = T$ if $\delta(T) = m$ and $T^* = \infty$ if $\delta(T) = k > 0, k \neq m$, and thus $P(T^* \leq t) = P(T \leq t, \delta = m)$ for all $t \geq 0$ and $P(T^* = \infty) = \sum_{k \neq m} P(\delta(T) = k)$, which causes technical difficulties when fitting models, as explained in the next section.

4.2.1 Proportional sub-distribution hazards model

The best known cumulative incidence model, commonly referred to as the Fine and Gray (FG) model (Fine and Gray, 1999), uses $g(t) = \log\{-\log(1-t)\}$ in Equation (4.22). This model was introduced by Gray (1988). Using this link, Fine and Gray (1999) incorporated covariates into r_m via the *sub-distribution hazard function* for the event m, defined as the probability that a subject fails from cause m in an infinitesimal time interval given that the subject has not experienced the event of type m up to t,

$$\begin{aligned} h_m(t, \mathbf{Z}) &= \lim_{\epsilon \to 0^+} \frac{1}{\epsilon} P\{t \leq T < t + \epsilon, \delta = m | T \geq t \cup (T \leq t \cap \delta \neq m), \mathbf{Z})\} \\ &= \lim_{\epsilon \to 0^+} \frac{1}{\epsilon} P(t \leq T^* < t + \epsilon | T^* \geq t, \mathbf{Z}) = \frac{\frac{d}{dt} r_m(t, \mathbf{Z})}{1 - r_m(t, \mathbf{Z})} = -\frac{d \log\{1 - r_m(t, \mathbf{Z})\}}{dt}. \end{aligned} \tag{4.23}$$

Fine and Gray (1999) assumed a proportional hazards model for the sub-distribution hazard,

$$h_m(t, \mathbf{Z}) = h_{m0}(t) \exp(\boldsymbol{\gamma}'\mathbf{Z}), \tag{4.24}$$

where $h_{m0}(t)$ is an unspecified non-negative function of t. Recalling that $g(t) = \log\{-\log(1-t)\}$ in (4.22), we see that $\psi_0(t) \equiv \log\{\int_0^t h_{0m}(s)ds\} = \log\{H_{0m}(t)\}$ and thus

$$r_m(t, \mathbf{Z}) = 1 - \exp\left\{-\int_0^t h_m(s, \mathbf{Z})ds)\right\} = 1 - \exp\{-H_{m0}(t)\exp(\boldsymbol{\gamma}'\mathbf{Z})\}. \quad (4.25)$$

If a binary covariate Z has a positive regression coefficient γ in (4.24), then the absolute risk $r_m(t, \mathbf{Z})$ is higher for individuals with $Z = 1$ than for those with $Z = 0$. In the cause-specific hazards formulation Z might increase λ_m, but its effect on r_m would depend on if and how Z affected other cause-specific hazards.

Fine and Gray (1999) proposed to estimate the parameters $\boldsymbol{\gamma}$ in (4.24) based on a partial likelihood that has the same form as the Cox partial likelihood. However, the risk set at the time t of a failure due to cause m is comprised of all the cohort members who have not failed from that cause, including those individuals who previously failed from other causes, namely the set of all individuals i with $\{(T_i \geq t) \cup (T_i < t \cap \delta_i \neq m)\}$. This definition of the risk set makes the analysis of time-dependent covariates challenging, as one has to define covariate values for those individuals who failed from causes other than cause m, but who are nevertheless technically still in the risk set (Beyersmann and Schumacher, 2008). For example, if we wish to assess the impact of hormone replacement therapy use as a time-dependent variable on absolute risk of incident breast cancer, a woman who died at age 60 from a non-breast cancer cause would still be in the risk set for breast cancer incidence at age 70, but her usage of hormone replacement therapy is not defined. This problem does not arise for fixed covariates. In the absence of censoring, an indicator of whether an individual is in the sub-distribution risk set is $Y_0^*(t) = I(T \geq t) + I(T < t, \delta(T) = k, k > 0, k \neq m)$.

In the presence of right censoring, the corresponding sub-distribution at risk process is given by $Y^*(t) = I(\min(T, C) \geq t) + I(T < t \leq C, \delta(T) = k, k > 0, k \neq m)$. As in general the second indicator function is unknown, Fine and Gray (1999) replaced $Y^*(t)$ by an "estimated" contribution to the risk set, $\widehat{Y}^*(t)$, by weighting the observable uncensored indicators $Y_0^*(t)$ with"inverse probability of censoring weights" (IPCW) (Robins and Rotnitzky, 1992). To obtain these weights, one needs to estimate the censoring distribution for each individual. Assuming censoring is completely at random, i.e., that censoring does not depend on any covariates, Fine and Gray (1999) estimated the censoring distribution by the Kaplan–Meier estimator $\hat{G}(t) = \hat{P}(C \geq t)$, and used the time-dependent weights $w_i(t) = I\{C_i \geq \min(T_i, t)\}\hat{G}(t)/\hat{G}(\min(C_i, T_i, t-))$ to obtain

$$\begin{aligned}\widehat{Y}^*(t) &= w(t)Y_0^*(t) = w(t)\{I(T \geq t) + I(T < t, \delta(T) = k, k > 0, k \neq m)\} \\ &= I(\min(T, C) \geq t) + \frac{I(C_i \geq T_i)\hat{G}(t)}{\hat{G}(T_i-)} I(T < t, \delta(T) = k, k > 0, k \neq m). \quad (4.26)\end{aligned}$$

This estimate is asymptotically unbiased, in the sense that $E\widehat{Y}^*(t) = Y^*(t)$.

Alternatively, the censoring distribution could be modeled parametrically or semi-parametrically and also be allowed to depend on covariates $\mathbf{Z}$.

An estimate $\hat{\gamma}$ is thus obtained by solving the weighted score equations

$$\vec{U}(\gamma) = \sum_{i=1}^{n} dN_{mi}(t)w_i(t)\left\{\mathbf{z}_i - \frac{\sum_{j=1}^{n} w_j(t)Y_{0j}^*(t)\exp(\boldsymbol{\gamma}'\mathbf{Z}_j)\mathbf{Z}_j}{\sum_{j=1}^{n} w_j(t)Y_{0j}^*(t)\exp(\boldsymbol{\gamma}'\mathbf{Z}_j)}\right\}. \quad (4.27)$$

Here N_{mi} is the counting process associated with events of type m, defined in the same way as for the cause-specific setting as $N_{mi} = I(\min(T_i, C_i) \leq t, \delta_i(t) = m)$. The estimated cumulative sub-distribution hazard function is given by

$$\hat{H}_m(t, \mathbf{Z}) = \int_0^t \exp(\hat{\boldsymbol{\gamma}}'\mathbf{Z})d\hat{H}_{m0}(t),$$

where $\hat{H}_{m0}(t)$ is a modified version of the Breslow estimator for a standard cumulative hazard function, given by

$$\hat{H}_{m0}(t) = \sum_{\min(T_i^*, C_i) \le t} \frac{\sum_{i=1}^n dN_{mi}\{\min(T_i^*, C_i)\}}{\sum_{i=1}^n Y_i^*\{\min(T_i^*, C_i)\} \exp(\hat{\gamma}'\mathbf{Z}_i)}.$$

Using $\hat{\gamma}$ and $\hat{H}_{m0}(t)$ in Equation (4.25) yields the estimate

$$\hat{r}_m(t, \mathbf{Z}) = \hat{P}(T \le t, \delta = m|\mathbf{Z}) = 1 - \exp\{-\hat{H}_m(t, \mathbf{Z})\}.$$

Fine and Gray (1999) prove consistency and asymptotic normality of $\hat{\gamma}$ based on weighted score equations, and show that $\hat{r}_m(t, \mathbf{Z})$ has an asymptotic normal distribution. They also provide point-wise confidence intervals and confidence bands.

The computation of $\hat{r}_m(t, \mathbf{Z})$ is implemented in the *R* package *cmprsk*, (https://cran.r-project.org/web/packages/cmprsk/index.html/), and also in the *STATA* software (StataCorp., 2015). One limitation is that the theory in Fine and Gray (1999) did not allow for left truncation or time-dependent covariates, nor does this software.

Only recently has the estimation of the sub-distribution hazards model been extended to accommodate left truncation as well as right censoring. Geskus (2011) showed that estimates of γ in (4.24) can be obtained by solving a weighted score equation where the time-dependent weights depend on the censoring and the truncation distribution. Letting L denote the left truncation variable, this can be done by noting that the sub-distribution risk set enumerator becomes $Y^*(t) = I\{L < t \le \min(T, C)\} + I\{\max(T, L) < t \le C, \delta(T) = k, k > 0, k \ne m\}$, which can be replaced in the score equation by the "estimated" risk set indicator $\widehat{Y}^*(t) = I\{L \le T \le \min(T, C)\} + I(C \ge T > L)\hat{G}(t)\hat{H}(t)/\{\hat{G}(T-)\hat{H}(T-)\}I(T < t, \delta(T) = k, k > 0, k \ne m)$, where $\hat{H}(t)$ is an estimator of $P(L \le t)$. Thus estimates of γ are obtained by solving the score Equations (4.27) with weights $w(t) = \hat{G}(t)\hat{H}(t)/\{\hat{G}(T-)\hat{H}(T-)\}$. Geskus (2011) derived asymptotic results for the proportional sub-distribution hazards model under left truncation using these time-dependent weights, and a corresponding *R* function is built into the *R* package *mstate* (https://cran.r-project.org/web/packages/mstate/mstate.pdf, (de Wreede et al., 2011)).

Contemporaneously, Zhang et al. (2011) also developed an approach to fitting the Fine–Gray proportional sub-distribution hazard model with left truncated and right censored observations. These authors start from the general case where the truncation and censoring distributions depend on covariates (but are independent conditional on these covariates), but then provide details only for non-parametric estimates of the weights using inverse probability weighting (IPW). Geskus (2011) argued that even if the censoring and/or truncation distribution depended on covariates it is not necessary to include these covariates in the weights. Zhang et al. (2011) used a stabilized weight rather than the IPW to reduce the variability in the original weight. These weights seem quite different from those of Geskus (2011) as they depend on an estimate of overall survival, and a careful comparison of the performance of these two approaches would be useful.

4.2.2 Other cumulative incidence regression models

Equation (4.22) allows for other link functions, such as the logit link function, $g(t) = \log\{t/(1-t)\}$ studied in (Fine, 2001). Scheike et al. (2008) also modeled the covariate effect for the absolute risk estimate via binomial regression. They also extended the FG model to allow for time-dependent effects of some of the covariates,

$$\text{logit}\{r_m(t)\} = \mathbf{Z}_1\gamma_1(t) + \mathbf{Z}_2'\gamma_2.$$

Scheike and Zhang (2011) gave software for fitting such models. Right censoring is accommodated using the probability of censoring as weights. The authors compared the performance of two estimates of the censoring distribution, the Kaplan–Meier survival function and a Cox regression model. They found in simulations that incorporating covariates into the estimation of the censoring distribution resulted in significant efficiency gains for the logistic cumulative incidence regression model. However, no such efficiency gain was seen when the FG sub-distribution hazard model was fit to r_m. Klein and Andersen (2005) described simple methods to estimate models (4.22) by applying generalized linear models to jackknife-like pseudo-values.

4.2.3 Relationship between the cause-specific and the proportional sub-distribution hazards models

Differentiating minus the logarithm of one minus Equations (4.1) and (4.25) and noting that $1 - P(T \leq t, \delta = m) = P(T > t) + \sum_{k \neq m} P(T \leq t, \delta = k) = P(T > t) + \sum_{k \neq m} r_k(t)$, we see that the cause-specific and the sub-distribution hazards functions are related through

$$\lambda_m(t) = \left[1 + \frac{\sum_{k \neq m} r_k(t)}{P(T > t)}\right] h_m(t). \tag{4.28}$$

Equation (4.28) highlights differences between the cause-specific and the sub-distribution hazard functions. First, $\lambda_m(t) \geq h_m(t)$. Second, as the first factor on the right hand side of (4.28) depends on t, proportionality over covariates cannot hold simultaneously for h_m and λ_m. Third, Equation (4.28) indicates how a covariate might increase λ_m but decrease h_m and hence r_m. Suppose a binary covariate increases λ_m by a factor of 1.5, but increases all the other cause-specific hazards functions $\lambda_k, k \neq m$, much more, so that $1+\sum_{k \neq m} r_k / P(T > t)$ increases by a factor of 2. The effect of the covariate is to multiply h_m by $1.5/2 = 0.75$. Thus the parameters $\boldsymbol{\gamma}$ describe the overall impact of a covariate on r_m. However, the cause-specific $\boldsymbol{\beta}$ parameters may offer insight into how the covariates impact r_m and also allow for an etiologic interpretation of the covariate effects, which may be preferred by some epidemiologists. Gerds et al. (2012) discuss potential problems of interpretation of various models for cumulative incidence regression including: absolute risk estimates may exceed 1.0 for some models; the sum of absolute risk projections over causes may exceed 1.0 (which cannot occur for cause-specific models); and the methods that require inverse probability weighting to account for censoring can yield biased results if the censoring model is misspecified. Andersen and Keiding (2012) question the interpretability of the sub-distribution hazard because the corresponding risk sets include persons who have had absorbing events.

4.3 Examples

4.3.1 Absolute risk of breast cancer incidence

Data

We illustrate the methods described above based on a slightly modified version of a recently developed absolute risk model for breast cancer (Pfeiffer et al., 2013). In that paper, we combined data from two large cohorts to estimate the model parameters. For ease of exposition, we only use one of the cohorts here, namely the National Institutes of Health-AARP Diet and Health Study (NIH-AARP), that is described in detail in Schatzkin et al. (2001). It included 567,169 men and women who, in 1995–1996, were 50–71 years old and resided in one of eight states. Participants returned a self-administered baseline questionnaire and a second more detailed questionnaire, sent 6 months after the baseline questionnaire. Cancer cases were identified through linkage with state cancer registries with 90% completeness of case ascertainment (Michaud et al., 2005). All invasive breast cancer cases had a histologic diagnosis. Vital status was ascertained through annual linkage to the Social Security Administration Death Master File and the National Death Index Plus.

We restrict the analysis to 191,604 non-Hispanic, white women who completed the baseline questionnaire, had follow-up information, and had no personal history of breast cancer at baseline. Among these women, $n = 5,905$ were diagnosed with invasive epithelial breast cancer during follow up, including 35 breast cancers that developed in women after a diagnosis of *in situ* breast cancer, and 12,383 women died from causes other than breast cancer.

Estimation of the cause-specific hazard function for breast cancer incidence

To build the absolute risk model, we first estimated the cause-specific hazard function for invasive breast cancer. We fit a Cox proportional hazards model to the data with age as the time scale, to estimate relative risk (RR) parameters, 95% confidence intervals (CIs) and the cause-specific baseline hazard function for invasive breast cancer. Women were considered at risk from the age at study entry (completion of baseline questionnaire) until the age at the earliest of the following: (1) diagnosis of invasive breast cancer, (2) death, or (3) administrative censoring on December 31, 2003. Thus the data were left truncated on the age scale. Death and administrative censoring were combined into a single censoring event for the purpose of estimating the cause-specific hazard (Prentice et al., 1978). Proportionality of the hazard functions was assessed by visual inspection of hazard plots and Schoenfeld residuals. Using *PROC PHREG*, SAS v9.2 software, and the function *coxph* in the R Package *survival* (Therneau and Grambsch, 2000), yielded virtually identical results. Late entry is accommodated using the *entry* option in the model statement of *PROC PHREG*, and in the specification of the survival object defined using *Surv* in R.

Details on variable coding and model building can be found in Pfeiffer et al. (2013). When building the model we considered the following risk factors: body mass index (BMI), age at menarche, number of live-born children (parity), age at first birth, duration of oral contraceptive (OC) use, menopausal status and age at natural menopause, status and duration of menopausal hormone therapy (MHT) use, status and duration of estrogen and progestin MHT use, duration of unopposed estrogen MHT use, history of benign breast disease and past breast biopsies, first-degree family history of breast cancer (first degree relatives defined as mother, daughters and sisters with a breast cancer diagnosis), first-degree family history of ovarian cancer, any previous gynecologic surgery (defined as hysterectomy and/or partial or bilateral oophorectomy), smoking status, cigarettes per day smoked and alcohol consumption. Table 4.1 describes some key variables with the number of cases, competing deaths and non-events in each category.

Information for benign breast disease was missing on more than 20% of the women in the dataset, and we thus created an indicator for missing values. We excluded 20,273 women who had missing information on family history, BMI, gynecologic surgery or age at first live birth, from the analysis, leaving 171,331 women in NIH-AARP to fit the final breast cancer RR model. Of those women 5,284 were diagnosed with invasive breast cancer and 10,610 died from other causes.

We first assessed the main effects of all risk factors listed above. The final model included only variables that were significant in multivariable models with $p < 0.01$. We chose a stringent p-value as we did not want to include variables with modest RRs that would not improve prediction. Model building was repeated using stepwise variable selection in Cox proportional hazards models and led to the same selection of variables. We also assessed the significance at $p < 0.01$ of all first-order interaction terms of variables included in the final model. We fitted variables with trends whenever appropriate (see Table 4.2). For all risk factors, the reference category was the lowest risk category.

Table 4.1: Numbers of invasive breast cancer cases and non-cases by selected characteristics of non-Hispanic, white women in the NIH-AARP cohort

			Number of	
		breast cancer cases (%)	**competing cause deaths (%)**	**no events (%)**
Characteristic	**Subcategory**	$n = 5,905$	$n = 12,383$	$n = 173,316$
BMI, kg/m^2	< 25	2,464 (41.7)	5,110 (41.3)	76,452 (44.1)
	25 to < 30	1,901 (32.2)	3,454 (27.9)	54,353 (31.4)
	30 to < 35	848 (14.4)	1,787 (14.4)	23,859 (13.8)
	≥ 35	510 (8.6)	1,291 10.43	12,935 (7.5)
	Missing	182 (3.1)	741 (6.0)	5,717 (3.3)
Family history of breast or ovarian cancer	No	4,554 (77.1)	10,204 (82.4)	142,970 (82.5)
	Yes	1,240 (21.0)	1,859 (15.0)	26,905 (15.5)
	Missing	111 (1.9)	320 (2.6)	3,441 (2.0)
Benign breast disease	No	1,947 (33.0)	4,392 (35.5)	65,091 (37.6)
	Yes	2,607 (44.1)	3,808 (30.8)	61,006 (35.2)
	Missing	1,351 (22.9)	4,183 (33.8)	47,219 (27.2)
Parity	Nulliparous	1,000 (16.9)	1,843 (14.9)	24,566 (14.2)
	1-2	2,134 (36.1)	4,049 (32.7)	62,975 (36.3)
	≥ 3	2,640 (44.7)	6,160 (49.8)	82,496 (47.6)
	Missing	131 (2.2)	331 (2.7)	3,279 (1.9)
Estrogen and progestin MHT use	0 years	1,301 (22.0)	3,369 (27.2)	42,862 (24.7)
	19	605 (10.2)	443 (3.6)	13,983 (8.1)
	≥ 10	322 (5.5)	247 (2.0)	5,034 (2.9)
	NA or missing	3,677 (62.3)	8,324 (67.2)	111,437 (64.3)
Alcohol consumption, drinks/day	0	1,573 (26.6)	4,764 (38.5)	48,059 (27.7)
	< 1	3,343 (56.6)	5,900 (47.7)	101,841 (58.8)
	≥ 1	989 (16.8)	1,719 (13.9)	23,416 (13.5)
Other MHT use	No	4,197 (71.1)	9,428 (76.1)	122,700 (70.8)
	Yes	1,708 (28.9)	2,955 (23.9)	50,616 (29.2)
Age at birth of first child, years	< 25	4,268 (72.3)	9,538 (77.0)	130,087 (75.1)
	$(25, 29]$	1,130 (19.1)	1,971 (15.9)	30,978 (17.9)
	≥ 30	410 (6.9)	644 (5.2)	9,854 (5.7)
	NA or missing	97 (1.6)	230 (1.9)	2,397 (1.4)
Gynecologic Surgery	No	3,406 (57.7)	6,310 (51.0)	92,035 (53.1)
	Yes	2,189 (37.1)	5,290 (42.7)	72,510 (41.8)
	Missing	310 (5.3)	783 (6.3)	8,771 (5.1)
Age at menopause, years	< 50	3,020 (51.1)	7,836 (63.3)	97,847 (56.5)
	$[50, 55)$	2,000 (33.9)	3,410 (27.5)	53,647 (31.0)
	≥ 55	545 9.23	766 (6.2)	11,703 (6.8)
	Premenopausal/ missing	340 (5.8)	371 (3.0)	10,119 (5.8)
Smoking	Never smoker	2,459 (41.6)	3,395 (27.4)	76,533 (44.2)
	Former smoker	856 (14.5)	3,219 (26.0)	23,738 (13.7)
	Current smoker	2,409 (40.8)	5,294 (42.8)	67,555 (39.0)
	Missing	181 (3.1)	475 (3.84)	5,490 (3.2)

The cases include 35 women who developed invasive breast cancer after a diagnosis of *in situ* breast cancer.

Table 4.2: Multivariable cause-specific relative risk (RR) estimates for invasive breast cancer and death from causes other than breast cancer among non-Hispanic, white women in the NIH-AARP cohort

Characteristic	Subcategory	Invasive breast cancer RR (95% CI)	Competing causes of death RR (95% CI)
BMI	$< 25kg/m^2$	1.0 (referent)	1.0 (referent)
	Per category increase	1.11 (1.08-1.15)	1.06 (1.04-1.08)
Estrogen and progestin	No MHT use	1.0 (referent)	1.0 (referent)
MHT use	Per category increase	1.42 (1.34-1.51)	0.75 (0.71-0.80)
Other/unknown	No	1.0 (referent)	1.0 (referent)
MHT use	Yes	1.22 (1.13-1.33)	0.80 (0.75-0.84)
Alcohol consumption	0 drinks/day	1.0 (referent)	1.0 (referent)
	Per category increase	1.12 (1.08-1.17)	0.80 (0.77-0.82)
Gynecologic Surgery	Yes	1.0 (referent)	
	No	1.14 (1.07-1.23)	
Parity	1+ children	1.0 (referent)	1.0 (referent)
	Nulliparous	1.32 (1.23-1.42)	1.13 (1.07-1.19)
Family history of breast or	No		
ovarian cancer	Yes	1.39 (1.30-1.49)	
Age at first live birth	< 25 years	1.0 (referent)	1.0 (referent)
	Per category increase	1.15 (1.10-1.20)	0.93 (0.89-0.96)
Age at menopause	< 50 years	1.0 (referent)	1.0 (referent)
	Per category increase	1.13 (1.07-1.18)	0.86 (0.83-0.88)
	NA/missing	1.04 (0.91-1.18)	0.61 (0.53-0.70)
Benign breast	No	1.0 (referent)	1.0 (referent)
disease/biopsy	Yes	1.41 (1.32-1.50)	0.88 (0.84-0.93)
	missing	1.30 (1.11-1.52)	0.84 (0.75-0.94)
Smoking	Never smoker		1.0 (referent)
	Per category increase		1.29 (1.27-1.32)

All variables are coded so that the lowest risk category for invasive breast cancer is the reference category.
Categories for variables fitted with a trend: BMI: $< 25, 25$ to $< 30, 30$ to < 35, and $\geq 35kg/m^2$; estrogen and progestin MHT use: never, $< 10, \geq 10$ years; age at first birth: $< 25, 25-29$, and ≥ 30 years; age at menopause: $< 50, 50-54, \geq 55$ years, missing; alcohol consumption: $0, < 1, \geq 1$ drinks/day; age menopause: 0: premenopausal or ≤ 49, $1: 50-54$ years, 2: ≥ 55 years; smoking: 0: never smoker, 1: former smoker, 2: current smoker.

The final RR model (Table 4.2) included: BMI ($< 25, 25$ to $< 30, 30$ to $< 35, \geq 35kg/m^2$), estrogen and progestin MHT use (never, $< 10, \geq 10$ years), other or unknown MHT use (no, yes), parity ($0, \geq 1$ children), age at first birth ($< 25, 25-29, \geq 30$ years), premenopausal (no, yes), age at menopause ($< 50, 50$ to $< 55, \geq 55$ years), benign breast diseases (no, yes), previous gynecologic surgery (no, yes), family history of breast or ovarian cancer (no, yes), and alcohol consumption ($0, < 1, \geq 1$ drinks/day). The largest RRs per category increase in the model were obtained for having used estrogen and progestin MHT, $RR = 1.42$ ($95\%CI : 1.34 - 1.51$) per category increase in duration, and having a history of benign breast disease/biopsy, $RR = 1.41$ ($95\%CI : 1.32 - 1.50$).

The only competing outcome in our example is death from causes other than breast cancer. Among the women in our cohort, we observed $11,092(6.2\%)$ deaths during follow-up. We estimated a cause-specific hazard function for death using a Cox- proportional hazards model. For this model we treated administrative censoring and breast cancer incidence as censoring events. The relative risk estimates are given in the fourth column of Table 4.2. For ease of comparison we used the same reference category for each variable as in the breast cancer relative risk model. Model selection was performed in the same manner as for the relative risk model for invasive breast cancer. Having a family history of breast or ovarian cancer and having had a prior gynecological surgery were not associated with the risk of dying. However, as expected, smoking increased risk of death from causes other than breast cancer, with $RR = 1.29$ $(95\%CI : 1.27 - 1.32)$

We estimated the baseline hazard function for each cause non-parametrically and then plugged them into Equation (4.13) to estimate the absolute risk of invasive breast cancer. Table 4.3 gives examples of 5 and 10 year projections of absolute risk of invasive breast cancer for three 60 year old women. Profile 1 corresponds to a low risk woman; her 5- and 10-year absolute risks of developing invasive breast cancer are 0.83% and 1.76%, respectively. Profile 2 is that of an intermediate risk women, and profile 3 shows a woman at somewhat elevated breast cancer risk. Her 5 and 10 year risks of developing invasive breast cancer are 6.60% and 13.88%, respectively. Had this woman been a current smoker, her absolute breast cancer risks would be slightly lower due to her increased risk of dying from causes other than breast cancer; her 5- and 10-year absolute breast cancer risks would be 6.57% and 13.77%. This calculation illustrates that changes in covariates that affect competing causes usually have little impact on the absolute risk of the cause of interest because they enter the integral expression (4.1) as a second order term.

Estimation of the sub-distribution hazard function for breast cancer incidence

We fit the proportional sub-distribution hazards regression model (Fine and Gray, 1999) to the breast cancer data in Section 4.3.1 to compare it with the cause-specific approach to estimation of absolute risk. We used the *R* function *crprep* in the package *mstate* (Geskus, 2011; de Wreede et al., 2011). This function uses an estimate of the survivor function of the censoring distribution to reweight contributions to the risk sets for failures from competing causes and time-dependent weights to accommodate left truncation. We first used all the covariates that were predictors for either the cause-specific hazard of breast cancer, or the cause-specific hazard of death in our model. However, in the Fine and Gray model the smoking variable was not statistically significantly associated with cumulative incidence of breast cancer ($p > 0.05$); thus we omitted it from the final model. The sub-distribution relative risk estimates for invasive breast cancer based on model (4.24) in Table 4.4 are very similar to the cause-specific relative risks for breast cancer ($m = 1$) in Table 4.2. This is because the absolute risk of death is small in this example (6.2%) so that $r_2(t)/P(T > t) << 1$ in Equation (4.28). It follows that the cause-specific hazard ratio

$$\exp(\boldsymbol{\beta}'\mathbf{z}) = \exp(\boldsymbol{\gamma}'\mathbf{z})\,[1 + r_2(t;\mathbf{z})/P(T > t|\mathbf{z})]\,[1 + r_2(t;\mathbf{z}_0)/P(T > t|\mathbf{z}_0)]^{-1} \approx \exp(\boldsymbol{\gamma}'\mathbf{z}),$$

provided the same covariates $\mathbf{z}$ are used to model λ and h.

4.3.2 Absolute risk of second primary thyroid cancer (SPTC) incidence

Our second example is based on a model that we developed to predict the absolute risk of second primary thyroid cancer (SPTC) among five-year survivors of a childhood cancer

Table 4.3: Projections from the cause-specific model of absolute risk of invasive breast cancer for three 60-year-old women with selected risk profiles

Characteristics	**Profile 1**	**Profile 2**	**Profile 3**
BMI, kg/m^2	24	36	41
Estrogen and progestin MHT use	No MHT use	12 years	11 years
Other/unknown MHT use	No	No	Yes
Parity	2 children	1 child	1 child
Age at first live birth	23	24	22
Age at menopause	< 50 years	52	58
Benign breast disease/biopsy	No	No	Yes
Family history of breast or ovarian cancer	No	No	Yes
Alcohol consumption	0 drinks/day	0 drink/day	2 drinks/day
Gynecologic Surgery	yes	no	no
Smoking	Never smoker	Never smoker	Never smoker
Relative risk estimate for breast cancer	1.0	3.22	10.71
Relative risk estimate for competing mortality	1.0	0.44	0.28
5-year absolute risk	0.83%	2.96%	6.60%
Influence based standard error	0.05%	0.25%	0.61%
Bootstrap based standard error	0.07%	0.31%	0.65%
10-year absolute risk	1.76%	6.36%	13.88%
Influence based standard error	0.10%	0.52%	0.76%
Bootstrap based standard error	0.14%	0.65%	1.18%

(Kovalchik et al., 2013a). The incidence of childhood cancers in developed nations has been increasing at a modest but consistent rate (Steliarova-Foucher et al., 2004). Owing to therapeutic advances, this rise has coincided with a significant decline in mortality, and 85% of five-year childhood cancer survivors diagnosed after 1970 are expected to survive another 30 years or more (Mertens et al., 2008). Despite its curative benefit, the treatment for childhood cancers can have adverse late effects on the health of long-term survivors, including an elevated risk of second primary malignancies and cardiac- or pulmonary-related mortality (Armstrong, 2010). Approximately 10% of subsequent primary malignancies among childhood cancer survivors are cancers of the thyroid gland (Reulen et al., 2011). This excess risk is largely attributable to prior radiotherapy and persists throughout the adult life of irradiated survivors.

In Kovalchik et al. (2013a), we combined data from a large cohort, the Childhood Cancer Survivor Study (CCSS) (Robison et al., 2009), and two case-control studies, the Late Effects Study Group (LESG) (Tucker et al., 1991) and the Nordic Childhood Cancer Survivor Study (Olsen et al., 2009; Svahn-Tapper et al., 2006). This example however, is based only on data from the CCSS cohort.

Data

CCSS included 11,997 five-year survivors of childhood cancer diagnosed between 1970 and 1986 at 26 medical centers in the US and Canada, with follow-up to January 1, 2010

Table 4.4: Multivariable sub-distribution relative risk (RR_s) estimates for invasive breast cancer among non-Hispanic, white women in the NIH-AARP cohort

Characteristic	**Subcategory**	**Invasive breast cancer RR_s (95% CI)**
BMI	$< 25kg/m^2$	1.0 (referent)
	Per category increase	1.10 (1.07-1.13)
Estrogen and progestin MHT use	No MHT use	1.0 (referent)
	Per category increase	1.43 (1.34-1.51)
Other MHT use	No	1.0 (referent)
	Yes	1.23 (1.13-1.34)
Age at first live birth	< 25 years	1.0 (referent)
	Per category increase	1.16 (1.11-1.22)
Parity	1+ children	1.0 (referent)
	Nulliparous	1.29 (1.20-1.39)
Age at menopause	< 50 years	1.0 (referent)
	Per category increase	1.14 (1.09-1.20)
	NA/missing	0.99 (0.87-1.14)
Benign breast disease/biopsy	No	1.0 (referent)
	Yes	1.41 (1.32-1.50)
Family history of breast or ovarian cancer	No	1.0 (referent)
	Yes	1.39 (1.30-1.49)
Alcohol consumption	0 drinks/day	1.0 (referent)
	Per category increase	1.13 (1.09-1.18)
Gynecologic Surgery	yes	1.0 (referent)
	No	1.14 (1.22-1.06)

Categories for variables fitted with a trend: BMI: $< 25, 25$ to $< 30, 30$ to < 35, and $\geq 35kg/m^2$; estrogen and progestin MHT use: never, $< 10, \geq 10$ years; age at first birth: $< 25, 25-29$, and ≥ 30 years; age at menopause: $< 50, 50-54, \geq 55$ years, missing; benign breast diseases/biopsy: no, yes, missing; alcohol consumption: $0, < 1, \geq 1$ drinks/day; age menopause: 0: premenopausal or ≤ 49, $1 : 50-54$ years, 2: ≥ 55 years.

for the present analysis. Subjects were eligible for inclusion in the analysis if they were (1) alive and at-risk of developing SPTC five years after a first cancer diagnosed before age 21 and (2) had a reconstructed radiation absorbed dose to the thyroid gland.

Estimation of the cause-specific hazard functions for second primary thyroid cancer (SPTC) incidence and for competing events

For the present example, we built an absolute risk model that includes variables from self-report and medical records, but not from reconstructed radiation dose. We used age as the time scale. The data were left truncated because cohort members first became eligible for inclusion at the age at which they had survived five years beyond their first primary cancer diagnosis. We fit Cox proportional cause-specific hazard models to estimate the relative risks for selected predictors for incidence of SPTC, defined as the first occurrence of a pathologically-confirmed thyroid malignancy, and for competing events. Competing events for SPTC were death (n = 1,403), self-reported complete removal of the thyroid gland (n = 115), and other second primary cancers (n = 965), which were determined from pathology reports with follow-up to January 1, 2010. During follow-up, n = 124 patients were diagnosed with SPTC, and n = 2,483(21%) of the patients experienced a competing event.

Patients provided self-reports of demographic information, medical conditions, and health behaviors. Factors obtained from medical records included use of radiation therapy, body regions irradiated, and use of chemo-therapeutic agents during the first 10 years following the childhood cancer diagnosis. Selected characteristics in groups of individuals defined by outcome are listed in Table 4.5.

Indicator variables for any radiation, radiation therapy to the neck, and the use of an alkylating agent were strong risk factors for SPTC (Table 4.6). Birth after 1970, age less than 15 years at first primary cancer diagnosis and female gender were also statistically significantly associated with SPTC risk. The strongest predictor in the model was having received radiation therapy that included the neck (RR = 7.64 with (95%CI: 4.81-12.14). In the competing events model, the strongest predictors were treatment-related variables, namely alkylating agents (yes/no) with RR = 1.60 (95%CI: 1.48-1.74), radiation (yes/no) with RR = 2.06 (95%CI: 1.83-2.32), and radiation to the neck (yes/no), with RR = 1.79 (95%CI: 1.64-1.96). This analysis gives some insight into how a given risk factor influences absolute risk. For example, female gender acts primarily though its effect on the hazard of SPTC, rather than through its small effect on the hazard of competing events.

We estimated the baseline hazard function for both the primary event, and the competing events non-parametrically. For illustrative purposes, we report 20-year SPTC risk for three selected childhood cancer survivor profiles (Table 4.7). The SPTC absolute risk for a survivor at the lowest level of all risk factors (Profile 1) was 0.04%, while it was 8.29% for an individual in the highest risk category (Profile 3, Table 4.7). A person with the same risk factor profile as Profile 3, except no radiation to the neck, had an absolute 20-year risk of SPTC of 1.36%, highlighting the importance of this predictor.

Estimation of the sub-distribution hazard function for second primary thyroid cancer (SPTC) incidence

The relative risk parameter estimates for the sub-distribution hazard function for SPTC given in Table 4.8 are somewhat different from those for the cause-specific hazard function in Table 4.6. For example, the estimate for the variable "radiation to the neck" has a sub-distribution relative risk estimate of 6.38 (95% CI:= 4.02-10.12) while the cause-specific relative risk estimate for SPTC was 7.64 (95%CI: 4.81-12.14). The lower effect of this predictor on the sub-distribution hazard stems from the fact that neck radiation is also associated with increased risk of competing events (cause-specific relative risk for the competing events hazard of 1.79), which lowers its impact on absolute risk of SPTC. Although the sub-distribution relative hazards (Table 4.8) summarize the overall impact of a covariate on absolute SPTC risk, they do not describe the separate effects of these covariates on SPTC risk and on the risk of competing events, as do the cause-specific relative risks (Table 4.6).

4.4 Estimating cause-specific hazard functions from sub-samples from cohorts

For large cohorts and rare outcomes, it may be more cost-effective to measure expensive covariates on all or most cases that occur during follow-up, i.e., subjects who experience the event of interest, but only on a small subset of the individuals who have not experienced the event ("controls"). The two most popular sub-sampling strategies are the nested case-control design and the case-cohort design, both of which permit efficient estimation of cause-specific hazards. We describe how one can estimate cause-specific hazard functions from these designs and use them to build absolute risk models in the next two sections. Although these designs do not require covariate information on all members of the cohort,

Table 4.5: Summary characteristics of the analytic sample stratified by second primary thyroid cancer (SPTC) case status

		Number of patients who experienced				
		SPTC(%)	**death (%)**	**other SPC [a](%)**	**thyroid removal (%)**	**no event (%)**
Characteristic	**Subcategory**	**n = 124**	**n = 1,403**	**n = 965**	**n = 115**	**n = 9,390**
Gender	Female	86 (69)	574 (41)	528 (55)	82 (71)	4,425 (47)
Type of first cancer	HD[b]	39 (31)	255 (18)	330 (34)	55 (48)	874 (9)
	Bone	19 (15)	204 (15)	83 (9)	20 (17)	1,354 (14)
	Leukemia	15 (12)	142 (10)	65 (7)	18 (16)	897 (10)
	Kidney	19 (15)	207 (15)	89 (9)	21 (18)	1,316 (14)
	Brain	11 (9)	118 (8)	60 (6)	15 (13)	979 (10)
	Brain & CNS[c]	13 (11)	169 (12)	80 (8)	17 (15)	1,220 (13)
	NHL[d]	18 (15)	206 (15)	82 (9)	18 (16)	1,357 (15)
Age at diagnosis, years	< 5	33 (27)	399 (28)	207 (22)	32 (28)	4,208 (45)
	$5 - 9$	27 (22)	305 (22)	163 (17)	16 (14)	2,115 (23)
	$10 - 14$	50 (40)	340 (24)	237 (25)	32 (28)	1,737 (19)
	15+	14 (11)	359 (26)	358 (37)	35 (30)	1,330 (14)
Year of birth	Before 1970	55 (44)	764 (55)	631 (65)	76 (66)	2,964 (32)
	1970-1986	69 (56)	639 (46)	334 (35)	39 (34)	6,426 (68)
Any radiation	Yes	112 (90)	1,173 (84)	831 (86)	106 (92)	5,786 (62)
	No	12 (10)	230 (16)	134 (14)	9 (8)	3,604 (38)
Chemotherapy	Alkylating agent	84 (68)	992 (71)	552 (57)	69 (60)	4,792 (51)
Radiation to neck	Yes	88 (71)	585 (42)	475 (49)	92 (80)	1,736 (19)
	No	36 (29)	818 (58)	490 (51)	23 (20)	7,654 (82)
	Missing	0 (0)	0 (0)	0 (0)	0 (0)	0 (0)
Any thyroid medication	Yes	11 (9)	193 (14)	84 (9)	9 (8)	1,408 (15)
	No	8 (7)	26 (2)	6 (1)	12 (10)	67 (1)
Any thyroid condition	Yes	8 (7)	31 (2)	12 (1)	19 (17)	107 (1)
	No	11 (9)	188 (13)	76 (8)	2 (2)	1,343 (14)

[a] SPC: second primary cancer; [b] HD: Hodgkin disease; [c] CNS: central nervous system; [d] NHL: Non-Hodgkin lymphoma. Numbers of patients are shown, with percentages in parentheses.

Table 4.6: Multivariable cause-specific relative risk (RR) estimates for second primary thyroid cancer (SPTC) and competing causes among 5-year survivors of a childhood cancer in the CCSS cohort

Characteristic	**Subcategory**	**SPTC RR (95% CI)**	**Competing causes RR (95% CI)**
Birth year after 1970	no	1.0 (referent)	1.0 (referent)
	yes	1.87 (1.24, 2.82)	0.74 (0.67, 0.82)
Age at FPC $<$ **15 years**	no	1.0 (referent)	1.0 (referent)
	yes	3.43 (1.88, 6.28)	0.82 (0.73, 0.91)
Female	no	1.0 (referent)	1.0 (referent)
	yes	2.79 (1.90, 4.09)	1.06 (0.98 1.14)
Any alkylating agent[a]	no	1.0 (referent)	1.0 (referent)
	yes	1.58 (1.08, 2.30)	1.60 (1.48, 1.74)
Any radiation[a]	no	1.0 (referent)	1.0 (referent)
	yes	1.37 (0.69, 2.75)	2.06 (1.83, 2.32)
Radiation treatment to neck[a]	no	1.0 (referent)	1.0 (referent)
	yes	7.64 (4.81, 12.14)	1.79 (1.64, 1.96)

[a]Within 10 years of first primary cancer.

Table 4.7: Examples of 20-year projections of absolute risk of second primary thyroid cancer from the cause-specific model for three 15-year-old childhood cancer survivors with selected risk profiles

Characteristic	**Profile 1**	**Profile 2**	**Profile 3**
Age at start of projection	15	15	15
Birth year after 1970	No	Yes	Yes
Age $<$ 15 years at first primary cancer diagnosis	No	Yes	Yes
Female	No	Yes	Yes
Any alkylating agent for FPC	No	Yes	Yes
Any radiation	No	Yes	Yes
Radiation treatment to neck	No	No	Yes
Absolute risk estimate (in %)	0.04%	1.36%	8.29%

they do require complete information on follow-up and event times. One of the attractive features of the cause-specific models of absolute risk is that they are estimable from sub-samples of cohorts.

4.4.1 Case-cohort design

The case-cohort design, introduced for time-to-event data by Prentice (1986) and further studied by Self and Prentice (1988), requires collecting covariate data for all cases and for a random sample of the entire cohort (the "subcohort"), which can include cases. The size

Table 4.8: Sub-distribution relative risk estimates (RR_s) for SPTC among 5-year survivors of a childhood cancer in the CCSS cohort

Characteristic	Subcategory	RR_s (95% CI)
Birth year after 1970	No	1.0 (referent)
	Yes	1.30 (0.87, 1.93)
Age at FPC $<$ 15 years	No	1.0 (referent)
	Yes	2.88 (1.58, 5.28)
Female	No	1.0 (referent)
	Yes	2.75 (1.87, 4.03)
Any alkylating agent[a]	No	1.0 (referent)
	Yes	1.30 (0.89, 1.91)
Any radiation[a]	No	1.0 (referent)
	Yes	1.24 (0.62, 2.47)
Radiation treatment to neck[a]	No	1.0 (referent)
	Yes	6.38 (4.02, 10.12)

[a] Within 10 years of first primary cancer diagnosis.

of the subcohort, $\tilde{n}$, is usually much smaller than the size of the cohort, n. This design is closely related to designs for dichotomous outcomes proposed earlier by Kupper et al. (1975) and Miettinen (1976). The case-cohort design can substantially reduce cost and effort of exposure assessment in epidemiologic cohort studies with only a small loss of efficiency compared to a full cohort design. It is most cost-effective when the most expensive part of the study is not in recruiting subjects, but in measuring exposures and predictors of interest. The case-cohort design is particularly suited to molecular epidemiologic studies in which biospecimens can be collected and stored for later analysis. For the cases and members of the subcohort, these specimen can then be analyzed to determine an individual's exposure at study entry when the samples were collected, and, if serial specimens were stored, the exposure levels over time. The case-cohort design has been applied in cancer, cardiovascular, and HIV research, and is popular for genetic epidemiologic studies.

An advantage of the case-cohort design over the nested case-control design (Section 4.4.2) is that the sub-cohort may serve as the comparison group for multiple disease outcomes, because it was chosen without regard to failure status. Sorensen and Andersen (2000) extended the pseudo-likelihood approach for analyzing case-cohort studies proposed by Self and Prentice (1988) to apply to a common control group for multiple event types and provided methods for variance estimation and hypothesis testing. They also developed cause-specific baseline hazard estimates for absolute risk estimation. We outline their approach here for cause-specific hazards that satisfy the proportional hazards model (4.3).

Let the sampling indicator V_i be one if person i is selected into the sub-cohort or 0 otherwise. With simple random sampling of sub-cohort members, $P(V_i = 1) = \tilde{n}/n$, i.e., the proportion of the cohort sampled into the subcohort. However, more complex sampling schemes, for example stratification or time dependent sampling, where $P(V = 1)$ varies with follow-up time, can also be accommodated (see Self and Prentice (1988)). In the pseudo-likelihood approach (Self and Prentice, 1988; Sorensen and Andersen, 2000), each time an event occurs a sampled risk set is formed by the case and the controls in the sub-cohort, i.e.,

$$PsL(\boldsymbol{\beta}) = \prod_{m=1}^{M} \prod_{i=1}^{n} \prod_{t \geq 0} \left(\frac{\exp(\boldsymbol{\beta}_m' \mathbf{Z}_i^m)}{(n/\tilde{n}) \sum_{j=1}^{n} \{V_j Y_j(t) + (1 - V_j) dN_{mj}(t)\} \exp(\boldsymbol{\beta}_m' \mathbf{Z}_j^m)} \right)^{dN_{mi}(t)}. \tag{4.29}$$

This pseudo-likelihood above differs from the partial likelihood (4.6) for a full cohort study in that the denominator is a weighted sum over the case and subjects at risk in the sub-cohort rather than a sum over all subjects at risk in the entire cohort. Numerical studies (Sorensen and Andersen, 2000) indicate that better estimates of $\boldsymbol{\beta}$ are obtained by including the case in the denominator of (4.29) as in the original proposal (Prentice, 1986), even though asymptotically equivalent methods use only the subcohort members in the denominator (Self and Prentice, 1988). In addition, because cases are added at the time of event, the risk sets are not nested. Sub-cohort members contribute to the analysis over their entire time on study, and some of them may in fact experience the event of interest, but the failures outside the sub-cohort contribute only at their failure times.

The score of the pseudo-likelihood (4.29) has expected value of zero at the true value of $\boldsymbol{\beta}_m$, but the inverse information matrix does not estimate the variance of the estimator due to sampling-induced covariances between the score terms. Self and Prentice (1988) and Sorensen and Andersen (2000) proved results on the asymptotic distribution of $\hat{\boldsymbol{\beta}}_m$ using a combination of martingale and finite population convergence results and provided variance estimators. Sorensen and Andersen (2000) gave variance estimates for multiple event types both for a pseudo-likelihood that includes the case in the denominator of Equation (4.29) and for the pseudo-likelihood that only includes subcohort members in the denominator.

As the subcohort is a random sample from the full cohort, the non-parametric baseline hazard, $\lambda_{0m}(t)$ can be estimated using a weighted Breslow estimator

$$\hat{\lambda}_{0m}(t) = \frac{\sum_{i=1}^{n} dN_{mi}(t)}{(n/\tilde{n}) \sum_{i=1}^{n} V_i Y_i(t) \exp(\hat{\boldsymbol{\beta}}_m' \mathbf{Z}_i^m)},$$

where $\tilde{n}/n$ is the proportion of the cohort sampled into the sub-cohort (Prentice, 1986; Self and Prentice, 1988).

If the components of $\boldsymbol{\beta}$ for the different event types are distinct (functionally independent), then standard Cox regression software can be used to estimate cause-specific parameters for the case-cohort samples by analyzing each event type separately while treating other events as independent censoring. However, variance computations need to be adapted to accommodate the design. For asymptotic derivations, a key assumption is that $\tilde{n}/n \to \pi$ for $0 < \pi < 1$ as $n \to \infty$, i.e., the cohort and the sub-cohort grow at the same rate. Using the same techniques as Self and Prentice (1988), Sorensen and Andersen (2000) derived the asymptotic distributions of $\hat{\boldsymbol{\beta}}_m$ and $\hat{\Lambda}_{0k}(t) = \int \hat{\lambda}_{0k}(u)du, k = 1, \ldots, M$, for the competing risk setting, when M event types are analyzed.

As for the full cohort, other hazard models can be used here as well. For example, Kang et al. (2013) fitted marginal additive hazards regression models for case-cohort studies with multiple disease outcomes using a weighted estimating equations approach for the estimation of model parameters.

4.4.2 Nested case-control design

Another approach to sub-sampling from a cohort is the nested case-control design (Liddell et al., 1977). At each time an event occurs, the full cohort risk set is replaced by a specified number $\tilde{n} - 1$ of controls selected from among those individuals in the cohort who are at risk and have not experienced the event by that time. If, for example, $\tilde{n} = 2$, each case is matched on time to one control, thereby drastically reducing the number of individuals for whom covariate information needs to be collected. A new set of controls is selected every time an event occurs, and cohort members can be selected repeatedly. A person who subsequently develops disease can serve as a control for an earlier event. Borgan et al. (1995) derived general asymptotic theory for the maximum partial likelihood estimator of the regression parameters and cumulative baseline hazard estimator under the Cox proportional hazards model for a single event type.

We briefly describe the estimation of the cause-specific hazard functions for M competing events when controls at event time t are selected randomly and without replacement from the $Y(t)-1$ individuals at risk in the cohort. However, more general sampling schemes also can be used, and Borgan et al. (1995) described methods to estimate the regression parameters and baseline hazard functions for the Cox proportional hazards model when a cohort is sub-sampled with more general sampling schemes. Those authors used marked point processes to model the occurrence of failures and the sampling of controls at each failure time simultaneously. The marked counting process records the time when failures occur and the individuals who fail. The authors provided a general approach that includes the nested case-control design as a special case. These results can also be found in Aalen et al. (2008) (Chapter 4.3). We adapt the notation used in Borgan et al. (1995) and assume for simplicity that for each failure type m the same number $\tilde{n}-1$ of controls is selected. We let $\mathcal{F}_t$ denote the information about the events in the cohort as well as the sampling of the controls up to but not including time t. Denote by $\mathcal{P}_{\tilde{n}}$ the collection of all possible subsets of $\{1,\ldots,Y(t)\}$ of size $\tilde{n}$ and by $\tilde{\mathcal{R}}(t)$ the risk set actually sampled at time t. If individual i fails at time t from event type m, the probability that a particular set $\mathbf{r}\in\mathcal{P}_{\tilde{n}}$ of size $\tilde{n}$ that includes the case i is sampled is given by

$$p(\mathbf{r}|t,i) = P(\tilde{\mathcal{R}}(t)=\mathbf{r}|dN_{mi}(t)=1,\mathcal{F}_t) = \frac{\tilde{n}}{Y(t)}\Big/\binom{Y(t)}{\tilde{n}} = \binom{Y(t)-1}{\tilde{n}-1}^{-1}.$$

The probability of a set $\mathbf{r}$ without regard to case status is

$$P(\mathbf{r}|t) = \binom{Y(t)}{\tilde{n}}^{-1}.$$

Thus the sampling weight defined as $w_i(t) = p(\mathbf{r}|t,i)/p(\mathbf{r}|t)$ is

$$w_i(t) = \frac{Y(t)}{\tilde{n}}. \tag{4.30}$$

For $\mathbf{r}\in\mathcal{P}_{\tilde{n}}$ and $i\in\mathbf{r}$ one can define a marked counting process $N_{i,\mathbf{r},m}(t) = I(X_i \leq t, \delta_i = m, \tilde{\mathcal{R}}(t)=\mathbf{r}), t\geq 0$, that indicates the failure of type m for individual i and with associated sampled risk set $\mathbf{r}$. If the sampling is independent, that indicates knowledge of which individuals were selected as controls before t does not alter their intensity of failure of any type at time t, then the intensity of the new process $N_{i,\mathbf{r},m}$ is

$$\lambda(t)Y_i(t)\binom{Y(t)-1}{\tilde{n}-1}^{-1} I(\mathbf{r}\in\tilde{\mathcal{R}}(t), \mathbf{r}\in\mathcal{P}_{\tilde{n}}, i\in\mathbf{r}).$$

If the cause-specific hazard functions $\lambda_k, k=1,\ldots,M$ each follow a Cox proportional hazards model, the partial likelihood is

$$PL(\boldsymbol{\beta}) = \prod_{m=1}^{M}\prod_{i=1}^{n}\prod_{t\geq 0}\left(\frac{w_i(t)\exp(\boldsymbol{\beta}_m'\mathbf{Z}_i^m)}{\sum_{j\in\tilde{\mathcal{R}}(t)} w_j(t)Y_j(t)\exp(\boldsymbol{\beta}_m'\mathbf{Z}_j^m)}\right)^{dN_{i,\mathbf{r},m}(t)}. \tag{4.31}$$

The partial likelihood for the full cohort is a special case of the partial likelihood (4.31) with all the weights w equal to one, as the whole risk set is used. The weights $w_i(t)$ in (4.30) are the same for all members of the risk set, and (4.31) simplifies to

$$PL(\boldsymbol{\beta}) = \prod_{m=1}^{M} \prod_{i=1}^{n} \prod_{t \geq 0} \left(\frac{\exp(\boldsymbol{\beta}_m' \mathbf{Z}_i^m)}{\sum_{j \in \tilde{\mathcal{R}}(t)} Y_j(t) \exp(\boldsymbol{\beta}_m' \mathbf{Z}_j^m)} \right)^{dN_{i,\mathbf{r},m}(t)} . \quad (4.32)$$

Thus, maximum likelihood estimates for $\boldsymbol{\beta}_m$ can be obtained by using standard statistical software for the Cox regression model for full cohort analysis, with modified risk sets.

The Breslow estimate for the nested case-control design is given by

$$\hat{\lambda}_{0m}(t) = \frac{\sum_{i=1}^{n} dN_{i,\mathbf{r},m}(t)}{\sum_{i \in \tilde{\mathcal{R}}(t)} w_i(t) Y_i(t) \exp(\hat{\boldsymbol{\beta}}_m' \mathbf{Z}_i^m)},$$

where $\hat{\boldsymbol{\beta}}_m$ maximizes (4.31) and w_i is given by (4.30). Langholz and Borgan (1997) described corresponding absolute risk estimates with variances.

Efficiency comparisons between the nested case-control design and the case-cohort design indicate that in many situations the former is slightly more efficient (Langholz and Thomas, 1990, 1991), but the choice of design is often determined by other factors. For example, if an exposure assay varies by day or plate, it may be desirable to put specimens from a case and its matched controls on the same plate; the nested case-control samples are well suited for this contingency. If a major goal is to study several different disease outcomes, the case-cohort design is preferred.

4.5 Estimating cause specific hazard functions from cohorts with complex survey designs

The methods in Sections 4.1, 4.2, and 4.4 assume that individuals in a cohort are simple random samples from the population. However, the methods can be extended to cohorts based on complex sample designs, such as mortality-linked data from national health surveys, that could be used to assess how demographic characteristics and health behaviors impact the risk of death from various causes.

We now summarize work (Kovalchik and Pfeiffer, 2013) that used methods to estimate hazard functions from survey data (Binder, 1992; Lin, 2000; Gray, 2009) to estimate absolute risk. These estimates are functions of design-based survey weights. If risk models were perfectly specified, ignoring the sampling design would also yield unbiased relative risk estimates, but using a weighted approach reduces dependence on model assumptions and thus improves model robustness (Patterson et al., 2002). Weighting is necessary, however, to obtain consistent estimates of absolute risk (Kovalchik and Pfeiffer, 2013). We now introduce an example of such survey data that we analyze later using survey-related methods to estimate absolute risk.

4.5.1 Example of survey design

We suppose that the cohort for the development of the absolute risk models comes from a complex multistage survey that is linked with outcome data. For example, individuals sampled into the National Health and Nutrition Examination Survey (NHANES) are linked to national mortality data in the NHANES Epidemiologic Followup studies (Cox et al., 1992).

NHANES samples are designed to be nationally representative of the civilian, non-institutionalized U.S. population. Participants for the surveys are selected using multistage probability sampling designs. In the first stage primary sampling units (PSUs) are selected with probability proportional to size (PPS) sampling from strata defined by geography and proportions of minority populations. For all NHANES surveys, the PSUs are single counties or, in a few cases, groups of contiguous counties. In the second stage the PSUs are divided into segments (usually city blocks or their equivalent) and sample segments are selected with PPS sampling. In stage 3, a random sample of households within each segment is drawn, and in stage 4 individuals from a list of all persons residing in selected households are chosen at random within designated age-sex-race/ethnicity screening subdomains. On average, 1.6 persons are selected per household.

For example, NHANES II, conducted from 1976 to 1980, had 32 strata with two PSUs sampled from each stratum. Survey sample weights are provided on the public use data files; the weights can be used to obtain nationally representative estimates.

Mortality follow-up was based on a probabilistic match with death certificate records from the National Death Index (NDI) for participants in NHANES II who were 30–75 years of age and completed a medical examination. Detailed information on the NHANES II survey, and the follow-up study can be found in McDowell et al. (1981). Thus, the ages and covariates of individuals in the sample are known at baseline, and ages at death and cause of death of individuals who died in or before 1993 are known. This information can be used to build models of absolute risk for various competing causes of death.

4.5.2 Data

In what follows, a superscript refers to cause-specific quantities and three sub-indices accommodate the sampling scheme. To summarize, the sampling frame of the survey is divided into I non-overlapping strata and J_i PSUs are selected from the ith stratum with inclusion probabilities $p_{i1}, \ldots, p_{iJ_i}$. There can be several additional stages of complex sampling after the first stage that we will not describe further. Cluster sampling can also be accommodated in this framework. At the end of the sampling, $k = 1, \ldots, n_{ij}$ individuals are sampled from the jth sampled PSU of the ith stratum, and the final inclusion probabilities p_{ijk} of the ijk-th individual are the products of the PSU level inclusion probabilities from the first stage times the conditional inclusion probabilities from the later stages. The sampling weights are $w_{ijk} = 1/p_{ijk}$, $k = 1, \ldots, n_{ij}$, with possible adjustment for nonresponse and non-coverage bias.

At baseline, the age of individual ijk in the sample, denoted by T_{0ijk}, and a vector of covariates $\mathbf{Z}_{ijk}$ are observed. Over the course of the study we also observe the minimum of the age at death or age at censoring, T_{ijk}, with censoring assumed to be non-informative. Again, the at-risk indicator at time t is $Y_{ijk}(t) = I(T_{ijk} \geq t)$, and $\delta_{ijk}(t) = m$ if an event of type m occurs at time t or zero otherwise. Thus, the data for the ijkth individual at time t are $(T_{0ijk}, T_{ijk}, \mathbf{Z}_{ijk}, w_{ijk}, \delta_{ijk}(t), Y_{ijk}(t))$.

4.5.3 Estimation of hazard ratio parameters and the baseline hazard function

Using a pseudo-likelihood formulation as suggested by Binder (1992), the formulas (4.8) and (4.9) can be extended to estimating equations for $\boldsymbol{\beta}^{(m)}$, $m = 1, \ldots, M$, given by

$$\vec{U}(\boldsymbol{\beta}_m) = \sum_{i=1}^{I} \sum_{j=1}^{J_i} \sum_{k=1}^{n_{ij}} w_{ijk} dN_{ijk}^m(t_{ijk}) \{\mathbf{z}_{ijk}^m - \vec{E}(\boldsymbol{\beta}_m, t_{ijk})\}, m = 1, \ldots, M, \tag{4.33}$$

and

$$\vec{E}(\boldsymbol{\beta}_m, t) = \frac{\sum_{i=1}^{I} \sum_{j=1}^{J_i} \sum_{k=1}^{n_{ij}} w_{ijk} Y_{ijk}(t) \exp(\boldsymbol{\beta}_m' \mathbf{Z}_{ijk}^m) \mathbf{Z}_{ijk}^m}{\sum_{i=1}^{I} \sum_{j=1}^{J_i} \sum_{k=1}^{n_{ij}} w_{ijk} Y_{ijk}(t) \exp(\boldsymbol{\beta}_m' \mathbf{Z}_{ijk}^m)}.$$

Standard optimization algorithms can be used to obtain the solution $\hat{\boldsymbol{\beta}}_m$ such that $\vec{U}(\hat{\boldsymbol{\beta}}_m) = 0$.

Nonparametric baseline hazard model

A weighted Nelson–Aalen estimator (Aalen, 1978) for the non-parametric cause-specific baseline hazard function is

$$\hat{\lambda}_{0m}(t) = \frac{\sum_{i=1}^{I}\sum_{j=1}^{J_i}\sum_{k=1}^{n_{ij}} w_{ijk} dN_{ijk}^m(t)}{\sum_{i=1}^{I}\sum_{j=1}^{J_i}\sum_{k=1}^{n_{ij}} w_{ijk} Y_{ijk}(t)\exp(\hat{\boldsymbol{\beta}}_m^{'}\mathbf{Z}_{ijk}^m)}.$$

Piecewise exponential baseline hazard model

Data from a complex survey sample can also be analyzed under a piecewise constant baseline hazard model (i.e., piecewise exponential model), as in for a standard cohort. Define a set of ordered t possibly unequally spaced time intervals $\mathcal{I}_1, \mathcal{I}_2, \ldots,$ with $\mathcal{I}_q = [\tau_{0q}, \tau_{1q})$ and $\tau_{1q} = \tau_{0(q+1)}$.

Letting t_{0ijk} be the time that the kth individual from the jth PSU and ith stratum is first at-risk, the at-risk time during the qth interval for that person is

$$\mathcal{A}_{ijk}(\tau_q) = I(t_{0ijk} < \tau_{1q} \cap t_{ijk} > \tau_{0q})\{\min(t_{ijk}, \tau_{1q}) - \max(t_{0ijk}, \tau_{0q})\}. \qquad (4.34)$$

Let $D^m(\mathcal{I}_q)$ equal to the total weighted person-time during the qth interval,

$$D^m(\mathcal{I}_q) = \sum_{i=1}^{I}\sum_{j=1}^{J_i}\sum_{k=1}^{n_{ij}} \mathcal{A}_{ijk}(\tau_q)\exp(\hat{\boldsymbol{\beta}}_m^{'}\mathbf{z}_{ijk}^m)w_{ijk},$$

and let $d^m(\mathcal{I}_q) = \sum_{i=1}^{I}\sum_{j=1}^{J_i}\sum_{k=1}^{n_{ij}} w_{ijk} I\{\delta_i(t_{ijk}) = m, \tau_{0q} \le t_{ijk} < \tau_{1q}\}$ be the observed events of type m in $(\tau_{0q}, \tau_{1q}]$. Then the estimate of $\lambda_{0m}(\mathcal{I}_q)$ is

$$\hat{\lambda}_{0m}(\mathcal{I}_q) = \frac{d^m(\mathcal{I}_q)}{D^m(\mathcal{I}_q)}.$$

The baseline cumulative hazard up to time t given survival to τ_{0q} is

$$\hat{\Lambda}_0^{(m)}(t) = \sum_{q:\tau_{0q}<t} \hat{\lambda}_0^{(m)}(\tau_q)\{\min(t, \tau_{1q}) - \tau_{0q}\}.$$

4.5.4 Example: absolute risk of cause-specific deaths from the NHANES I and II

To illustrate our methodology, we built population-based cause-specific models for various causes of death from NHANES I and II, pooling data from the two surveys to increase sample size and improve the precision of our estimates. The designs for these surveys are described in Section 4.5.1.

We classified underlying causes of death as cancer, cardiovascular disease, or "other causes," according to International Classification of Diseases, Ninth Revision. In the pooled NHANES I/II sample of 23,659 individuals, who were followed up to December 31, 1993, cardiovascular disease accounted for 49% of observed deaths in men and 51% in women, while cancer was the underlying cause for 25% of observed deaths in men and 24% in women. Although the overall proportions dying of cardiovascular disease and cancer were similar in men and women, there were notable gender differences in distributions of subtypes of cardiovascular deaths and cancer deaths (Table 4.9). Therefore, we built separate cause-specific absolute risk models for men and women.

When the absolute risk is estimated in subpopulation A, estimates are derived with the modified sampling weights $w_{ijk}^A = I_{ijk}^A w_{ijk}$, where I_{ijk}^A is an indicator for the kth individual's membership in subpopulation A, and the n_{ij} are replaced with $n_{ij}^A = \sum_{k=1}^{n_{ij}} I_{ijk}^A$. The computations are otherwise unchanged (Korn and Graubard, 1999, Chapter 5.4).

The covariates examined were baseline race, income, martial status, body mass index (BMI; kg/height in meters squared), smoking, diabetes diagnosis, hypertension, alcohol consumption, and serum cholesterol level. BMI, hypertension, and serum cholesterol levels were based on physical measurements conducted as part of NHANES; all remaining variables were self-reported.

For analyses with the piecewise exponential model, the baseline hazard function was divided into the seven age intervals $[30, 55)$, $[55, 60)$, $[60, 65)$, $[65, 70)$, $[70, 75)$, $[75, 80)$, $[80, 100)$.

Using the weighted pseudo-likelihood described in Section 4.1.1, we selected risk factors with backward stepwise regression and the design-based significance test suggested by Rao and Scott (1987) with a significance level of 0.10. Confidence intervals for the hazard ratios were constructed by exponentiating the lower and upper endpoints for the corresponding large-sample confidence interval of the log-hazard ratios. For men and women, smoking was significantly associated with increased risk for every cause of death (Table 4.10). Alcohol consumption was protective for CVD in women. Having a $BMI > 30kg/m^2$ was significantly associated with increased risk of death from CVD in men and women. Having a $BMI < 18kg/m^2$ was strongly associated with increased risk from "other causes" in men and women. The final gender- and outcome-specific models included the risk factors indicated in Table 4.10.

Table 4.11 gives estimates of the 10-year absolute risks of dying from CVD and from cancer for a 65 year old man, depending on smoking status and with all other risk factors at their reference levels. Results are shown both for piecewise exponential and for semi-parametric Cox models. This table also shows estimated standard errors for the absolute risk estimates computed by the influence function approach in Section 4.6 and, for comparison, by jackknife resampling. For computational efficiency we used a subsample of 20 randomly selected males from each of the 169 stratum-PSUs in the NHANES I/II dataset. Letting i index the full sample and j the subsample, population estimates were obtained from the subsample by modifying the weight of the kth individual in the subsample to $w_k^* = w_k(\sum_i w_i / \sum_j w_j)$. Estimates of absolute risk agreed well between the piecewise exponential and semi-parametric models. Current smokers had much higher absolute risks than never or former smokers, not only for cancer but also for cardiovascular disease. There was good agreement between the influence function-based and jackknife estimates of standard error (Table 4.11), both for the piecewise exponential and semi-parametric models. For cancer outcomes, the standard errors are slightly smaller under the piecewise exponential model than under the semi-parametric model.

A useful application of population-based risk models is to estimate the number of cause-specific deaths that might be prevented by changes in population exposures to risk factors. For example, one might want to estimate the numbers of deaths that could be prevented in the male US population aged 35–75 over a 10-year period under two smoking intervention scenarios (Table 4.12). For the "cessation" scenario, we treated current smokers as former smokers at the beginning of the projection period (Table 4.12). For the "no exposure" scenario, all former and current smokers were regarded as never smokers, leaving other covariates unchanged. We do not consider the feasibility of interventions leading to these scenarios, nor whether the interventions would have the effects estimated from the observational data. However, if these exposure reductions could be achieved, and if the risks were thereby reduced by amounts suggested by the observational data, then smoking cessation

Table 4.9: Numbers of deaths (and percentages[a]) by selected causes of death and gender in NHANES I/II

Cardiovascular		**Cancer**		Other	
Cause	**No. (%)**	**Cause**	**No. (%)**	**Cause**	**No. (%)**
Men					
Myocardial infarction	647 (35.8)	Lung	295 (32.6)	Chronic lower respiratory	140 (14.7)
Other ischemic heart disease	575 (31.8)	Prostate	121 (13.4)	Pneumonia	133 (14.0)
Cerebrovascular disease	229 (12.7)	Colon	87 (9.6)	Emphysema	54 (5.7)
Other heart disease	127 (7.0)	Pancreas	44 (4.9)	Diabetes	50 (5.2)
Heart failure	47 (2.6)	Leukemia	42 (4.6)	Liver disease	46 (4.8)
Hypertensive heart disease	45 (2.5)	Esophegeal	32 (3.5)	Unspecified disease	46 (4.8)
Aneurysm	37 (2.0)	Stomach	29 (3.2)	Suicide	30 (3.1)
Atherosclerosis	32 (1.8)	Kidney	27 (3.0)	Septicemia	29 (3.0)
Diseases of the pericardium	15(0.8)	Non-Hodgkin lymphoma	26 (2.9)	Alzheimer	19 (2.0)
Hypertension and renal disease	15(0.8)	Bladder	25 (2.8)	Nephritis	14 (1.5)
Total	1,805		906		953
Women					
Other ischemic heart disease	444 (29.7)	Breast	131 (18.3)	Diabetes	83 (11.5)
Myocardial infarction	418 (27.9)	Lung	115 (16.1)	Pneumonia	83 (11.5)
Cerebrovascular disease	312 (20.9)	Colon	109 (15.3)	Chronic lower respiratory	54 (7.5)
Other heart disease	111 (7.4)	Ovarian	36 (5.0)	Septicemia	31 (4.3)
Heart failure	54 (3.6)	Pancreatic	35 (4.9)	Liver disease	30 (4.1)
Hypertensive heart disease	35 (2.3)	Non-Hodgkin lymphoma	25 (3.5)	Unspecified disease	23 (3.2)
Atherosclerosis	28 (1.9)	Leukemia	22 (3.1)	Emphysema	20 (2.8)
Diseases of the pericardium	21 (1.4)	Brain/CNS	21 (2.9)	Nephritis	18 (2.5)
Diseases of arteries	17 (1.1)	Multiple myeloma	21 (2.9)	Kidney infection	16 (2.2)
Aneurysm	15 (1.0)	Stomach	19 (2.7)	Nutritional deficiency	15 (2.1)
Total	1,492		714		723

[a]The percentages are obtained by dividing by the total numbers of deaths, including some deaths from unlisted causes. Thus, the percentages do not sum to 100.

Table 4.10: Selected risk factors for gender- and cause-specific weighted Cox regression analyses in NHANES I/II

Characteristic	Women			Men		
	CVD[a]	Cancer	Other	CVD	Cancer	Other
	RR (95% CI)	RR (95% CI)	RR (95% CI)	RR (95% CI)	RR (95% CI)	RR (95% CI)
Race						
White	1.00 (referent)				1.00 (referent)	
Black	1.27 (1.05, 1.55)				1.10 (0.84, 1.43)	
Other)	0.96 (0.44, 2.07)				0.35 (0.14, 0.85)	
Annual income						
<10,000				1.42 (1.23, 1.64)	1.29 (1.07, 1.56)	1.99 (1.59, 2.46)
≥10,000				1.00 (referent)	1.00 (referent)	1.00 (referent)
Marital status						
Divorced or separated	1.28 (0.99, 1.66)				1.56 (1.14, 2.13)	1.70 (1.26, 2.29)
Other	1.00 (referent)				1.00 (referent)	1.00 (referent)
BMI[b]						
<18			4.34 (3.01, 6.25)		1.91 (1.04, 3.49)	3.21 (2.22, 4.65)
18-30	1.00 (referent)		1.00 (referent)	1.00 (referent)	1.00 (referent)	1.00 (referent)
>30	1.46 (1.25, 1.71)			1.35 (1.12, 1.62)	1.27 (0.99, 1.63)	
Smoking status						
Never	1.00 (referent)	1.00 (referent)	1.00 (referent)	1.00 (referent)	1.00 (referent)	1.00 (referent)
Former	1.28 (1.03, 1.60)	1.06 (0.78, 1.43)	1.34 (1.00, 1.81)	1.09 (0.92, 1.28)	1.15 (0.89, 1.49)	1.21 (0.95, 1.56)
Current	2.08 (1.74, 2.48)	1.87 (1.48, 2.368)	2.34 (1.83, 3.01)	1.90 (1.61, 2.25)	2.37 (1.84, 3.07)	2.11 (1.66, 2.67)
Unknown	2.35 (1.79, 3.08)	1.64 (1.06, 2.53)	2.54 (1.67, 3.87)	4.05 (3.03, 5.40)	2.48 (1.65, 3.73)	3.55 (2.46, 5.12)
Hypertensive (≥160/90)						
No	1.00 (referent)		1.00 (referent)	1.00 (referent)		
Yes	1.97 (1.66, 2.33)		1.55 (1.18, 2.04)	1.92 (1.60, 2.29)		
Alcohol consumption						
<1 drinks per week	1.00 (referent)	1.00 (referent)	1.00 (referent)	1.00 (referent)	1.00 (referent)	1.00 (referent)
1 – 7 drinks per week	0.84 (0.68, 1.03)	1.26 (1.00, 1.59)	0.74 (0.56, 0.98)	0.76 (0.65, 0.89)	1.00 (0.82, 1.22)	0.97 (0.79, 1.19)
> 7 drinks per week	0.70 (0.49, 1.01)	0.99 (0.65, 1.52)	0.95 (0.62, 1.45)	0.83 (0.69, 0.99)	1.29 (1.02, 1.63)	1.60 (1.27, 2.01)
Serum cholesterol (mg), Mean (SD)	1.002 (1.000, 1.003)			1.003 (1.002, 1.005)		0.998 (0.996, 1.000)
Diabetic						
No	1.00 (referent)		1.00 (referent)	1.00 (referent)		1.00 (referent)
Yes	2.30 (1.81, 2.92)		1.97 (1.40, 2.77)	1.89 (1.47, 2.44)		2.20 (1.59, 3.05)
Unknown	1.26 (1.08, 1.48)		1.06 (0.83, 1.35)	0.89 (0.76, 1.04)		1.20 (0.96, 1.49)

[a] Cardiovascular disease
[b] Body mass index

Table 4.11: Estimated 10-year absolute risk $\hat{r}$ of cause-specific death (%) by smoking status for a 65-year-old male with all other risk factors at their reference levels

	Piecewise exponential	**Estimated standard error**		**Semi-parametric**	**Estimated standard error**	
Smoking status	$\hat{r}$(%)	Influence	Jackknife	$\hat{r}$(%)	Influence	Jackknife
Cardiovascular						
Never	23.1	5.5	5.6	23.2	5.7	5.4
Former	29.2	7.8	7.6	29.3	7.3	7.2
Current	37.6	9.9	10.0	37.8	9.2	9.3
Unknown	55.8	11.1	11.1	55.7	11.0	11.2
Cancer						
Never	6.8	2.5	2.7	6.9	2.6	2.8
Former	8.0	3.3	2.9	8.2	3.4	3.3
Current	12.5	4.5	4.4	12.7	4.6	4.6
Unknown	8.6	6.4	6.6	8.7	6.7	6.8

could prevent over one million deaths over ten years, and societal changes that eliminated smoking altogether might prevent over three million deaths (Table 4.12).

Table 4.12: Expected number of cause-specific deaths in 10 years for the US male population sampled by NHANES I/II aged 35–75 under different smoking intervention scenarios

Cause of death	**No intervention**	**Smoking intervention, N (Prevented deaths)** Cessation	No exposure
	Deaths	Deaths (deaths prevented)	Deaths (deaths prevented)
Cancer	3,088,427	2,610,800 (477,627)	1,868,455 (1,219,972)
Cardiovascular	5,173,242	4,757,214 (416,028)	3,814,235 (1,359,007)
Other	2,785,291	2,548,402 (236,889)	2,109,647 (675,643)
Total	11,046,960	9,916,416 (1,130,544)	7,792,337 (3,254,623)

"Cessation" refers to the deaths (and deaths prevented) if current smokers were former smokers. "No exposure" refers to the deaths (and deaths prevented) if current and former smokers were never smokers.

4.6 Variance estimation

The following sections on variance estimation include details needed to compute confidence intervals on absolute risk estimates. Skipping this section will not impact readability of later sections.

The literature gives variance estimates for various models for r_m and estimators of r_m, some of which were mentioned earlier in this chapter. We review them briefly for the cause-specific proportional hazards model (4.4) and the Fine-Gray model before presenting an influence function based approach that is applicable to many designs for estimating the cause-specific proportional hazards model. In particular, it can be applied to each of the designs mentioned in this chapter, including complex survey sampling, as well as to an approach in Chapter 5 that combines estimates of relative and attributable risk from cohort or case-control data with external registry data.

Variance estimators given by Cheng et al. (1998) yield pointwise confidence intervals and simultaneous confidence bands as t varies for the cause-specific proportional hazards model. The software described by Rosthoj et al. (2004) estimates the variance of r_m under this model using general Markov methods (Andersen et al., 1993, Chapter VII 2.9). The Nelson–Aalen survival estimate in Equation (4.1), namely $\exp\{-\sum_{i=1}^{m}\hat{\Lambda}_i(t;\mathbf{z}_m)\}$, is replaced by the asymptotically equivalent Johansen-Aalen continued product, which reduces to a Kaplan-Meier estimate in the absence of covariates. Beyersmann et al. (2012) described how these calculations can be performed with the *R* package *mstate*. Langholz and Borgan (1997) described variance calculations for absolute risk with nested case-control sampling. Gerds et al. (2017) developed the *R* package *riskRegression* that gives variance estimates for r_m with $t_0 = 0$ under proportional cause-specific hazards.

Variance estimates for $\hat{r}_m$ for the Fine-Gray model are given in Fine and Gray (1999) with the accompanying *R* package, *cmprsk*, but left truncation is not accommodated. Klein and Andersen (2005) and Binder et al. (2014) jackknifed pseudovalues to estimate the variance of $\hat{r}_m$ but did not discuss left truncation. Geskus (2011) developed theory, including variance estimates, that allows for left truncation and cites an *R* package, *crhaz* in the Biometrics Supplemental Material. A version of this package, *crprep*, is used within the program *mstate* that is available at https://cran.r-project.org/web/packages/mstate/index.html.

4.6.1 Approaches to variance estimation

A general analytic approach to computing the variance of a statistic, T, is linearization, by which T is approximated by a linear function of random variable(s), whose variances can often be easily obtained. A well known linearization is the parametric delta method, for which $T(\hat{\theta}) \approx T(\theta) + T'(\theta)(\hat{\theta} - \theta)$. This approach requires that θ be finite dimensional. Benichou and Gail (1995) used this approach for the variance computation of absolute risk with discrete covariates.

Instead, we obtain variance estimates from influence functions for Taylor linearization. Taylor linearization is a non-iterative method to obtain the variance of complex estimators that can be expressed as sums of differentiable functions of parameters and observed data, and it has been widely applied to survey statistics for design-based inference (Woodruff, 1971; Demnati and Rao, 2010). The Taylor-linearized variance can be estimated from the empirical influence function $\Delta\{.\}$, which yields the analytic jackknife residual, or Taylor deviate, for each observation. Influence functions have been used to estimate the variance of M-estimators (Hampel, 1974), complex survey statistics (Graubard and Fears, 2005), and the hazard ratios of the proportional hazards model for cohort data (Reid and Crepeau, 1985). Key properties of the influence operator have been previously discussed by Shah (2002) and Deville (1999).

Although we illustrate the influence functions for a cohort obtained by simple random sampling, a great advantage of this approach is that is simple, easy to implement, and can easily be extended to accommodate complex sampling designs. Mark and Katki (2001) and Mark and Katki (2006) used influence functions to compute variances for the case-cohort design and for two-stage cohort samples, respectively. Results are also available for linearization methods for estimates defined as the solution of estimating equations (Binder, 1983).

Alternatively one could use resampling approaches, such as the jackknife and bootstrap, to estimate the variance of absolute risk. The jackknife is based on repeated computation of the statistic for a dataset that omits one of the observations or groups of observations at a time. Jackknife and linearization methods are similar in that analytical derivatives in the linearization are replaced by numerical approximation in the jackknife (Davison and Hinkley, 1997). The bootstrap recomputes the statistic based samples drawn with replacement from the original dataset, and in a manner that reflects the sampling design. The bootstrap requires considerable computation, and the resulting variance estimates are not deterministic functions of the data, unlike the jackknife or influence function estimates.

In our example we compare the influence function based variance estimates to those obtained from a bootstrap.

4.6.2 Influence function based variance of the absolute risk estimate from cohort data

We base our variance derivation on a linearization approach, that allows one to obtain variance estimates of a statistic T through a first order approximation of T, such that

$$\mathrm{var}(T) \approx \mathrm{var}\{\sum_{i=1}^{n} \Delta_i(T)\}, \tag{4.35}$$

where $\Delta_i(T)$ denotes the influence function operator that captures the influence of observation i on T. In what follows $T = \hat{r}_m(t_0, t_1, \mathbf{z})$ and we assume simple random sampling of cohort members. Extensions for complex sampling are in Kovalchik and Pfeiffer (2013).

Recall that the estimate of the absolute risk (4.1) can be written as a sum over the distinct observed event times $u_1, \ldots, u_L$ for the primary cause m occurring within $(t_0, t_1]$, as

$$\hat{r}_m(t_0, t_1; \mathbf{z}) = \sum_{l=1}^{L} \hat{\lambda}_{0m}(u_l) \exp(\hat{\boldsymbol{\beta}}_m' \mathbf{z}^m) \exp\left[-\sum_{k=1}^{M} \{\hat{\Lambda}_k(u_l; \mathbf{z}^k) - \hat{\Lambda}_k(t_0; \mathbf{z}^k)\}\right] =$$
$$\sum_{l=1}^{L} \hat{\lambda}_{0m}(u_l) \exp(\hat{\boldsymbol{\beta}}_m' \mathbf{z}^m) \prod_{k=1}^{M} \exp\left[-\{\hat{\Lambda}_{0k}(u_l) - \hat{\Lambda}_{0k}(t_0)\} \exp(\hat{\boldsymbol{\beta}}_k' \mathbf{z}^k)\right] = \sum_{l=1}^{L} \prod_{k=1}^{M} \theta^k(u_l),$$

where

$$\theta^m(u_l) = \hat{\lambda}_{0m}(u_l) \exp(\hat{\boldsymbol{\beta}}_m' \mathbf{z}^m) \exp\left[-\{\hat{\Lambda}_{0m}(u_l) - \hat{\Lambda}_{0m}(t_0)\} \exp(\hat{\boldsymbol{\beta}}_m' \mathbf{z}^m)\right]$$

and for all competing events, $k \neq m$,

$$\theta^k(u_l) = \exp\left[-\{\hat{\Lambda}_{0k}(u_l) - \hat{\Lambda}_{0k}(t_0)\} \exp(\hat{\boldsymbol{\beta}}_k' \mathbf{z}^k)\right].$$

The Taylor deviates for the absolute risk estimate are weighted sums of the deviates of θ, weighted by the partial derivatives of the absolute risk with respect to θ. The form of the ith deviate is

$$\Delta_i\{\hat{r}_m(t_0, t_1; \mathbf{z})\} = \sum_{l=1}^{L} \sum_{k=1}^{M} \frac{\partial \hat{r}_m(t_0, t_1; \mathbf{z})}{\partial \theta^k(u_l)} \Delta_i\{\theta^k(u_l)\} = \sum_{k=1}^{M} \Delta_i^k\{\hat{r}_m(t_0, t_1; \mathbf{z})\}, \tag{4.36}$$

where $\Delta_i^k\{\hat{r}_m(t_0, t_1; \mathbf{z})\}$ is the total influence due to a specific cause k on the absolute risk for event m, and $\Delta_i\{\theta^k(u_l)\}$ will be given later for piecewise constant and non-parametric hazard models. Given the Taylor deviates (influences) $\Delta_i\{\hat{r}_m(t_0, t_1; \mathbf{z})\}$ in (4.36), the variance estimate for the absolute risk is

$$\widehat{\mathrm{var}}(\hat{r}_m(t_0, t_1; \mathbf{z})) = \frac{n}{n-1} \sum_{i=1}^{n} [\Delta_i\{\hat{r}_m(t_0, t_1; \mathbf{z})\} - \bar{\Delta}\{\hat{r}_m(t_0, t_1; \mathbf{z})\}]^2 \tag{4.37}$$

where $\bar{\Delta}\{\hat{r}_m(t_0, t_1; \mathbf{z})\} = n^{-1} \sum_{i=1}^{n} \Delta_i\{\hat{r}_m(t_0, t_1; \mathbf{z})\}$ is the average of these individual influences. Note that (4.37) is a variance estimate for a simple random sample but could be generalized for complex sampling by treating Δ_i as a random sample from the complex design.

Influences for the piecewise exponential hazard function

We express the absolute risk estimate (4.14) in a more compact form,

$$\hat{r}_m(\tau_{0n_0}, \tau_{1n_1}; \mathbf{z}) = \sum_{q=n_0}^{n_1} \hat{S}(\mathcal{I}_q) A_q (1 - B_q)$$

where

$$A_q = \frac{\hat{\lambda}_{0m}(\mathcal{I}_q) \exp(\hat{\boldsymbol{\beta}}_m' \mathbf{z}^m)}{\sum_k \hat{\lambda}_{0k}(\mathcal{I}_q) \exp(\hat{\boldsymbol{\beta}}_k' \mathbf{z}^k)},$$

$$B_q = \exp\{-\sum_k \hat{\lambda}_{0k}(\mathcal{I}_q) \exp(\hat{\boldsymbol{\beta}}_k' \mathbf{z}^k)(\tau_{1q} - \tau_{0q})\},$$

and $\hat{S}(\mathcal{I}_q)$ is defined in Equation (4.15). Then the influences for $\hat{r}_m(\tau_{0n_0}, \tau_{1n_1}; \mathbf{z})$ are

$$\begin{aligned} \Delta_i\{\hat{r}_m(\tau_{0n_0}, \tau_{1n_1}; \mathbf{z})\} = \; & \textstyle\sum_{q=n_0}^{n_1} \Big[\hat{S}(\mathcal{I}_q)(1 - B_q)\Delta_i\{A_q\} \\ & + A_q(1 - B_q)\Delta_i\{\hat{S}(\mathcal{I}_q)\} - A_q \hat{S}(\mathcal{I}_q)\Delta_i\{B_q\} \Big]. \end{aligned} \tag{4.38}$$

Taking each component in turn, the deviates for A_q are

$$\Delta_i\{A_q\} = T_q^{-1}\Delta_i\{T_q^{(1)}\} - \frac{T_q^{(1)}}{T_q^2} \sum_{k=1}^{M} \Delta_i\{T_q^{(k)}\}$$

where $T_q^{(m)} = \hat{\lambda}_{0m}(\mathcal{I}_q) \exp(\hat{\boldsymbol{\beta}}_m' \mathbf{z}^m)$ and $T_q = \sum_{k=1}^{M} T_q^{(k)}$, with deviates

$$\Delta_i\{T_q^{(m)}\} = \exp(\hat{\boldsymbol{\beta}}_m' \mathbf{z}^m)\Delta_i\{\hat{\lambda}_{0m}(\mathcal{I}_q)\} + \mathbf{z}^m T_{1q} \Delta_i\{\hat{\boldsymbol{\beta}}_m\}.$$

The deviates for B_q are

$$\Delta_i\{B_q\} = -\sum_{m=1}^{M} \left[\exp(\hat{\boldsymbol{\beta}}_m' \mathbf{z}^m)(\tau_{1q} - \tau_{0q}) B_q \left(\mathbf{z}^m \hat{\lambda}_{0m}(\mathcal{I}_q)\Delta_i\{\hat{\boldsymbol{\beta}}_m\} + \Delta_i\{\hat{\lambda}_{0m}(\mathcal{I}_q)\} \right) \right].$$

For $q > n_0$, we note that $\hat{S}(\mathcal{I}_q) = \prod_{l=n_0}^{q-1} B_l$ so that

$$\Delta_i\{\hat{S}(\mathcal{I}_q)\} = \hat{S}(\mathcal{I}_q) \sum_{l=n_0}^{q-1} B_l^{-1} \Delta_i\{B_l\},$$

and $\Delta_i\{\hat{S}(\mathcal{I}_q)\}$ is zero when $q = n_0$. The Taylor deviates for A_q, B_q and $\hat{S}(\mathcal{I}_q)$ are each functions of $\hat{\lambda}_{0m}$ and $\hat{\boldsymbol{\beta}}_m$. For $\hat{\lambda}_{0m}$, we have

$$\Delta_i\{\hat{\lambda}_{0m}(\mathcal{I}_q)\} = D^{(m)}(\mathcal{I}_q)^{-1} \left[dN_i^m(t_i) I(\tau_{0q} \le t_i < \tau_{1q}) - \hat{\lambda}_{0m}(\mathcal{I}_q)\Delta_i\{D^{(m)}(\mathcal{I}_q)\} \right]$$

where

$$\begin{aligned} \Delta_i\{D^{(m)}(\mathcal{I}_q)\} = \; & \mathcal{A}_i(\mathcal{I}_q) \exp(\hat{\boldsymbol{\beta}}_m' \mathbf{z}_i^m) \\ & + \left[\textstyle\sum_i \mathbf{z}_i^m \mathcal{A}_i(\mathcal{I}_q) \exp(\hat{\boldsymbol{\beta}}_m' \mathbf{z}_i^m) \right] \Delta_i\{\hat{\boldsymbol{\beta}}_m\}, \end{aligned} \tag{4.39}$$

and where $\mathcal{A}_i(\mathcal{I}_q)$ is defined in Equation (4.16). Here we let $\hat{\boldsymbol{\beta}}^m$ be the estimate from the partial likelihood and $\sum_t$ denote summation over all event times. Then the Taylor deviates for each $\hat{\boldsymbol{\beta}}_m$ (Reid and Crepeau, 1985) are

$$\Delta_i\{\hat{\boldsymbol{\beta}}_m\} = \mathcal{E}(\hat{\boldsymbol{\beta}}_m)^{-1} \sum_t \left[\{\mathbf{z}_i^m - \vec{E}(\hat{\boldsymbol{\beta}}_m, t)\} \left(dN_i^m(t) - y_i(t)\exp(\hat{\boldsymbol{\beta}}_m' \mathbf{z}_i^m) \frac{\sum_l dN_l^m(t)}{\sum_l y_l(t)\exp(\hat{\boldsymbol{\beta}}_m' \mathbf{z}_l^m)} \right) \right], \tag{4.40}$$

where $\mathcal{E}(\hat{\boldsymbol{\beta}}_m)$ is minus the second partial derivative of the log-pseudo-likelihood,

$$\mathcal{E}(\hat{\boldsymbol{\beta}}_m) = \sum_t \left[\sum_i \mathbf{z}_i^m \mathbf{z}_i^{m\prime} e_i^{(m)}(t) - \vec{E}(\hat{\boldsymbol{\beta}}_m, t)\vec{E}(\hat{\boldsymbol{\beta}}_m, t)' \right], \tag{4.41}$$

where $\vec{E}(\hat{\boldsymbol{\beta}}_m, t)$ is defined in Equation (4.9), and

$$e_i^{(m)}(t) = y_i(t)\exp(\hat{\boldsymbol{\beta}}_m' \mathbf{z}_i^m) / \sum_i y_i(t)\exp(\hat{\boldsymbol{\beta}}_m' \mathbf{z}_i^m).$$

The first term inside the summation in Equation (4.40), $dN_i^m(t)\{\mathbf{z}_i^m - \vec{E}(\hat{\boldsymbol{\beta}}_m, t)\}$, is non-zero only if person i has an event. Thus, the deviates for $\hat{\boldsymbol{\beta}}_m$ are equivalent to the per-observation update in a Newton-Raphson optimization algorithm where the objective function is the weighted pseudo-likelihood of the Cox regression model. By successively substituting these expressions we obtain $\Delta_i\{\hat{r}_m(\tau_{0n_0}, \tau_{1n_1}, \mathbf{z})\}$ in (4.38) and hence the needed influences for Equation (4.37).

We could have used maximum likelihood estimates of $\boldsymbol{\beta}_m$ and λ_{0m} based on the full likelihood (Friedman, 1982) instead of estimating $\boldsymbol{\beta}_m$ from the partial likelihood (Section 4.1.1) and then estimating λ_{0m} as in Section 4.1.4. Here λ_{0m} is a vector of interval-specific baseline hazards in terms of which the baseline hazard function $\lambda_{0m}(t)$ is defined as in Section 4.1.4. Letting $\lambda_m(t;\mathbf{z}^m) = \lambda_{0m}(t)\exp(\boldsymbol{\beta}_m' \mathbf{z}^m)$, $\lambda(t;\mathbf{z}) = \sum_{m=1}^{M} \lambda_m(t;\mathbf{z}^m)$, and $S(t;\mathbf{z}) = \exp\{-\int_0^t \lambda(u;\mathbf{z})du\}$, we can write the likelihood as follows. A person with an event of type m at time t contributes $\lambda_m(t;\mathbf{z})S(t)$ to the likelihood for $\{\lambda_{0m}\}$ and $\{\boldsymbol{\beta}_m\}$. If the person survives to time t without any event, the contribution is $S(t)$. If $\mathbf{I}$ is the estimated Fisher information from the full likelihood in $\{\boldsymbol{\beta}_m\}$ and $\{\lambda_{0m}\}$, which are concatenated into column vectors $\boldsymbol{\beta}$ and $\boldsymbol{\lambda}_0$, and if $\mathbf{U}_i$ is the vector of contributions to the log-likelihood score equations from the ith subject, then, from standard results for scores, the influences for the respective components of the maximum likelihood estimates $(\hat{\boldsymbol{\beta}}^T, \hat{\boldsymbol{\lambda}}_0^T)^T$ are $-\mathbf{I}^{-1}\mathbf{U}_i$. These influences can be substituted for $\Delta_i\{\hat{\boldsymbol{\beta}}_m\}$ and $\Delta_i\{\hat{\lambda}_{0m}(\mathcal{I}_q)\}$ in previous expressions to compute the variance of $\hat{r}_m(\tau_{0n_0}, \tau_{1n_1}; \mathbf{z})$.

Derivatives and Taylor deviates for the semi-parametric hazard model

Denote $\hat{S}_{0k}(t) = \exp\{-\hat{\Lambda}_{0k}(t)\}$ and the $N_k, k = 1, \ldots, M$ ordered observed event times occurring within $(t_0, t_1]$ for the kth cause as $t_0 < u_1^k < u_2^k < \cdots < u_{N_k}^k \le t_1$. In terms of these event times, Equation (4.1) becomes

$$\begin{aligned} \hat{r}_m(t_0, t_1; \mathbf{z}) &= \sum_{j=1}^{N_m} \exp(\hat{\boldsymbol{\beta}}_m' \mathbf{z}^m)\hat{\lambda}_{0m}(u_j^m) \prod_{k=1}^{M} \left(\frac{\hat{S}_{0k}(u_j^m)}{\hat{S}_{0k}(t_0)} \right)^{\exp(\hat{\boldsymbol{\beta}}_k' \mathbf{z}^k)} \\ &= \sum_{j=1}^{N_m} \exp(\hat{\boldsymbol{\beta}}_m' \mathbf{z}^m)\hat{\lambda}_{0m}(u_j^m) \prod_{k=1}^{M} \left\{ \hat{R}_{0k}(u_j^m) \right\}^{\exp(\hat{\boldsymbol{\beta}}_k' \mathbf{z}^k)} = \sum_{j=1}^{N_m} \hat{r}_m(u_j^m), \end{aligned} \tag{4.42}$$

where $\hat{R}_{0k}(u_j^m) = \hat{S}_{0k}(u_j^m)/\hat{S}_{0k}(t_0) = \exp\{-\hat{\Lambda}_{0k}(u_j^m) + \hat{\Lambda}_{0k}(t_0)\}$. As with the piecewise exponential model, we determine the derivative and deviates for each component of (4.42). For the $\hat{\boldsymbol{\beta}}_k$, the derivative is

$$\frac{\partial \hat{r}_m(t_0,t_1;\mathbf{z})}{\partial \hat{\boldsymbol{\beta}}_k} = \mathbf{z}^k \left[\hat{r}_m(t_0,t_1;\mathbf{z}) + \exp(\hat{\boldsymbol{\beta}}_k'\mathbf{z}^k) \sum_{j=1}^{N_m} \log\left\{\hat{R}_{0k}(u_j^m)\right\} \hat{r}_m(u_j^m) \right]$$

for $k = m$, and

$$\frac{\partial \hat{r}_m(t_0,t_1;\mathbf{x})}{\partial \hat{\boldsymbol{\beta}}_k} = \mathbf{z}^k \exp(\hat{\boldsymbol{\beta}}_k'\mathbf{z}^k) \sum_{j=1}^{N_m} \log\left\{\hat{R}_{0k}(u_j^m)\right\} \hat{r}_m(u_j^m)$$

for competing causes $k \neq m$. The Taylor deviates for each $\hat{\boldsymbol{\beta}}_k$ are the same as given by Equation (4.40) for the piecewise exponential model. The derivatives for the baseline hazard components are

$$\frac{\partial \hat{r}_m(t_0,t_1;\mathbf{x})}{\partial \hat{\lambda}_{0m}(u_j^m)} = \hat{\lambda}_{0m}(u_j^m)^{-1}\hat{r}_m(u_j^m).$$

Recalling from (4.10) that the baseline hazard functions $\hat{\lambda}_{0j}(t)$ are estimated as

$$\hat{\lambda}_{0k}(t) = \frac{\sum_{l=1}^n dN_{kl}(t)}{\sum_{l=1}^n y_l(t)\exp(\hat{\boldsymbol{\beta}}_k'\mathbf{z}_l^k)} = \frac{N_k(t)}{G_k(t)},$$

the Taylor deviates for the baseline hazard of cause m at observed event time t are

$$\Delta_i\{\hat{\lambda}_{0m}(t)\} = \frac{\partial \hat{\lambda}_{0m}(t)}{\partial N_m(t)}\Delta_i\{N_m(t)\} + \frac{\partial \hat{\lambda}_{0m}(t)}{\partial G_m(t)}\Delta_i\{G_m(t)\}.$$

In terms of these quantities, the Taylor deviates are

$$\Delta_i\{\hat{\lambda}_{0m}(t)\} = G^m(t)^{-1}\left[dN_{mi}(t) - \hat{\lambda}_{0m}(t)\Delta_i\{G_m(t)\}\right]$$

with

$$\begin{aligned}\Delta_i\{G_m(t)\} = \; & y_i^m(t)\exp(\hat{\boldsymbol{\beta}}_m'\mathbf{z}_i^m) \\ & + \left[\textstyle\sum_l \mathbf{z}_l^m y_l^m(t)\exp(\hat{\boldsymbol{\beta}}_m'\mathbf{z}_l^m)\right]\Delta_i\{\hat{\boldsymbol{\beta}}_m\}.\end{aligned}$$

We note that the hazard deviates for the piecewise and semiparametric model in Equation (4.39) are equivalent when each interval of the piecewise model contains exactly one observed event time.

The final components are the survival functions. The derivatives for each $\hat{R}_{0j}(u_k^m)$ are

$$\frac{\partial \hat{r}_m(t_0,t_1;\mathbf{x})}{\partial \hat{R}_{0k}(u_j^m)} = \exp(\hat{\boldsymbol{\beta}}_k'\mathbf{z}^k)\hat{R}_{0k}(u_j^m)^{-1}\hat{r}_m(u_j^m).$$

From the semiparametric estimate of Equation (4.11), the Taylor deviates for $\hat{R}_{0j}(u_k^m)$ are

$$\Delta_i\{\hat{R}_{0k}(u_j^m)\} = \Delta_i\{\exp[-\hat{\Lambda}_{0k}(u_j^m) + \hat{\Lambda}_{0k}(t_0)\} = -\hat{R}_{0k}(u_j^m) \sum_{t_0 < u_l^k \leq u_j^m} \Delta_i\{\hat{\lambda}_{0k}(u_l^k)\}.$$

To simplify the computation, we use that

$$\frac{\hat{r}_m(t_0,t_1;\mathbf{z})}{\partial \hat{R}_{0k}(u_j^m)}\Delta_i\{\hat{R}_{0k}(u_j^m)\} = -\exp(\hat{\boldsymbol{\beta}}_k'\mathbf{z}^k)\hat{r}_m(u_j^m) \sum_{t_0 < u_l^k \leq u_j^m} \Delta_i\{\hat{\lambda}_{0k}(u_l^k)\}.$$

Combining these results, we obtain the expression for the Taylor deviates of $\hat{r}_m(t_0, t_1; \mathbf{x})$ for individuals $i = 1, \ldots, n$ in the cohort as

$$\begin{aligned}\Delta_i\{\hat{r}_m(t_0, t_1; \mathbf{x})\} = & \sum_{k=1}^{M} \frac{\hat{r}_m(t_0,t_1;\mathbf{z})}{\partial \hat{\boldsymbol{\beta}}_k} \Delta_i\{\hat{\boldsymbol{\beta}}_k\} + \sum_{j=1}^{N_m} \frac{\hat{r}_m(t_0,t_1;\mathbf{z})}{\partial \hat{\lambda}_{0m}(u_j^m)} \Delta_i\{\hat{\lambda}_{0m}(u_j^m)\} \\ & - \sum_{j=1}^{N_m} \sum_{k=1}^{M} \left[\exp(\hat{\boldsymbol{\beta}}_k' \mathbf{z}^k) \hat{r}_m(u_j^m) \sum_{t_0 < u_l^k \leq u_j^m} \Delta_i\{\hat{\lambda}_{0k}(u_l^k)\}\right].\end{aligned}$$

Chapter 5

Estimating absolute risk by combining case-control or cohort data with disease registry data

Equation (4.1) expresses absolute risk in terms of cause-specific hazards. If the cause-specific hazards depend on covariates through a proportional hazards relationship, Equation (4.4), it is possible to estimate covariate- and cause-specific hazards by combining relative and attributable risk estimates from case-control or cohort data or subsamples of cohorts, as in the case-cohort design (Prentice, 1986), with estimates of age-specific incidence from a registry. This approach is applicable even if the covariates in Equation (4.4) are time-dependent. The ability to combine information on relative and attributable risk with registry data to estimate absolute risk is one of the major advantages of the cause-specific formulation of absolute risk, Equation (4.1).

This approach is particularly appealing in the setting of rare outcomes, where association parameters are often estimated from case-control studies that do not provide any information on disease incidence. It also allows one to obtain more stable and efficient estimates of the hazards when cohort data or subsamples from cohorts are available because the registry rates are usually known with good precision. The use of registry rates, which are often population-based, calibrates the model to the general population from which the registry derives. The gain in information from the use of registry data depends, however, on the size and quality of the available registry data.

5.1 Relationship between attributable risk, composite age-specific incidence, and baseline hazard

Disease registries usually cover a well defined population and collect information on the characteristics of persons diagnosed with a particular disease. These characteristics typically include age at diagnosis, sex, race/ethnicity, and features of the disease, such as cancer stage. For example, the National Cancer Institute's Surveillance, Epidemiology and End Results (SEER) program attempts to ascertain all cancers (with a few exceptions such as non-melanoma skin cancers) diagnosed in defined geographic areas each year. SEER now covers about 28% of the US population (http://seer.cancer.gov/registries/data.html). By combining such information with data on population size, SEER publishes gender-, race/ethnicity-, calendar year- and age-specific cancer rates. For example, from 2009–2013 SEER data, the breast cancer incidence rate for white women aged $60 - 64$ is $\lambda_1^*(t) = 340$ per 10^5 women-years (http://seer.cancer.gov/faststats), where the subscript 1 indicates the incidence rate of the outcome of principal interest, t is age, and the asterisk indicates that this is a "composite" rate, because it reflects the experience of a population of women with various combinations of risk factors. In Equation (4.4), we require the baseline hazard rate $\lambda_{01}(t)$ for a woman with relative risk 1.0, i.e., who has all covariates at their lowest levels,

$\mathbf{z}^1 = \mathbf{0}$. To avoid confusion in any computation, we assume that all covariates $\mathbf{z}^1$ are coded so that relative risks are greater or equal to one, i.e., all non-null factors increase risk, but cannot lower it. Depending on the example, this may require changes of baseline or referent categories compared to some commonly used risk factor coding.

For a population aged t, the *attributable hazard function* (Chen et al., 2006b; Samuelsen and Eide, 2008) for outcome 1, the fraction of the incidence that is explained by the risk factors $\mathbf{z}^1$ in the model, is

$$AR(t) = \frac{\lambda_1^*(t) - \lambda_{01}(t)}{\lambda_1^*(t)}. \tag{5.1}$$

The quantity $AR(t)$ in Equation (5.1) can be approximated by the attributable risk in a set of subjects in an age interval near t. We use the notation $AR(t)$ to refer to the outcome of main interest, $m = 1$, but the same approach could be used for other outcomes. Hence the baseline hazard satisfies

$$\lambda_{01}(t) = \{1 - AR(t)\}\lambda_1^*(t). \tag{5.2}$$

The needed covariate- and cause-specific hazard is estimated under Equation (4.3) as

$$\hat{\lambda}_1(t; \mathbf{z}^1) = \hat{\lambda}_{01}(t) rr(\hat{\boldsymbol{\beta}}_1' \mathbf{z}^1) = \{1 - \widehat{AR}(t)\}\lambda_1^*(t) rr(\hat{\boldsymbol{\beta}}_1' \mathbf{z}^1), \tag{5.3}$$

where rr denotes the relative risk. The SEER composite rate $\lambda_1^*(t)$ is usually based on large samples and is thus assumed to be known without error, but the random variation in $\{1 - \widehat{AR}(t)\} rr(\hat{\boldsymbol{\beta}}_1' \mathbf{z}^1)$ needs to be taken into account, as described in Section 5.8. Sometimes it may be necessary to accommodate the variability in the composite hazard, $\lambda_1^*(t)$, but we do not consider this in what follows. Equation (5.1) was used by Gail et al. (1989) but called the "population attributable risk fraction for women of age t".

5.2 Estimating relative risk and attributable risk from case-control data

Suppose for a rare outcome one has conducted a population-based case-control study and focuses on cases ($D = 1$) and controls ($D = 0$) in a given age interval $[\tau_{0t}, \tau_{1t})$, that could be a single year or an age interval, such as ages 60–64 years. We sometimes use the shorthand notation $t_i = t$ to mean $t_i \in [\tau_{0t}, \tau_{1t})$. Over short time periods, the probability of disease is usually small. Thus relative odds from case-control data approximate relative risks, and log relative odds from case-control data estimate $\boldsymbol{\beta}_1$ in model (5.3) with $rr(u) = exp(u)$. Here an estimate $\hat{\boldsymbol{\beta}}_1$ is obtained from unconditional or conditional logistic regression. If cases are representative of all cases in the population of interest, they can be used to estimate attributable risk from the Bruzzi formula (Bruzzi et al., 1985)

$$1 - \widehat{AR}(t) = \frac{1}{\sum_{i=1}^n d_i I(t_i = t)} \sum_{i=1}^n \frac{d_i I(t_i = t)}{rr(\hat{\boldsymbol{\beta}}_1' \mathbf{z}_i^1)}, \tag{5.4}$$

where n is the total sample size in the case-control study, d is the observed case indicator, I denotes the indicator function, and $\mathbf{z}_i^1$ and t_i are the covariates and age for person i, respectively. Thus $d_i I(t_i = t) = 1$ only if person i is a case diagnosed in age interval t. Greenland and Drescher (1993) showed that the maximum likelihood estimate of $AR(t)$ was scarcely more efficient than Equation (5.4) and required stronger assumptions.

Sometimes there are nuisance variables, $\mathbf{Z}^0$, such as study center or year of enrollment into a study, that are not going to be part of the actual risk model but have to be accounted for in the model fitting to yield unbiased estimates of $\boldsymbol{\beta}_1$ for the variables of interest, $\mathbf{Z}^1$, that will be in the risk model. To obtain estimates $\hat{\boldsymbol{\beta}}_1$, one can adjust for $\mathbf{Z}^0$ by stratification or by including it in a joint relative risk model such as $rr(\hat{\boldsymbol{\beta}}_1' \mathbf{Z}^1, \hat{\boldsymbol{\gamma}}_1' \mathbf{Z}^0) = \exp(\hat{\boldsymbol{\beta}}_1' \mathbf{Z}^1 + \hat{\boldsymbol{\gamma}}_1' \mathbf{Z}^0)$. Assuming that the cases in the study are similar to cases in a target population, Equation

(5.4) should be used with $rr(\hat{\boldsymbol{\beta}}_1'\mathbf{Z}^1) = \exp(\hat{\boldsymbol{\beta}}_1'\mathbf{Z}^1)$. Here we are not trying to estimate the adjusted attributable risk (see Bruzzi et al. (1985)) that describes the fractional reduction in risk in the study population if $\mathbf{Z}^1$ is set to 0 but $\mathbf{Z}^0$ is unchanged.

Often controls are matched to cases on age and other factors and are therefore not representative of the entire population. However, if controls are a simple random sample of non-cases, they can also be used to estimate the attributable risk under the rare disease assumption via

$$1 - \widehat{AR}(t) = \frac{\sum_{i=1}^{n}(1-d_i)I(t_i = t)}{\sum_{i=1}^{n}(1-d_i)I(t_i = t)rr(\hat{\boldsymbol{\beta}}_1'\mathbf{z}_i^1)}. \tag{5.5}$$

Benichou and Gail (1990b) discussed estimation of attributable risk for four ways of choosing controls: simple random sampling; stratified random sampling; frequency matching controls to cases within strata; and individual matching of controls to cases. They gave corresponding methods for inference for the attributable risk, but not for the product $\{1-\widehat{AR}(t)\}\exp(\hat{\boldsymbol{\beta}}_1'\mathbf{z}^1)$. Graubard and Fears (2005) used used a linearization approach based on influence functions to obtain the variance of $\widehat{AR}(t)$ for various study designs. Pfeiffer and Petracci (2011) extended the influence function based variance computation for the attributable risk and provided variances for the absolute risk $\hat{r}_1(t)$ estimated from case-control data combined with registry information on incidence. We present that approach to variance estimation in detail in Section 5.8.

Equations like (5.4) and (5.5) can be expressed in terms of averages with respect to the empirical distribution of covariates in cases or in the population, respectively. The latter distribution can be estimated from controls in a case-control study if the disease is rare. For example, if $\hat{F}$ is the empirical distribution of covariates among cases diagnosed at age t, $1 - \widehat{AR}(t) = \int\{rr(\hat{\boldsymbol{\beta}}_1'\mathbf{z}^1)\}^{-1}d\hat{F}(\mathbf{z}^1)$. Thus these expressions generalize to combinations of discrete and continuous covariates (Benichou and Gail, 1990b).

5.3 Estimating relative risk and attributable risk from cohort data

Equation (5.3) can also be used for cohort data by modifying the estimators. Log relative hazards $\boldsymbol{\beta}_1$ can be estimated with the methods in Chapter 4, either based on the full cohort, on nested case-control samples within the cohort, or on case-cohort samples. Although absolute risk can be estimated directly from the cohort data (Chapter 4), cohorts may provide imprecise estimates of $\lambda_{01}(t)$, even though estimates of relative and absolute risk have adequate precision. In this setting, using composite age-specific hazards $\lambda_1^*(t)$ from registry data can improve the precision of estimates of absolute risk $r_1(t_0,t_1;\mathbf{Z}^1 = \mathbf{z}^1)$. If censoring is independent of covariates and failure time, attributable risks can be estimated as in Chen et al. (2006b) by summing over all cohort members at risk in age interval t, i.e., those for whom the at risk process $Y(t)$ defined in Section 2.6. equals 1,

$$1 - \widehat{AR}(t) = \frac{\sum_{i=1}^{n} Y_i(t)}{\sum_{i=1}^{n} Y_i(t)rr(\hat{\boldsymbol{\beta}}_1'\mathbf{z}_i^1)}. \tag{5.6}$$

Again, it is important that all covariates in the above formula are coded so that all coefficients β_i are non-negative. Graubard et al. (2007) described how to estimate attributable risks and standard errors from simple and complex sampled cohorts, including multistage stratified cluster samples, which are used in national household surveys. We derive the variance of $1 - \widehat{AR}(t)$ in Section 5.8 following the approach by Graubard et al. (2007).

As for the case-control setting in Section 5.2, when nuisance variables $\mathbf{Z}^0$ such as study center or year of accrual are included in the joint relative risk model $rr(\hat{\boldsymbol{\beta}}_1'\mathbf{z}^1, \hat{\gamma}_1'\mathbf{z}_i^0)$, one obtains an adjusted estimate $\hat{\boldsymbol{\beta}}_1$. Provided the distribution of $\mathbf{Z}^1$ is similar to that in the target population, however, Equation (5.6) still applies with the adjusted estimate $\hat{\boldsymbol{\beta}}_1$. Here we are assuming that the adjusted log relative risks from the study population approximate the log relative risks that would have been obtained by applying the model based only on $\mathbf{Z}^1$ to the target population.

Liu et al. (2014) provided rigorous theory for estimating the functions $\phi(t) = \{1-AR(t)\}$ and $r_1(t_{0,} = 0, t_1 = t; \mathbf{Z}^1 = \mathbf{z}^1)$, regarded as a function of continuous time t, from survival data in a cohort, such as women followed in the Women's Health Initiative (WHI). Because women entered the cohort at various ages, and the analysis was done on the age scale, they allowed for left-truncation as well as for right-censoring. Under the Cox proportional hazards model with fixed covariates,

$$1 - AR(t) = \frac{\int \exp\{-\Lambda_0(t)\exp(\boldsymbol{\beta}_1'\mathbf{z}^1)\}dF(\mathbf{z}^1)}{\int \exp(\beta_1'\mathbf{z}^1)\exp\{-\Lambda_0(t)\exp(\boldsymbol{\beta}_1'\mathbf{z}^1)\}dF(\mathbf{z}^1)}, \tag{5.7}$$

where F is the distribution of $\mathbf{Z}^1$ in the cohort. If the cohort is representative of the registry population, such as SEER, then F also describes the distribution of risk factors in the registry population, and letting $\phi(t) = 1 - AR(t)$, one can use $\lambda_{01}(t) = \phi(t)\lambda_1^*(t)$ to compute absolute risks in the registry population. For models that are to be used for the general population, a registry like SEER is likely to be more representative of the general population than a particular cohort, justifying this approach. Liu et al. (2014), however, were interested in estimating absolute risk for the WHI population, not the SEER registry population. They therefore re-calibrated the SEER rates by multiplying by a constant factor ρ to obtain $\lambda_{01,WHI}(t) = \rho\phi(t)\lambda_1^*(t)$ and estimated $\boldsymbol{\beta}_1'$ from maximum partial likelihood, $\Lambda_0(t)$ from the Breslow estimator, and ρ from the ratio of observed to expected events in the WHI cohort. They used martingale theory to prove consistency and asymptotic normality for $\hat{\rho}$ and the processes $\hat{\phi}(t)$ and $\hat{r}_1(t_0, t_1; \mathbf{Z}^1 = \mathbf{z}^1)$, together with needed variance and covariance estimates. The marginal normal theory for $\hat{\phi}(t)$ and $\hat{r}_1(t_0, t_1; \mathbf{Z}^1 = \mathbf{z}^1)$ supports inference for risk projection in the general population (ρ =1). Equation (5.7) relies strongly on the proportional hazards assumption, but only requires that censoring be independent of failure time conditional on all covariates used for modeling the competing risks. The estimator of $\phi(t)$ in Equation (5.6) is less model-based and can be used to estimate $\lambda_{01}(t) = \phi(t)\lambda_1^*(t)$. The variability of λ_1^* is often negligible compared to that of $\hat{\phi}(t)$. One can also use the estimators of $\boldsymbol{\beta}_1'$ and $\Lambda_0(t)$ with Equation (5.7) for nested case-control designs and case-cohort designs (Chapter 4), instead of for the full cohort, and increase the efficiency of absolute risk estimates by employing $\lambda_{01}(t) = \phi(t)\lambda_1^*(t)$. However, additional theoretical work, or a bootstrap procedure, would be needed to provide confidence intervals for the resulting absolute risk estimates.

5.4 Estimating the cause-specific hazard of the competing causes of mortality, $\lambda_2(t; \mathbf{z}^2)$

To estimate the absolute risk of incidence of disease 1, the only competing risk is death from other causes, with cause-specific hazard $\lambda_2(t; \mathbf{z}^2)$. Data from the National Center for Health Statistics of the Centers for Disease Control and Prevention are accessible through SEER and give estimates of the composite hazard, $\lambda_2^*(t)$ for the general US population. Often cohort studies are too small to provide reliable covariate models for competing mortality, and the cohort may not provide reliable cause-of-death data. Thus, one often ignores covariates and sets $\lambda_2(t; \mathbf{z}^2) = \lambda_2^*(t)$ in applications of Equation (4.2) with M =2 causes. This is often a good approximation, because allowing for covariates in modeling the competing risk 2 may have little impact on estimates of the absolute risk of incident disease 1, as Liu et al. (2014) found in their analyses of colorectal cancer risk in WHI.

In some applications, where the competing mortality has a large hazard and where

$\lambda_2(t; \mathbf{z}^2)$ is strongly influenced by covariates, it is essential to include covariates in $\lambda_2(t; \mathbf{z}^2)$. In the example presented in Section 4.3.2, to estimate the absolute risk of a second primary thyroid cancer in long term survivors of other types of childhood cancer, Kovalchik et al. (2013a) modeled the risk of competing mortality. This more detailed modeling was necessary to capture the strong impact of treatments for the first cancer on competing mortality. Special cohort data from childhood cancer survivors were needed to model the competing risk of mortality from causes other than thyroid cancer. In this example, covariates describing the initial treatment were needed to model competing mortality because the hazard of competing mortality was high and strongly associated with the initial treatment.

5.5 Some strengths and limitations of using registry data

The use of registry data is appealing because it increases the precision of absolute risk estimates when combined with cohort data, and it allows one to compute absolute risks even with case-control data. Moreover, if the registry is representative of the target population for which the risk model is designed, use of the registry composite rates calibrates the model to the target population. There are some limitations of this approach, however. First, representative registry data may not be available for the desired disease outcome. For example there are no national registries for incident stroke. One needs to rely on selected cohorts or on less comprehensive registries instead. Second, the approach implicit in Equation (5.3) also assumes that relative risk parameters and attributable hazard functions estimated from the case-control or cohort study are appropriate for the catchment population for the registry.

If incidence information from registries is based on small numbers of events, the variation in λ_1^* needs to be accounted for in any variance computation. This occurs, for example, with very rare outcomes, or outcomes in small subgroups of a population. One usually assumes that estimates of $\boldsymbol{\beta}_1$ and AR are independent of λ_1^*. If the numbers of events in registries are small and these events are included in the studies used to estimate $\boldsymbol{\beta}_1$ and AR, covariances need to be taken into account.

5.6 Absolute risk estimate

Recall from Chapter 4 that the absolute risk in the age interval $(t_0, t_1]$ for a person who has survived event free to age t_0 is defined as

$$r_1(t_0, t_1; \mathbf{Z} = \mathbf{z}) = P(t_0 < T \leq t_1, \delta = 1 | T > t_0) = \int_{t_0}^{t_1} \lambda_1(u, \mathbf{z}^1) S(u-) du =$$
$$\int_{t_0}^{t_1} \lambda_1(u; \mathbf{z}^1) \exp\{-\int_{t_0}^{u} \sum_{k=1}^{M} \lambda_k(s; \mathbf{z}^k) ds\} du. \quad (5.8)$$

In what follows we assume $M = 2$, and piecewise exponential models, where $\lambda_{10}(t) = \lambda_{1j0}$ and $\lambda_2(t) = \lambda_{2j0}$ are constant over single year age intervals $[t_j, t_{j+1}), j = 1, \ldots, J$. For example, if $t_0 = 50$ and $t_1 = 55$, the projection is over (50.0, 55.0], a span of five years. After integration, (5.8) simplifies to

$$r_1(t_0, t_1; \mathbf{Z} = \mathbf{z}) = \sum_{j=t_0}^{t_1-1} \frac{\lambda_{1j0} rr_j(\mathbf{z}^1, \boldsymbol{\beta}_1)}{\lambda_{1j0} rr_j(\mathbf{z}^1, \boldsymbol{\beta}_1) + \lambda_{2j0} rr_j(\mathbf{z}^2, \boldsymbol{\beta}_2)} [1 - \exp\{-\lambda_{1j0} rr_j(\mathbf{z}^1, \boldsymbol{\beta}_1)$$
$$- \lambda_{2j0} rr_j(\mathbf{z}^2, \boldsymbol{\beta}_2)\}] \exp\left[-\sum_{l=t_0}^{j-1} \{\lambda_{1l0} rr_l(\mathbf{z}^1, \boldsymbol{\beta}_1) + \lambda_{2l0} rr_l(\mathbf{z}^2, \boldsymbol{\beta}_2)\}\right], \quad (5.9)$$

where λ_{1j0} and λ_{2j0} are computed based on Equation (5.2) using the attributable risk, i.e., $\lambda_{mj0} = \lambda^*_{mj}(1 - \widehat{AR}_j)$. Note that if $j - 1 < t_0$, the sum within the exponential argument in (5.9) is 0. If intervals of different length, such as 5 years, are used, formula (5.9) can be modified by replacing $\lambda_{mj0}, m = 1, 2$ by e.g., $5\lambda_{mj0}$. Estimates of absolute risk are obtained by inserting estimates of $rr_{1j}(\mathbf{z}^1)$ and $rr_{2j}(\mathbf{z}^2)$ in Equation (5.9). Here $rr(\mathbf{z}^m)$ are general relative risk functions of $\mathbf{z}^m$ and $\boldsymbol{\beta}_m$ with values in $[0, \infty)$. The quantities $\lambda^*_{mj}, m = 1, 2$ are regarded as constants in the variance calculations in the following examples. Variance calculations are deferred to Section 5.8.

5.7 Example: estimating absolute risk of breast cancer incidence by combining cohort data with registry data

In Chapter 4 we estimated relative risks of invasive breast cancer from the AARP cohort (Table 4.2) and estimated absolute risk using internal cohort estimates of the baseline hazard and cumulative hazard. Here we use the AARP data to estimate relative risks and attributable risks (from Equation (5.6)) and combine them with SEER registry data via Equation (5.3) to estimate absolute breast cancer risk. We computed attributable risk estimates in the AARP cohort separately in four age categories: < 55, $[55, 60)$, $[60, 65)$, and 65+ years at baseline. The corresponding attributable risk estimates $\widehat{AR}(t)$ were $0.648, 0.656, 0.651$, and 0.642. As there was no appreciable heterogeneity by age, we combined all ages and used the overall attributable risk estimate $\widehat{AR} = 0.649$. We present examples of 5- and 10-year projections of absolute risk of invasive breast cancer for three 60 year old women with the same risk profiles as in Table 4.3. For comparison, we present the absolute risk estimates that used non-parametric internal cohort estimates of the cause-specific baseline hazard function for each cause. We modeled the hazard of competing mortality with covariates for the internal cohort analysis, but not for the analysis based on SEER rates. These hazards were then plugged into Equation (4.13) to estimate the absolute risk of invasive breast cancer.

For Profiles 1 and 2, the estimates from the model that used SEER data were somewhat lower than those based on AARP data alone, for both 5- and 10-year projections, but for Profile 3, the model that used SEER data had higher projections, both at 5 and 10 years. (Table 5.1). Standard errors of absolute risk estimates were smaller for the SEER-based model than for the model with internal cohort estimates of cause-specific hazards, except in one instance. The same pattern was observed whether one used influence-function based estimates of standard error or bootstrap estimates of standard error. However, for analysis based on smaller cohorts than AARP with fewer events, the gain in precision from using registry rates would be more pronounced.

5.8 Variance computations

This section describes variance calculations suited to whether the cause-specific log relative hazards and attributable risks come from case-control or cohort designs. Skipping this section will not impact the readability of later sections. We describe the linearization approach (see also Section 4.6), that allows one to obtain variance estimates of a statistic $\hat{T}$ through a first order approximation of $\hat{T}$, such that for a simple random sample

$$\text{var}(\hat{T}) \approx \text{var}\{\sum_1^n \Delta_i(\hat{T})\}, \tag{5.10}$$

where $\Delta_i(\hat{T})$ denotes the influence function operator that captures the influence of observation i on $\hat{T}$. Graubard and Fears (2005) summarize the properties of $\Delta_i(.)$, and further details can be found in Deville (1999). The variance estimate for $\hat{T}$ can be generalized for

Table 5.1: Projections of 5- and 10-year absolute risk of invasive breast cancer for three 60-year-old women with different risk profiles

Characteristics	Profile 1	Profile 2	Profile 3
BMI, kg/m^2	24	36	41
Estrogen and progestin MHT use	No MHT use	12 years	11 years
Other MHT use	No	No	Yes
Parity	2 children	1 child	1 child
Age at first live birth	23	24	22
Age at menopause	< 50 years	52	58
Benign breast disease/biopsy	No	No	Yes
Family history of breast or ovarian cancer	No	No	Yes
Alcohol consumption	0 drinks/day	0 drink/day	0.5 drink/day
Gynecologic surgery	Yes	No	No
Smoking	Never smoker	Never smoker	Never smoker
Relative risk estimate for breast cancer	1.0	3.22	10.71
Relative risk estimate for competing mortality	1.0	0.44	0.28
Absolute risk estimates (and standard errors) with internal AARP cohort baseline rates[a]			
5-year absolute risk	0.83%	2.96%	6.60%
Influence based standard error	0.05%	0.25%	0.61%
Bootstrap based standard error	0.07%	0.31%	0.65%
10-year absolute risk	1.76%	6.36%	13.88%
Influence based standard error	0.10%	0.52%	0.76%
Bootstrap based standard error	0.14%	0.65%	1.18%
Absolute risk estimates (and standard errors) that use SEER rates to estimate baseline rates			
5-year absolute risk	0.69%	2.20%	7.14%
Influence based standard error	0.04%	0.15%	0.56%
Bootstrap based standard error	0.04%	0.15%	0.58%
10-year absolute risk	1.43%	4.53%	14.29%
Influence based standard error	0.09%	0.31%	1.12%
Bootstrap based standard error	0.09%	0.31%	1.12%

[a] Competing mortality modeled with covariates for this analysis but not for the analysis with SEER rates.

complex sampling by treating Δ_i as a random sample from the complex design. We also describe resampling approaches to variance estimation (Section 5.8.4).

To to obtain an estimate $\widehat{\text{var}}(\hat{r})$, we first derive the influence $\Delta_i(\hat{r})$ of the i-th individual in the study used to estimate needed parameters on the absolute risk estimate $\hat{r}$. We assume that the competing mortality risk does not depend on covariates and has piecewise constant hazards. The extension to a covariate-dependent competing hazard is straightforward. Applying the Δ operator to (5.9), we get

$$\Delta_i(\hat{r}) = \Delta_i\{r(t_0, t_1, \mathbf{z}, \widehat{\boldsymbol{\beta}})\} =$$

$$\sum_{j=t_0}^{t_1-1} \Delta_i \left(\frac{\lambda_{1j0} rr_j(\mathbf{z}, \widehat{\boldsymbol{\beta}})}{\lambda_{1j0} rr_j(\mathbf{z}, \widehat{\boldsymbol{\beta}}) + \lambda_{2j0}} [1 - \exp\{-(\lambda_{1j0} rr_j(\mathbf{z}, \widehat{\boldsymbol{\beta}}) + \lambda_{2j0})\}] \exp\{-\sum_{l=t_0}^{j-1} (\lambda_{1l0} rr_l(\mathbf{z}, \widehat{\boldsymbol{\beta}}) + \lambda_{2l0})\} \right) =$$

$$\sum_{j=t_0}^{t_1-1} \Delta_i (\theta_{1j}\theta_{2j}\theta_{3j}), \quad (5.11)$$

where $\theta_{1j} = \lambda_{1j0} rr_j(\mathbf{z},\widehat{\boldsymbol\beta})/\{\lambda_{1j0} rr_j(\mathbf{z},\widehat{\boldsymbol\beta}) + \lambda_{2j0}\}$, $\theta_{2j} = 1 - \exp\{-(\lambda_{1j0} rr_j(\mathbf{z},\widehat{\boldsymbol\beta}) + \lambda_{2j0})\}$, and $\theta_{3j} = \exp\{-\sum_{l=t_0}^{j-1}(\lambda_{1l0} rr_l(\mathbf{z},\widehat{\boldsymbol\beta}) + \lambda_{2l0})\}$. Applying the chain rule, we express the Taylor deviates for the absolute risk estimate as weighted sums of the deviates of $\lambda_{1j0} rr_j(\mathbf{z},\widehat{\boldsymbol\beta})$, weighted by the partial derivatives of the absolute risk with respect to $\lambda_{1j0} rr_j(\mathbf{z},\widehat{\boldsymbol\beta})$,

$$\Delta_i\{r(t_0,t_1,\mathbf{z},\widehat{\boldsymbol\beta})\} = \sum_{j=t_0}^{t_1-1}\left(\theta_{3j}\Delta_i\{\lambda_{1j0} rr_j(\mathbf{z},\widehat{\boldsymbol\beta})\}\left[\frac{\partial\theta_{1j}}{\partial\{\lambda_{1j0} rr_j(\mathbf{z},\widehat{\boldsymbol\beta})\}}\theta_{2j} + \frac{\partial\theta_{2j}}{\partial\{\lambda_{1j0} rr_j(\mathbf{z},\widehat{\boldsymbol\beta})\}}\theta_{1j}\right]\right.$$
$$\left. - \theta_{1j}\theta_{2j}\theta_{3j}\sum_{l=t_0}^{j-1}\Delta_i\{\lambda_{1l0} rr_l(\mathbf{z},\widehat{\boldsymbol\beta})\}\right), \quad (5.12)$$

similar to (4.36). In the above equation

$$\frac{\partial\theta_{1j}}{\partial\{\lambda_{1j0} rr_j(\mathbf{z},\widehat{\boldsymbol\beta})\}} = \frac{\lambda_{2j0}}{\{\lambda_{1j0} rr_j(\mathbf{z},\widehat{\boldsymbol\beta}) + \lambda_{2j0}\}^2} \quad \text{and}$$
$$\frac{\partial\theta_{2j}}{\partial\{\lambda_{1j0} rr_j(\mathbf{z},\widehat{\boldsymbol\beta})\}} = \exp\{-(\lambda_{1j0} rr_j(\mathbf{z},\widehat{\boldsymbol\beta}) + \lambda_{2j0})\}.$$

Note that when AR and $rr(\mathbf{z},\widehat{\boldsymbol\beta})$ do not depend on time, then because $\Delta_i\{\lambda_{1j0} rr_j(\mathbf{z},\widehat{\boldsymbol\beta})\} = \lambda^*_{1j}\Delta_i\{(1-\widehat{AR}_j) rr_j(\mathbf{z},\widehat{\boldsymbol\beta})\}$, Equation (5.12) simplifies to

$$\Delta_i\{r(t_0,t_1,\mathbf{z},\widehat{\boldsymbol\beta})\} = \Delta_i\{(1-\widehat{AR}) rr(\mathbf{z},\widehat{\boldsymbol\beta})\}$$
$$\times\sum_{j=t_0}^{t_1-1}\left(\theta_{3j}\lambda^*_{1j}\left[\frac{\partial\theta_{1j}}{\partial\{\lambda_{1j0} rr_j(\mathbf{z},\widehat{\boldsymbol\beta})\}}\theta_{2j} + \frac{\partial\theta_{2j}}{\partial\{\lambda_{1j0} rr_j(\mathbf{z},\widehat{\boldsymbol\beta})\}}\theta_{1j}\right] - \theta_{1j}\theta_{2j}\theta_{3j}\sum_{l=t_0}^{j-1}\lambda^*_{1l}\right).$$

In the following sections we compute

$$\Delta_i\{\lambda_{1j0} rr_j(\mathbf{z},\widehat{\boldsymbol\beta})\} = \lambda^*_{1j}\Delta_i\{(1-\widehat{AR}_j) rr_j(\mathbf{z},\widehat{\boldsymbol\beta})\} \quad (5.13)$$

for various study designs when rr depends on the predictors through the linear function $\boldsymbol\beta'\mathbf{z}$.

5.8.1 *Relative risk parameters and attributable risk estimated from a case-control study*

We assume relative risk parameters and attributable risks are estimated from population-based case-control data and combined with age-specific disease incidence and mortality rates from registries. As registries have large samples and are typically independent from the case-control data, the incidence and mortality rates can be treated as fixed, and the variability of the absolute risk estimates arises solely from the estimation of the relative risk parameters and attributable risks.

We assume that age is a categorical variable, indexed by $j \in \{1,\ldots,J\}$. Let d_{ij} be one if individual i is a case of age j and zero otherwise and let $\mathbf{z}_{ij}$ denote a $1\times p$ vector containing the covariate information for the i-th individual that may also include interaction terms with age. The total sample size of the case control study is denoted by $n = n_1 + n_0$, where n_1 is the number of cases and n_0 the number of controls. We obtain relative risk estimates from the case-control data assuming that the probability of disease is given by a logistic model,

$$\ln\frac{P(D_{ij}=1|\mathbf{z}_{ij})}{1-P(D_{ij}=1|\mathbf{z}_{ij})} = \ln\frac{p(\mathbf{z}_{ij},\mu,\boldsymbol\beta)}{1-p(\mathbf{z}_{ij},\mu,\boldsymbol\beta)} = \mu + \boldsymbol\beta'\mathbf{z}_{ij}, \quad (5.14)$$

where $\boldsymbol\beta$ is a vector of regression parameters and all risk factors $\mathbf{z}$ are coded such that the components of $\boldsymbol\beta$ are positive, $\beta_k > 0$. Thus the relative risk associated with $\mathbf{z}$ is $\exp(\boldsymbol\beta'\mathbf{z})$.

Under model (5.14) the attributable risk formula given in (5.4) corresponds to

$$1 - \widehat{AR}_j = \frac{\sum_{i=1}^{n} \exp(-\widehat{\boldsymbol{\beta}}'\mathbf{z}_{ij})d_{ij}}{\sum_{i=1}^{n} d_{ij}}. \tag{5.15}$$

While n_1 and n_0 are fixed by design, the number of cases in a specific age category is typically a random quantity, which is reflected in the denominator of the expression above.

If cases and controls are sampled based on complex designs, for example from surveys, then each d_{ij} would be multiplied by a sampling weight w, the inverse of the probability of being included in the sample. While all our computations generalize to unequal weights, we omit the weights for ease of notation.

Here, we compute $\Delta_i\{\lambda_{1j0}rr_j(\mathbf{z}, \widehat{\boldsymbol{\beta}})\}$ in (5.13) from

$$\lambda_{1j0}rr_j(\mathbf{z}, \widehat{\boldsymbol{\beta}}) = \lambda_{1j}^*(1 - AR_j)rr_j(\mathbf{z}, \widehat{\boldsymbol{\beta}}) = \frac{\lambda_{1j}^* \sum_{k=1}^{n} d_{kj} \exp\{-\widehat{\boldsymbol{\beta}}'(\mathbf{z}_{kj} - \mathbf{z})\}}{\sum_{k=1}^{n} d_{kj}} = \frac{P_{1j}}{P_{2j}}. \tag{5.16}$$

Thus

$$\Delta_i\{\lambda_{1j0}rr_j(\mathbf{z}, \widehat{\boldsymbol{\beta}})\} = [\frac{\partial\{\lambda_{1j0}rr_j(\mathbf{z}, \widehat{\boldsymbol{\beta}})\}}{\partial P_{1j}}\Delta_i(P_{1j}) + \frac{\partial\{\lambda_{1j0}rr_j(\mathbf{z}, \widehat{\boldsymbol{\beta}})\}}{\partial P_{2j}}\Delta_i(P_{2j})]. \tag{5.17}$$

Differentiation yields

$$\frac{\partial\{\lambda_{1j0}rr_j(\mathbf{z}, \widehat{\boldsymbol{\beta}})\}}{\partial P_{1j}} = \frac{1}{\sum_{k=1}^{n} d_{kj}} \text{ and } \frac{\partial\{\lambda_{1j0}rr_j(\mathbf{z}, \widehat{\boldsymbol{\beta}})\}}{\partial P_{2j}} = -\frac{\sum_{k=1}^{n} \lambda_{1j}^* d_{kj} \exp\{-\widehat{\boldsymbol{\beta}}'(\mathbf{z}_{kj} - \mathbf{z})\}}{(\sum_{k=1}^{n} d_{kj})^2}. \tag{5.18}$$

The corresponding influences are

$$\Delta_i(P_{1j}) = \lambda_{1j}^* d_{ij} \exp\{-\widehat{\boldsymbol{\beta}}'(\mathbf{z}_{ij} - \mathbf{z})\} + (\frac{\partial P_{1j}}{\partial \widehat{\boldsymbol{\beta}}})'\Delta_i(\widehat{\boldsymbol{\beta}}) =$$

$$= \lambda_{1j}^* d_{ij} \exp\{-\widehat{\boldsymbol{\beta}}'(\mathbf{z}_{ij} - \mathbf{z})\} - \sum_{k=1}^{n} \lambda_{1j}^* d_{kj}[(\mathbf{z}_{kj} - \mathbf{z}) \exp\{-\widehat{\boldsymbol{\beta}}'(\mathbf{z}_{kj} - \mathbf{z})\}]'\Delta_i(\widehat{\boldsymbol{\beta}}) \tag{5.19}$$

and $\Delta_i(P_{2j}) = d_{ij}$. The influence $\Delta_i(\widehat{\boldsymbol{\beta}})$ is obtained from the estimating equation for the logistic regression model by solving $0 = \Delta_i[\sum_{k=1}^{n} \mathbf{z}_{kj}\{d_{kj} - p(\mathbf{z}_{kj}, \hat{\mu}, \widehat{\boldsymbol{\beta}})\}]$, where p stands for the logistic probability given in (5.14), to yield

$$\Delta_i(\widehat{\boldsymbol{\beta}}) = \Big[\sum_{k=1}^{n} \mathbf{z}_{kj}\mathbf{z}_{kj}' p(\mathbf{z}_{kj}, \hat{\mu}, \widehat{\boldsymbol{\beta}})\{1 - p(x_{kj}, \widehat{\boldsymbol{\beta}})\}\Big]^{-1} \mathbf{z}_{ij}\{d_{ij} - p(\mathbf{z}_{ij}, \hat{\mu}, \widehat{\boldsymbol{\beta}})\}. \tag{5.20}$$

To accommodate the case-control design, the variance of $\hat{r}$ is computed by treating cases and controls as separate strata and combining their empirical variance estimates,

$$\widehat{\text{var}}(\hat{r}) = \frac{n_0}{n_0 - 1}\sum_{i=1}^{n}(1 - d_i)\{\Delta_i(r) - \bar{\Delta}_{i0}(r)\}^2 + \frac{n_1}{n_1 - 1}\sum_{i=1}^{n} d_i\{\Delta_i(r) - \bar{\Delta}_{i1}(r)\}^2, \tag{5.21}$$

where $\bar{\Delta}_{i0}(r)$ and $\bar{\Delta}_{i1}(r)$ denote the empirical means over the influences $\Delta_i(r)$ in controls and cases, respectively.

5.8.2 *Relative risk parameters and attributable risk estimated from a cohort study*

When relative risk parameters $\boldsymbol{\beta}$ are estimated from a population-based cohort study, attributable risks can be estimated as in Chen et al. (2006b) by using Equation (5.5) but summing over all cohort members at risk in age interval t, rather than over controls, resulting in

$$(1-\widehat{AR}_t)rr_t(\mathbf{z},\hat{\boldsymbol{\beta}}) = \frac{\sum_{j=1}^{n} Y_j(t)}{\sum_{j=1}^{n} Y_j(t) rr_t(\hat{\boldsymbol{\beta}}'\mathbf{z}_j)} rr_t(\hat{\boldsymbol{\beta}}'\mathbf{z}). \tag{5.22}$$

For ease of exposition we will omit the subscript t in what follows. However, the formulas can easily be extended to relative risk expression that vary by age or time.

If disease is rare and we assume $rr(u) = \exp(u)$, Equation (5.22) is given by

$$(1-\widehat{AR})\exp(\hat{\boldsymbol{\beta}}'\mathbf{z}) = \frac{\sum_{j=1}^{n} Y_j(t)}{\sum_{j=1}^{n} Y_j(t)\exp\{\hat{\boldsymbol{\beta}}'(\mathbf{z}_j-\mathbf{z})\}}.$$

Letting $A = \sum_{j=1}^{n} Y_j(t)\exp\{\hat{\boldsymbol{\beta}}'(\mathbf{z}_j-\mathbf{z})\}$ and applying the chain rule yields

$$\begin{aligned}\Delta_i\{(1-\widehat{AR}_t)\exp(\hat{\boldsymbol{\beta}}'\mathbf{z})\} &= \frac{Y_i(t)}{A} \\ &- \frac{\sum_{j=1}^{n} Y_j(t)}{A^2}\left\{Y_i(t)\exp\{\hat{\boldsymbol{\beta}}'(\mathbf{z}_i-\mathbf{z})\} + \sum_{j=1}^{n} Y_j(t)\exp\{\hat{\boldsymbol{\beta}}'(\mathbf{z}_j-\mathbf{z})\}(\mathbf{z}_j-\mathbf{z})'\Delta_i(\hat{\boldsymbol{\beta}})\right\}. \end{aligned}\tag{5.23}$$

An explicit expression for the Taylor deviates of the relative risk parameters $\Delta_i(\hat{\boldsymbol{\beta}})$ is given in Equation (4.40).

5.8.3 *Variance computation when an external reference survey is used to obtain the risk factor distribution*

Suppose that a special cohort study yields valid estimates of relative risks that are applicable to the SEER population, but that its distribution of risk factors is not representative of the population in SEER. Suppose also that a representative survey in a SEER catchment area yields information on the distribution of risk factors, but no information on disease outcomes. One can combine the relative risk information from the special cohort with the risk factor distribution from the survey to estimate attributable risk in the SEER catchment area. Then, using Equation (5.3) with the composite hazard from SEER, one obtains the cause-specific hazard needed to compute absolute risk.

Here we let n^c denote the sample size of the cohort from which the relative risk parameters were estimated, and n^e is the sample size for the survey that provides information on the distribution of risk factors. Then similar to Equation (5.22), the external-sample estimate of $(1-\widehat{AR}_t)rr(\mathbf{z}^1,\widehat{\boldsymbol{\beta}})$ is

$$(1-\widehat{AR}_t)rr(\mathbf{z},\widehat{\boldsymbol{\beta}}) = \frac{\sum_{j=1}^{n^e} w_j I(t_j=t)}{\sum_{j=1}^{n^e} w_j I(t_j=t) rr(\hat{\boldsymbol{\beta}}'\mathbf{z}_j)} rr(\hat{\boldsymbol{\beta}}'\mathbf{z}),$$

where $I(t_j = t)$ is one if the jth respondent in the external survey has age in interval t and zero otherwise, and w_j are the external survey sampling weights, that are known without error.

Let $rr(u) = \exp(u)$, $B = \sum_{j=1}^{n^e} w_j I(t_j = t)$ and $A = \sum_{j=1}^{n^e} w_j I(t_j = t)\exp\{\hat{\boldsymbol{\beta}}'(\mathbf{z}_j - \mathbf{z})\}$.

For individuals $i = 1, 2, ..., n^c$ in the study cohort, the influences are

$$\Delta_i\{(1 - \widehat{AR}_t)\exp\{\hat{\boldsymbol{\beta}}'\mathbf{z}\}\} = -\frac{B}{A^2}\left\{\sum_{j=1}^{n^e} w_j I(t_j = t)\exp\{\hat{\boldsymbol{\beta}}'(\mathbf{z}_j - \mathbf{z})\}(\mathbf{z}_j - \mathbf{z})'\Delta_i(\hat{\boldsymbol{\beta}})\right\}, \tag{5.24}$$

where $\Delta_i(\hat{\boldsymbol{\beta}})$ is computed from the original cohort as in Equation (4.40). For individuals $j = 1, \ldots, n^e$ in the external survey,

$$\Delta_i\{(1 - \widehat{AR}_t)\exp(\hat{\boldsymbol{\beta}}'\mathbf{z})\} = -\frac{I(t_i = t)}{A} + \frac{B}{A^2}\left\{I(t_i = t)\exp\{\hat{\boldsymbol{\beta}}'(\mathbf{z}_i - \mathbf{z})\}\right\}.$$

5.8.4 Resampling methods to estimate variance

The bootstrap and jackknife methods can be used to estimate the variance of an estimate of absolute risk based partly on registry data. For example, suppose a cohort study is used to estimate log relative risks $\boldsymbol{\beta}$ and attributable risk $AR(t)$. Suppose we obtain B bootstrap samples from the cohort and obtain corresponding estimates $\hat{\boldsymbol{\beta}}_b, \widehat{AR}_b(t)$ for $b = 1, 2, ..., B$. For a given set of covariates $\mathbf{z}$ and time interval, we can compute the estimated absolute risk $\hat{r}_b$ by using $\hat{\beta}_b$ and $\widehat{AR}_b(t)$ in Equations (5.3) and (5.8). Confidence intervals on the absolute risk can be obtained from the quantiles of the bootstrap distribution of $\hat{r}_b$, and $\text{var}(\hat{r})$ can be estimated from $\sum_{b=1}^{B}(\hat{r}_b - \bar{r}_b)^2/(B-1)$. For case-control data, the same approach can be used, except the bootstrap proceeds by sampling the n_1 cases with replacement and the n_0 controls with replacement separately. The same sets of $\hat{\beta}_b$ and $\widehat{AR}_b(t)$ can be used repeatedly for various choices of $\mathbf{z}$ and time intervals, which reduces the computational burden.

The jackknife method is similar and has the advantage that the resulting variance estimate is a deterministic function of the data, whereas different bootstrap samples yield slightly different variance estimates. The computational burden can be greater for the jackknife, however. Suppose for a fixed $\mathbf{z}$ and time interval that $\hat{r}_{(-j)}$ for $i = 1, 2, ..., n$ is the estimate of absolute risk based on the registry data and on all members of the cohort except member i . Then the jackknife estimate of variance is $\{(n-1)/n\}\sum_{j=1}^{n}(\hat{r}_{(-j)} - \bar{r}_{(-j)})^2$, where $\bar{r}_{(-j)} = \sum_{j=1}^{n}\hat{r}_{(-j)}/n$. For case-control samples, the variance is $\{(n_1-1)/n_1\}\sum_{j=1}^{n_1}(\hat{r}_{(-j)} - \bar{r}_{(-j)})^2 + \{(n_0-1)/n_0\}\sum_{j=n_1+1}^{n_1+n_0}(\hat{r}_{(-j)} - \bar{r}_{(-j)})^2$, where the first summation is over the n_1 cases and the second summation is over the n_0 controls.

For individuals $i = 1, 2, \ldots, n$ in the study [illegible], the influences are

$$\Delta_i(U_2; \hat{\Lambda}, \exp(\hat{\beta}x)) = [illegible]$$

where $\hat{\Lambda}_0(t)$ is computed from the [illegible] as in Equation (4.10). For individuals [illegible] in the control group,

$$\Delta_i(U_2; \hat{\Lambda}, \exp(\hat{\beta}x)) = [illegible]$$

5.3.2 Bootstrapping [illegible]

The bootstrap and jackknife methods can be used to estimate the variance of an estimator [illegible]. For example, suppose a [illegible] study is used to estimate log relative risk β and [illegible] risk $\Lambda(t)$. [illegible] samples [illegible] and [illegible] corresponding [illegible] for [illegible] and [illegible] and then [illegible] the [illegible] by using [illegible] Equations [illegible]. Confidence intervals [illegible] can be obtained [illegible] the quantiles of the [illegible] distribution [illegible]

[illegible] For [illegible], the same approach [illegible]

[illegible] sampling with replacement [illegible] [illegible] choice of [illegible] intervals, which [illegible]

[illegible] function of the data [illegible] estimates. [illegible] can be [illegible] for the [illegible]

[illegible] For [illegible] control samples [illegible]

[illegible]

[illegible] summation is over the [illegible] cases [illegible] summation is over the [illegible] controls.

Chapter 6

Assessment of risk model performance

6.1 Introduction

Before a risk prediction model can be recommended for clinical or public health applications, one needs to assess how good the predictions are. In this chapter we consider various criteria for assessing the performance of a risk model. Although the criteria apply to absolute risk, many are also useful for other types of risk, such as the pure risk of an event or the risk of having prevalent screen-detectable disease.

Unless otherwise stated, we assume that we have developed a risk model on "training data" and assess the performance of the model on independent "test" or "validation" data. This approach, termed "external validation", provides a more rigorous assessment of the model than testing the model on the training data ("internal validation"), even though cross-validation techniques are available to reduce the "over-optimism" bias that can result from testing the model on the training data (Efron, 1986). If the test and training data are independent, one can regard the model as fixed. Random variation in the evaluation criteria derives from random variation of covariates and outcomes in the test data, not from variation in the model. This gives rise to simple distribution theory for the evaluation criteria. The distribution theory becomes much more complicated and even intractable if the model is evaluated in the training data and complex procedures were used to fit the model (see Section 6.3.4). This complication also arises when comparing two models (Chapter 7). We also assume that the validation data are observations from a cohort, i.e., that prospective follow-up information is available. This setting allows the most comprehensive assessment of model performance. However, some criteria can also be assessed based on case-control samples; we explicitly identify those criteria in this chapter.

Assume we have developed an absolute risk model, $r_1(t_0,t_1;\mathbf{Z})$, where $\mathbf{Z}$ denotes covariates. Sometimes $\mathbf{Z}$ contains only covariates pertaining to the cause of interest in the cause-specific hazard model $\lambda_1(t;\mathbf{z}^1)$, but $\mathbf{Z}$ might also include covariates for competing cause-specific hazards, and in cumulative incidence regression, $\mathbf{Z}$ would modulate the absolute risk itself, rather than the underlying cause-specific hazards. For ease of notation, let $R_i = r_1(t_{0i}, t_{1i}; \mathbf{Z}_i = \mathbf{z}_i)$ be the model-based estimate of risk for the ith member in the validation data. For the most part we regard the times (t_{0i}, t_{1i}) as fixed for each individual, but we mention some adaptations for the setting of varying t_1 in Section 6.4.4. For analysis on the age scale, t_{0i} would be the age of an individual at entry into a cohort and t_{1i} the age on the date when cohort follow-up ends. If the time scale is time on study, $t_{0i} = 0$ and t_{1i} is the duration of time until the cohort follow-up ends. Sometimes t_{1i} is defined in terms of the desired length of the risk projection interval, τ_i, i.e., $t_{1i} = t_{0i} + \tau_i$. For example, 5- or 10-year projections of absolute risk correspond to $\tau_i = 5$ or 10.

The outcome of interest for the ith person is occurrence of an event of type 1 in the projection interval, $O_i = I(t_{0i} < T_i \leq t_{1i}, \delta(T_i) = 1)$, where T_i is the time at which the first event occurs, $\delta(T)$ is the state at time T, and the indicator $I(\text{arg}) = 1$ if arg is true and 0 otherwise. If person i experiences a competing event, i.e., $\delta(T_i) = j \neq 1$, such as death from a competing cause, $O_i = 0$.

For most of this discussion we define t_{1i} in such a way that the outcome O_i is observed. In particular, if the end of potential follow-up for an individual occurs at the administrative censoring time C_i, we define $t_{1i} = \min(t_{0i} + \tau_i, C_i)$, where τ_i is the risk projection interval. For example, if individual i begins follow-up at age $t_{0i} = 50$ years on January 1,1996 and follow-up ends on December 31, 2000, then on the age scale $C_i = 55$ years, and if the desired projection interval were $\tau_i = 10$ years, $t_{1i} = \min(t_{0i} + \tau_i, C_i) = 55$ years. If the time scale is time on study with $t_{0i} = 0$, then C_i is the time from entry until administrative censoring. We refer to methods for right censored data in which O_i is not observed because $t_{0i} + \tau_i > C_i$ and no event occurs in $(t_{0i}, C_i]$ in Section 6.3.3, but we do not elaborate on these methods.

Model assessment can be based on general criteria, such as calibration (Section 6.3), predictive accuracy and classification accuracy (Sections 6.4.1 and 6.4.2), and discriminatory accuracy (Section 6.4.3). Another approach is to tailor the criterion to the particular application. Criteria for screening applications or high risk interventions are presented in Section 6.5. If losses can be specified in a well-defined decision problem, models can be assessed with respect to how much they reduce expected loss (or increase expected utility) (Section 6.6).

A key concept in formalizing all these criteria is the distribution of risk, that we define in the next section.

6.2 The risk distribution

Let $\mathbf{V} = (t_0, t_1, \mathbf{Z})$ denote the vector of risk predictors, $\mathbf{Z}$, and the risk projection interval delimiters, $(t_0, t_1]$. We let $\mathbf{v}$ be a realized value of $\mathbf{V}$ and use the notation $R(\mathbf{v}) = r_1(t_0, t_1; \mathbf{Z} = \mathbf{z})$ in the remainder of this chapter. If $\mathbf{Z}$ is discrete, $\mathbf{V}$ might also be discrete, but often the space of $\mathbf{V}$ is large and $\mathbf{V}$ is continuous.

In a specific population, in our case the validation cohort, the distribution of $\mathbf{V}$, $F_{\mathbf{V}}(\mathbf{v})$, induces the distribution F of risk R through

$$F(r) = P(R \leq r) = \int I(\mathbf{v} : R(\mathbf{v}) \leq r) dF_{\mathbf{V}}(\mathbf{v}). \tag{6.1}$$

The support of $F(r)$ may be a subset of $[0, 1]$ because R may be bounded below 1.

There is great advantage in reducing the information in $F_{\mathbf{V}}$ to the univariate distribution F. If we assume that the validation cohort of size n is a simple random sample from some larger population, we can estimate the distribution of risk F in that population based on the observed risks $r_1, \ldots, r_n$ by the empirical distribution function

$$\hat{F}(r) = F_n(r) = \frac{1}{n} \sum_{i=1}^{n} I(r_i \leq r). \tag{6.2}$$

Throughout this chapter we will use data from a validation study of the absolute risk model for invasive breast cancer with potentially modifiable risk factors, which we call "BC2013", for white women ages 50 or older as an example (Pfeiffer et al., 2013), that we mentioned earlier in Chapter 4. In Pfeiffer et al. (2013), we combined relative risk and attributable risk estimates from two large prospective cohort studies, the Prostate, Lung, Colorectal, and Ovarian Cancer Screening Trial (PLCO) and the National Institutes of Health-American Association of Retired Persons (NIH-AARP) Diet and Health Study, with incidence and competing mortality rates from the NCI's Surveillance, Epidemiology, and End Results Program (SEER) to estimate absolute risk of breast cancer. The general approach that incorporates registry data to develop an absolute risk model is described in Chapter 5. A SAS macro and R code that implement this model can be found at the web site (https://dceg.cancer.gov/tools/risk-assessment/).

In Pfeiffer et al. (2013), we validated BC2013 in independent data from the Nurses Health Study (NHS) cohort from July 1990 to June 2004 to cover the same calendar period as the training cohorts used for model development. The NHS cohort included 121,701 women aged 30 to 55 years in 1976 (Colditz and Hankinson, 2005). We applied the same exclusion criteria to women from the NHS that we had used for building the breast cancer model and excluded the following categories of women: age at entry younger than 50 years, non-whites, prevalent breast cancer, no follow-up time after baseline, missing birth year or covariates. The remaining validation cohort had 57,906 women. We computed the breast cancer absolute risk R for each woman from her baseline covariate values $\mathbf{Z}$ and from the projection interval defined by her age at entry (July 1990) into the NHS cohort and her later age on June 1, 2004. The projection lengths ranged from 13.42 to 14.33 years, with a median of 13.83 years, and the absolute breast cancer risk estimates ranged from 2.0% to 17.9%, with a mean of 5.1% and median of 4.75%.

The histogram of these risks in Figure 6.1 approximates the density of the distribution function F in Equation (6.1).

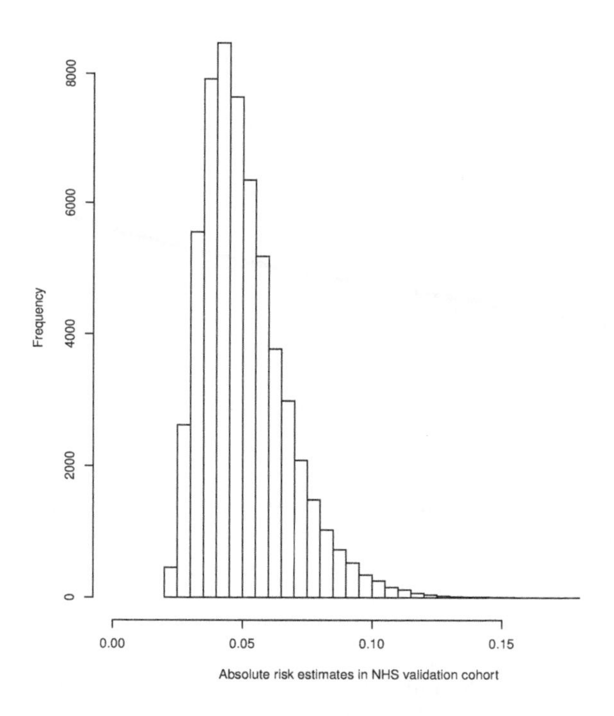

Figure 6.1: Histogram of absolute breast cancer risk estimates from the BC2013 model in the NHS validation cohort.

The histogram of risk estimates R indicates whether risks are large or small and whether there is large variation in risk. A risk distribution with some members at very high risk and the rest at very low risks indicates that the model will discriminate diseased from non-diseased populations well, as discussed in detail in Section 6.4.3.

6.2.1 The predictiveness curve

The "predictiveness curve" (Pepe et al., 2008) is a plot of the risk quantiles $t = \hat{F}^{-1}(p)$ against the corresponding cumulative proportion of the population with risks $\leq t$, namely

p where $0 \leq p \leq 1$. To create the predictiveness curve for the NHS validation cohort, we ordered the estimated absolute breast cancer risks from lowest to highest and plotted their values against p. As an example, the predictiveness curve allows one to read off the 90th percentile of risk, namely the level of risk above which 10% of the population have higher risks. At $p = 0.90$ the risk value is $\hat{F}^{-1}(p) = 0.073$. This indicates that 90% of subjects in the cohort have calculated risks at or below 0.073 and only 10% have risks above 0.073.

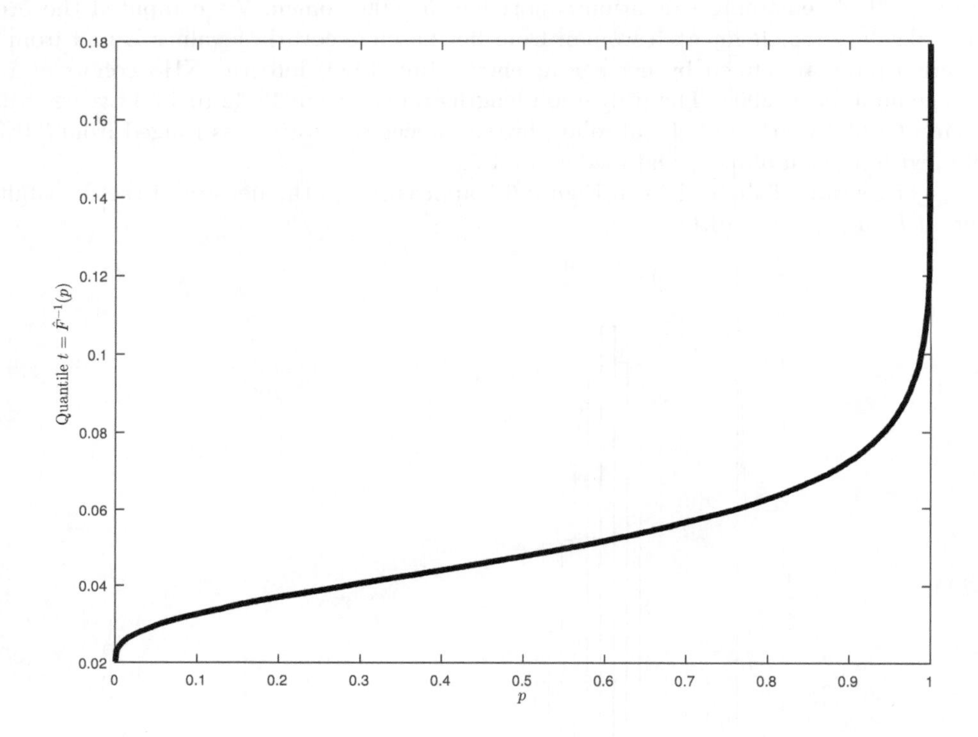

Figure 6.2: Predictiveness curve of absolute breast cancer risk estimates from the BC2013 model in the NHS validation cohort.

6.3 Calibration

Calibration measures how well the numbers of events predicted by a model agree with the observed events that arise in a cohort. Calibration is the most important general criterion, because if a model is not well calibrated, other criteria, such as discrimination, can be misleading. To test calibration, one requires cohort data, whereas some other criteria discussed later can be estimated from case-control data only.

6.3.1 Definition of calibration and tests of calibration

In addition to the covariates $\mathbf{V}$ that are used to compute the predicted risk R, there may be other information available in the validation cohort. In what follows we denote the vector of all available covariates in the validation cohort by $\mathbf{U}$. $\mathbf{U}$ contains all the covariates $\mathbf{V}$, but also includes variables that are not part of $\mathbf{V}$. We thus assess calibration of a model based on cohort observations $(R_i, O_i, \mathbf{U}_i), i = 1, \ldots, n$. Recall that R depends on $\mathbf{U}$ only through $\mathbf{V}$ but we use the notation $R(\mathbf{U})$ nonetheless.

A risk model $R(\mathbf{U})$ taking a set of values r is *well calibrated* if, for every such r

$$P(O = 1|r) = r, \tag{6.3}$$

i.e., among individuals with risk $R(\mathbf{U}) = r$, the fraction with $O = 1$ is r. If the model is well calibrated, then $\mu \equiv P(O = 1) = E(R) = \int_0^1 r dF(r)$. If risks are continuously distributed, some type of grouping or regression approach is needed to assess Equation (6.3).

One approach to assess overall calibration was proposed by (Cox, 1958), who used the regression

$$\text{logit}\{P(O_i = 1|r_i)\} = \nu_0 + \nu_1 w_i, \tag{6.4}$$

where $w_i = \log\{r_i/(1 - r_i)\}$. If the model fits perfectly, $\nu_0 = 0$ and $\nu_1 = 1$. The data $(O_i, R_i), i = 1, \ldots, n$ in the validation cohort can be used to estimate ν_0 and ν_1 and to test various hypotheses. Values $\hat{\nu}_0 < 0$ indicate that the model overestimates risk, $\hat{\nu}_0 > 0$ that the model underestimates risk, $\hat{\nu}_1 > 1$ that the model risks are not as spread out as the true risks but correctly order risks (i.e., cases have higher risks than those who do not experience the event), $0 < \hat{\nu}_1 < 1$ that the model risks are too spread out (which often happens in the context of over-fitting) but ordered correctly, and $\hat{\nu}_1 < 0$ that the model orders the true probabilities in the wrong direction, i.e., that individuals experiencing an event tend to have a lower modeled risk than those who do not.

In the NHS validation cohort, use of r from BC2013 in Equation (6.4) yielded estimates $\hat{\nu}_0 = -0.298$ with standard error 0.166, that was not significantly different from zero ($p =$ 0.07), and $\hat{\nu}_1 = 0.896$ with standard error 0.057 ($p < .0001$). These estimates indicate that the average risk projections are slightly (but not statistically significantly) too large, and that the model slightly overestimates high risks and/or underestimates low risks.

We call a risk model *strongly calibrated* if for every value of the measured covariates, $\mathbf{U}$, $E(O|\mathbf{U}) = R(\mathbf{U})$. Recall that $\mathbf{U}$ may contain covariates not used in the risk model. If $\mathbf{U}$ is discrete, it might be possible to test strong calibration by comparing the observed proportion of subjects with $O = 1$ among those with a particular value $\mathbf{U} = \mathbf{u}$ with the corresponding value of $R(\mathbf{u}) = r$. Usually, however, it is not possible to test strong calibration for every value of $\mathbf{U}$, because $\mathbf{U}$ is not discrete or the data are too sparse. In this case one can define a partition $\mathbf{S}$ of the space of $\mathbf{U}$ into G mutually exclusive and exhaustive subsets $\mathbf{S} = \{S_1, S_2, \ldots, , S_G\}$. Then the model R is *calibrated with respect to the partition* $\mathbf{S}$ if

$$E(O|\mathbf{U} \in S_g) = E(R|\mathbf{U} \in S_g) \text{ for each } S_g \in \mathbf{S}. \tag{6.5}$$

Strong calibration implies that R is calibrated with respect to $\mathbf{S}$ because

$$E\{OI(\mathbf{U} \in S_g)\} = E[E\{OI(\mathbf{U} \in S_g)|\mathbf{U}\}] = E[E\{RI(\mathbf{U} \in S_g)|\mathbf{U}\}] = E\{RI(\mathbf{U} \in S_g)\}.$$

The expectations on the left- and right-hand sides of Equation (6.5) can be estimated in the validation cohort from

$$\hat{E}(O|\mathbf{U} \in S_g) = \frac{\sum_{i=1}^n O_i I(\mathbf{U}_i \in S_g)}{\sum_{i=1}^n I(\mathbf{U}_i \in S_g)} \text{ and } \hat{E}(R|\mathbf{U} \in S_g) = \frac{\sum_{i=1}^n R_i I(\mathbf{U}_i \in S_g)}{\sum_{i=1}^n I(\mathbf{U}_i \in S_g)},$$

respectively. The number of observed events in subset g, $O^g = \sum_{i=1}^{n} O_i I(\mathbf{U_i} \in S_g)$ can be compared to the expected counts $E^g = \sum_{i=1}^{n} R_i I(\mathbf{U_i} \in S_g)$.

A crucial issue is how to define the partition $\mathbf{S}$. One approach is to focus on individual risk factors and stratify on them. For example, Pfeiffer et al. (2013) assessed the agreement between observed and expected breast cancer incidence counts in women whose first live births were at ages <25 years or nulliparous, ages 25–29 years, and ages 30 years or older (Table 6.1).

Table 6.1: Comparison of observed (O) and expected (E) incident breast cancers and the corresponding 95% confidence intervals (CIs) based on predictions from the BC2013 model in Pfeiffer et al. (2013) in women in the NHS validation cohort

	Number of women	Observed (O)	Expected (E)	E/O (95% CI)
All women	57,906	2,934	2,930	1.00 (0.96, 1.04)
Variable				
Age at first live birth				
<25 or nulliparous	33,863	1,601	1,586	0.99 (0.94–1.04)
25–29	18,923	1,024	1,021	1.00 (0.94–1.06)
≥ 30	5,120	309	323	1.05 (0.94–1.17)
BMI				
$< 25kg/m^2$	30,259	1,447	1,492	1.03 (0.98–1.09)
25 to $< 30\ kg/m^2$	18,219	971	935	0.96 (0.90–1.03)
30 to $< 35\ kg/m^2$	6,581	368	349	0.95 (0.86–1.05)
35 to $< 40\ kg/m^2$	2,847	148	154	1.04 (0.89–1.22)
Duration of EPT MHT use[a]				
0 years	49,511	2,367	2,402	1.01 (0.97–1.06)
1–9 years	8,380	567	527	0.93 (0.86–1.01)
10+ years	15	0	2	NA
Alcohol consumption				
0 drinks/day	23,314	1,139	1,091	0.96 (0.90–1.02)
< 1 drink/day	27,316	1,389	1,418	1.02 (0.97–1.08)
1+ drinks/day	7,276	406	421	1.04 (0.94–1.14)

[a] EPT MHT = estrogen and progestin menopausal hormone replacement therapy

Among the 33,863 women in the first category, O^1 =1,601 incident breast cancer cases were observed, compared to E^1 =1,586 expected (with rounding to the nearest integer). Because events are rare, we assume the observed count is a Poisson random variable. Thus, the variance of $\log(E^1/O^1)$ is estimated by $1/O^1$, and a 95% confidence interval on the log scale is $\log(E^1/O^1) \pm 1.96 \times (O^1)^{-0.5}$. By exponentiation, we obtain a confidence interval on the ratio E^1/O^1 = 1,586/1,601=0.99, namely (0.94–1.04). Based on the confidence intervals in Table 6.1, there is no statistically significant evidence of mis-calibration for women in any of the categories defined by age at first life birth and among all women. A global test could be based on

$$Q = \sum_{g=1}^{G} (O^g - E^g)^2/E^g \sim \chi^2_G. \tag{6.6}$$

In this case, Q =(1,601–1,586)^2/1,586 + (1,024–1,021)^2/1,021+ (309–323)^2/323=0.757, which is not significant when compared to a chi-squared distribution with G =3 degrees of freedom (p =0.86). For an overall assessment of calibration one can ignore subsets and simply compute $(O - E)^2/E \sim \chi^2_1$, where O = 2,934 is the total number of observed events in the whole population and E = 2,930 is the total expected events, resulting in a chi-square of 0.0055 (p = 0.94).

When the event is not rare, we can instead consider logistic regression (similar to Cox (1958)), where for subset S_g, $\text{logit}\{P(O_i = 1|r_i)\} = w_i + \gamma_g$, and where $w_i = \log\{r_i/(1-r_i)\}$. The corresponding log-likelihood for all the observations in S_g is $l = \sum_{i:\mathbf{V}_i \in S_g} O_i(w_i + \gamma_g) -$

$\sum_{i:\mathbf{V}_i \in S_g} \log\{1+\exp(w_i+\gamma_g)\}$. Here $\exp(\gamma_g)$ corresponds to O^g/E^g, and inference on γ_g provides a test of calibration in S_g. The score test of the null hypothesis of no lack of calibration, $H_0 : \gamma_g = 0$, from this likelihood is

$$U_g^2 = (O^g - E^g)^2 / \sum_{i:\mathbf{V}_i \in S_g} r_i(1-r_i) \sim \chi_1^2. \tag{6.7}$$

The analogous global test is $Q = \sum_{g=1}^{G} U_g^2 \sim \chi_G^2$. If $r_i << 1$, this Q is the same as Equation (6.6) and, for a single subset S_g, the test based on U_g^2 reduces to $(O^g - E^g)^2/E^g$. A test for overall calibration based on this statistic is simply $(O-E)^2/\sum_{i=1}^{n} r_i(1-r_i) \sim \chi_1^2$, where O is the total number of observed events in the population and E is the total expected events.

A common practice is to compute the deciles of the empirical distribution of R_i in the test data and let $S_g = \{\mathbf{V}_i : \xi_{0.1(g-1)} \leq R_i < \xi_{0.1g}\}$, where $\xi_{0.1g}$ are the deciles, $g = 1, 2, ..., 10$, and $\xi_0 = 0$. Thus $\mathbf{S}$ is a partition of the set of values $\mathbf{V}_i$ in the test data. The previous distribution theory applies without change, conditional on the partition. Model assessment based on dividing test data into risk deciles requires a sufficiently large validation sample, however. Hosmer and Lemeshow (1980) and Lemeshow and Hosmer (1982) used a statistic that is very similar to Equation (6.7), namely

$$HL = \sum_{g=1}^{G} (O^g - E^g)^2/\{E^g(1 - E^g/N^g)\}, \tag{6.8}$$

where N^g is the number of subjects in group g.

One can extend the idea of partitioning by risk deciles by plotting a kernel smoother of the O_i against risk (e.g., (Gerds et al., 2014)). Point-wise variances can be computed because the O_i are independent with Bernoulli variance in the independent test data.

Table 6.2 gives the observed and expected events (rounded to the nearest integer) by deciles of risk in the NHS validation cohort. The BC2013 model underestimated the number of events in the lower deciles; for example, in the first decile group, the model predicted 169 events while 179 were observed, with $E/O = 0.95$. The model slightly over predicted risk in the high-risk deciles. In decile 10, the number of expected events was 495 while 482 were observed, with $E/O = 1.03$. Overestimation of high risks and underestimation of low risks is consistent with the estimate $\hat{\nu}_1 = 0.896 < 1$ in Equation (6.4), which indicates that model risks are over-dispersed. The statistics Q, U and HL corresponding to Equations (6.6), (6.7), and (6.8) were respectively 6.9, 7.3, and 7.3. None of these statistics was statistically significant based on G=10 degrees-of-freedom (p = 0.73, 0.70, 0.70, respectively). (The Hosmer-Lemeshow test with $G - 2 = 8$ degrees-of-freedom and $p = 0.50$ seems less appropriate for an independent validation sample.)

6.3.2 Reasons for poor calibration and approaches to recalibration

There are several reasons why a risk model may show poor calibration in an independent validation cohort. An implicit assumption is that the population used to assess model performance is similar to the population used to develop the model. That assumption is violated when the validation cohort has different disease incidence rates from the training cohort, even after the differing distributions of covariates in the two populations are taken into account. Such differences could be due to secular changes in disease incidence rates or to differences in screening procedures or in procedures used to diagnose the disease outcome. For example, if one validates a breast cancer model in a cohort of women who are screened

Table 6.2: Comparison of observed (O) and expected (E) incident breast cancers in the NHS validation cohort by deciles of risk R

Decile	**R interval**	**N**	**E**	**O**	**E/O**
1	≤ 0.032	5788	169	179	0.95
2	$(0.032, 0.037]$	5790	202	206	0.98
3	$(0.037, 0.041]$	5802	225	231	0.97
4	$(0.041, 0.044]$	5785	244	269	0.91
5	$(0.044, 0.048]$	5788	264	265	1.00
6	$(0.048, 0.051]$	5791	286	302	0.95
7	$(0.051, 0.056]$	5790	312	292	1.07
8	$(0.056, 0.063]$	5791	343	340	1.01
9	$(0.063, 0.073]$	5790	388	368	1.06
10	> 0.073	5791	495	482	1.03

more frequently with mammography than the average US woman, then a model based on national breast cancer rates would likely underestimate risks in the validation cohort. Likewise, if the risk model was based on national rates from the 1980s but the validation data came from a later period when breast cancer risks were higher, the model would underestimate risk. A second reason for poor model calibration may be that predictors (covariates) in the model are specified differently in the training and validation data, due to differences in questionnaires between the two data sources. For example, the BC2013 breast cancer model in Pfeiffer et al. (2013) requires information on menopausal hormone replacement therapy (MHT) categorized into "Estrogen and progestin MHT" and "other MHT". If that level of detail on MHT use is not available in the validation cohort, there can be misspecification of the MHT variable and lack of fit in the validation cohort. An extreme type of misspecification occurs if a covariate is completely missing in the validation data. This problem often arises when molecular markers, such as single nucleotide polymorphisms (SNPs), are included as predictors and not measured on members of a validation cohort.

In addition to differences in specification of predictors or population differences, the modeling process itself can lead to biased prediction models and poor fit in validation data. If the model-fitting process involves selecting predictor variables from a large number of possible predictors and including a large number of the selected variables in a regression, it is likely that the model will be "over-fitted" and will tend to give a wider spread in risk predictions than will be observed in independent validation data ($0 < \hat{\nu}_1 < 1$ in Equation (6.4)). One can reduce or avoid such over-fitting by employing a heuristic shrinkage factor that applies equally to all coefficients β_i in the linear predictor portion of the risk model, $\sum Z_j \beta_j$, (Van Houwelingen and Le Cessie, 1990), or by estimating the required shrinkage factor using the bootstrap (Van Houwelingen and Le Cessie, 1990; Harrell, 2001; Steyerberg, 2009) or cross-validation (Copas, 1987; Van Houwelingen and Le Cessie, 1990; van Houwelingen, 2000, 2001) when building models with the training data. Another approach to avoid such over-fitting based solely on training data is to "penalize" the model for including too many risk factors or too large parameter estimates (Hastie et al., 2009; Steyerberg, 2009; Harrell, 2001). See Section 8.2 for additional discussion and references.

Suppose that one needs a model for a target population like the validation cohort, but that the original model based on the training data was not well calibrated in the validation cohort. Rather than build an entirely new model for the target population from which the validation sample came, one can *recalibrate* the risk estimates from the original model. For example the original risk estimates r_i with logit w_i can be transformed to new risk estimates with logit $\hat{\nu}_0 + \hat{\nu}_1 w_i$ via Equation (6.4) (Steyerberg et al., 2004; Steyerberg, 2009). Another approach might be to group the original risks into e.g., deciles as in Table 6.2 and to use the E/O ratios as non-parametric correction factors. For example, an original risk r_i falling in the tenth decile would be divided by the factor $E/O = 1.03$. More refined kernel smoother methods could also be used as in Li et al. (2011). The key is to recalibrate the scalar absolute risks non-parametrically. This approach avoids the "curse of dimensionality" that arises when trying to model the underlying multivariate predictors non-parametrically.

6.3.3 Assessing calibration with right censored data

Methods are available to evaluate calibration when the outcome O_i is subject to right censoring. Typically the analysis is on the time scale of time on study and $(t_{0i}, t_{1i}) = (0, \tau)$ with, for example, $\tau = 5$ years. However, some individuals are administratively censored at $C_i < \tau$ before any event has occurred. For such individuals, O_i is not observed (i.e., censored). For pure risk, Viallon et al. (2009) showed how appropriate E/O ratios are obtained by replacing O by the sample size times the Kaplan-Meier estimate of cumulative pure risk to time τ, and they discussed how to adapt this idea for absolute risk. Another approach for absolute risk (Gerds et al., 2014) replaces O_i by a pseudo-value $O_i^{pseudo} = n\hat{F}_n(\tau) - (n-1)\hat{F}_{n-1}^{(i)}(\tau)$, where $\hat{F}_n$ is the non-parametric estimate of absolute risk (Aalen, 1978; Gaynor et al., 1993) from the n subjects and $\hat{F}_{n-1}^{(i)}(\tau)$is the corresponding estimate with subject i omitted. In the absence of censoring, $O_i^{pseudo} = O_i$. Gerds et al. (2014) did not provide variance estimates, however. Another approach tests the underlying cause-specific hazards by comparing observed cumulative events against modeled cumulative hazard functions (Gong et al., 2014), but this approach does not test the validity of the absolute risk model directly and could not be used for the cumulative incidence regression models in Section 4.2.

6.3.4 Assessing calibration on the training data, that is, internal validation

Sometimes an appropriate independent validation cohort may not be available. This is often the case when a risk prediction model includes factors that are not measured in routine clinical practice, such as mammographic density or molecular or genetic biomarkers. In that situation *internal validation* is a first step toward assessing bias in the model predictions.

The distribution theory is more complex if the model is tested on the same data used to fit it, however. Tsiatis (1980) partitioned the covariate space into G groups and gave a valid theory if the risks R_i are estimated by logistic regression in training data and comparisons of O^g with E^g are made within the training data. The corresponding quadratic form is based on a score statistic but has $G - k$ degrees of freedom, where k is the degrees-of-freedom associated with the risk model. For a partitioning based on deciles of predicted risk, Hosmer and Lemeshow (1980) and Lemeshow and Hosmer (1982) computed a statistic (Equation (6.8)) but argued that it should be compared to a chi-square distribution with $G-2$ degrees of freedom. These methods, however, were investigated for logistic models, not for models of absolute risk. Moreover, variable selection and other features of model fitting, even for the logistic model, are often more complex than entertained in Tsiatis (1980), who assumed the variables in the model were known *a priori*. Thus the accuracy of the available distribution theory for evaluation of absolute risk models in the training data remains to be demonstrated. In contrast, the distribution theory above for assessing calibration of absolute risk models in independent test data is valid, regardless of the complexity of the fitting process in the training data, because the model is fixed and hence r_i are known constants in the test data.

6.4 Accuracy measures

6.4.1 Predictive accuracy: the Brier score and the logarithmic score

Calibration is concerned with bias in the predictions from a model R. Even if a prediction R is unbiased and has small variance, the difference $O - R$ can be quite variable for a particular individual because O is a binary outcome, i.e., a Bernoulli random variable. A measure of the predictive accuracy is based on the Brier score (Brier, 1950), $(O-R)^2$. The mean squared error of prediction (MSE) is the expected value of the Brier score.

The MSE can also be viewed as an expected loss for binary outcomes, and thus is related to a scoring rule. Scoring rules are functions that assign rewards for good predictions. An important class is *proper scoring rules*, i.e., rules $Sc(R,O)$ such that the expectation of $Sc(R,O)$ is maximal if $R = P(O = 1)$ (see, e.g., Gneiting and Raftery (2007)). The Brier score is an affine transformation of the quadratic score (a proper scoring rule) that decreases as the quadratic score increases; hence the expected Brier score is minimized if $R = P(O = 1)$.

Suppose that individual i has a true (unknown) absolute risk $\pi_i = E(O_i)$. Then the expected Brier score is

$$\begin{aligned} MSE = E(O-R)^2 = E(O-\pi+\pi-R)^2 &= E_\pi E_{O|\pi}(O-\pi)^2 + E_\pi E_{R|\pi}(\pi - R)^2 \\ &= E_\pi Var(O|\pi) + E_\pi(bias^2|\pi). \quad (6.9) \end{aligned}$$

We call MSE the Brier criterion because it is the expectation of the Brier score. The Brier criterion is the expected conditional variance of O_i given π_i plus the expected conditional squared bias of R_i given π_i. Thus, even if $R(\mathbf{V})$ is perfectly calibrated such that $R_i = \pi_i$ for every individual i, MSE is not equal to zero, as it still reflects the expected conditional variance in the outcome O given the true risk π. Perfect calibration is an even stronger condition than strong calibration, defined in Section 6.3.1, because perfect calibration requires that the risk factors in $\mathbf{V}$ fully define the risk for each individual. If $R(\mathbf{V})$ is perfectly calibrated, $MSE = \int_0^1 u(1-u)dF(u)$.

The MSE is estimated from the validation cohort with n observations as

$$\widehat{MSE} = n^{-1}\sum_{i=1}^{n}(O_i - r_i)^2.$$

In the NHS validation cohort, the estimated mean Brier score for the absolute breast cancer risk model was $\widehat{MSE} = 0.0480$. The expected root mean square error of prediction is $\widehat{MSE}^{0.5} = 0.22$. For rare outcomes with low predicted risks and few events, $\widehat{MSE}$ tends to be very low, regardless of the quality of the prediction. To illustrate that point assume that a model predicts every woman's breast cancer risk to be $r_i = 0$. In the NHS validation cohort the estimated mean Brier score for this model is $\widehat{MSE} = 0.0507$ which is not substantially larger than $\widehat{MSE} = 0.0480$ for the BC2013 breast cancer absolute risk model.

Another proper score (Gneiting and Raftery, 2007) for Bernoulli outcomes is minus half the Bernoulli deviance or the logarithmic score,

$$LS = -O\log(R) - (1-O)\log(1-R).$$

The expectation of this score is $E(LS) = E_\pi\{-\pi E_{R|\pi}\log(R) - (1-\pi)E_{R|\pi}\log(1-R)\}$. For a perfectly calibrated model, this expectation is $E(LS) = \int_0^1 \{-u\log(u) - (1-u)\log(1-u)\}$ $dF(u)$, whose integrand is the entropy of a Bernoulli distribution. Thus $E(LS) > 0$, even for a perfectly calibrated model, because O varies (Efron, 1978; Liao and McGee, 2003). An empirical estimate of the average entropy or average logarithmic score is $n^{-1}\sum_{i=1}^{n}\{-O_i\log(R_i)-(1-O_i)\log(1-R_i)\}$. For the breast cancer absolute risk model BC2013, the estimated mean logarithmic score was 0.1983. This estimate is difficult to interpret on its own but can be used for comparison against another model applied to the same validation data.

6.4.2 Classification accuracy

For many clinical decisions, such as whether or not to give an intervention or treatment, models are used to classify an individual as a case or not from

$$\hat{O}=\begin{cases}0 & \text{if } R\leq r^*\\ 1 & \text{if } R>r^*\end{cases} \tag{6.10}$$

where r^* is a risk or decision threshold. Thus, rather than giving a risk estimate R, one is forced to guess the outcome.

Classification accuracy measures how well this rule identifies those who will and will not experience the event.

6.4.2.1 Distribution of risk in cases and non-cases

In discussing classification accuracy, it helps to define two more distributions of risk, namely G, the distribution of risk in those who experience the event during follow-up (cases, $O=1$), given by

$$G(r)=P(R\leq r|O=1)=\frac{1}{P(O=1)}\int I\{\mathbf{v}:R(\mathbf{v})\leq r,O=1\}dF_{\mathbf{V}}(\mathbf{v}), \tag{6.11}$$

and K, the distribution of risk in non-cases or controls ($O=0$), given by

$$K(r)=P(R\leq r|O=0)=\frac{1}{P(O=0)}\int I\{\mathbf{v}:R(\mathbf{v})\leq r,O=0\}dF_{\mathbf{V}}(\mathbf{v}). \tag{6.12}$$

When needed to avoid confusion we will denote risk realizations from F by r^F, and risk realizations from cases and non-cases by r^G and r^K, respectively. The histograms of estimated breast cancer risk from the BC2013 model in cases and non-cases in the NHS validation cohort are given in Figure 6.3.

As in Equation (6.2) for the risk distribution F, we can estimate the distributions of risk in cases and non-cases from the observed risks and the corresponding event outcomes in the validation population $(r_i,O_i), i=1,\ldots,n$, by the empirical distribution functions

$$\hat{G}(r)=\frac{1}{n\bar{O}}\sum_{i=1}^{n}I(r_i\leq r,O_i=1) \text{ and } \hat{K}(r)=\frac{1}{n(1-\bar{O})}\sum_{i=1}^{n}I(r_i\leq r,O_i=0) \tag{6.13}$$

where $\bar{O}=\sum O_i/n$ denotes the sample mean of O.

Alternatively, G and K can be estimated from a case-control sample by the empirical distributions of risks $r_i^G\sim G, i=1,\ldots,m$, in cases and $r_j^K\sim K, j=1,\ldots,l$, in non-cases. We denote these distributions by G_m and K_l, respectively. In contrast to expression (6.13), the number of cases and controls is fixed, and the case-control sampling needs to be accommodated in variance calculations. If additionally the population event probability $\mu=P(O=1)$ is known, we can estimate the distribution of risk in the general population as $\hat{F}(r^*)=\mu G_m(r^*)+(1-\mu)K_l(r^*)$.

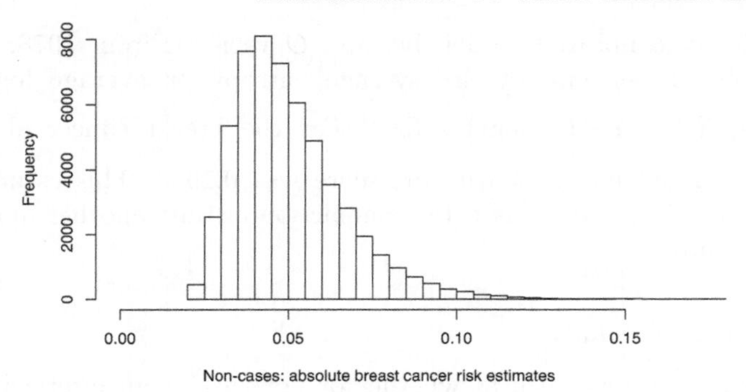

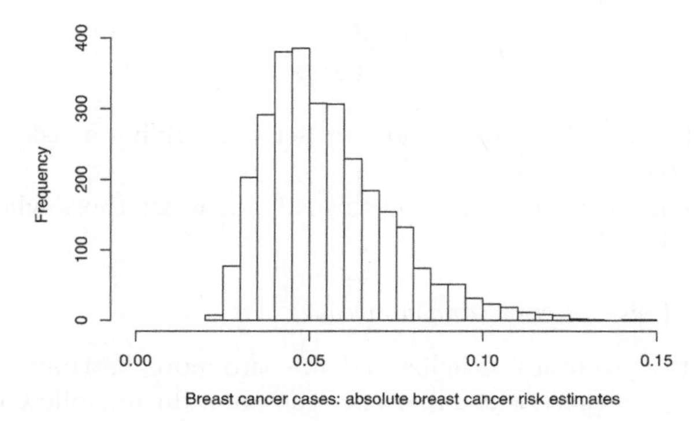

Figure 6.3: Histograms of absolute breast cancer risk estimates from the BC2013 model in the NHS validation cohort for breast cancer cases ($\hat{G}$) and non-cases ($\hat{K}$).

If the model is well calibrated, the average risk in the population is $\mu = \int rdF(r)$ and we can derive the distributions G and K from the distribution F in Equation (6.1) as described in Gail and Pfeiffer (2005). In particular, from Bayes theorem,

$$G(r) = \mu^{-1} \int_0^r udF(u). \tag{6.14}$$

Likewise for a well calibrated model we have (Gail and Pfeiffer, 2005)

$$K(r) = (1-\mu)^{-1} \int_0^r (1-u)dF(u). \tag{6.15}$$

These relationships can be exploited when estimating G and K.

6.4.2.2 Accuracy criteria

Several measures of accuracy can be calculated for the decision rule given in Equation (6.10) that defines $\hat{O} = 1$ if $R > r^*$. These include:

1. The positive predictive value (Vecchio, 1966),

$$PPV = P(O=1|\hat{O}=1) = P(O=1|R>r^*) = \frac{P(O=1)\{1-G(r^*)\}}{1-F(r^*)}. \tag{6.16}$$

2. The negative predictive value,

$$NPV = P(O=0|\hat{O}=0) = P(O=0|R \le r^*) = \frac{P(O=0)K(r^*)}{F(r^*)}. \tag{6.17}$$

3. The probability of correct classification,

$$\begin{aligned} PCC &= P(\hat{O}=0)P(O=0|\hat{O}=0) + P(\hat{O}=1)P(O=1|\hat{O}=1) \\ &= P(R \le r^*)P(O=0|R \le r^*) + P(R > r^*)P(O=1|R > r^*) \\ &= P(R \le r^*) \times NPV + P(R > r^*) \times PPV \\ &= P(O=0)K(r^*) + P(O=1)\{1 - G(r^*)\}, \end{aligned} \tag{6.18}$$

   or its complement,

4. The probability of misclassification,

$$\begin{aligned} PMC = 1 - PCC &= P(R \le r^*)P(Y=1|R \le r^*) + P(R > r^*)P(O=0|R > r^*) \\ &= P(R \le r^*) \times (1 - NPV) + P(R > r^*) \times (1 - PPV). \end{aligned} \tag{6.19}$$

   These quantities are all "prospective" in that they involve probabilities of the outcome O given the classification.
   The following quantities are retrospective and can be estimated from cases and controls only. In that sense, they are not "predictive".

5. $Sensitivity = P(\hat{O}=1|O=1) = P(R > r^*|O=1)$ = true positive probability (TP).
6. $Specificity = P(\hat{O}=0|O=0) = P(R \le r^*|O=0)$ = 1-false positive probability (FP).

We now illustrate these criteria with an example. Current American Society of Clinical Oncology guidelines indicate that premenopausal women and postmenopausal women with low risk of side effects and a 5-year projected risk $\geq$ 1.66% based on a well-established breast cancer model, the NCI's publicly available Breast Cancer Risk Assessment Tool (BCRAT; http://www.cancer.gov/bcrisktool) or "Gail model 2" (Costantino et al., 1999), may benefit from tamoxifen and/or raloxifene for breast cancer prevention (Visvanathan et al., 2009). This threshold was chosen as it corresponded to the average breast cancer risk of a 60-year-old woman (Redmond and Costantino, 1996). Using a 5-year breast cancer risk threshold of $r^* = 0.0166$, we classified the 17,085 women aged 50–55 years at baseline in the NHS cohort based on their 5-year BC2013 risk and computed the criteria (Table 6.3). Out of 252 women who developed breast cancer within 5 years of entry on study, only 84

Table 6.3: Accuracy measures for the absolute breast cancer risk model BC2013 based on a 5-year absolute risk threshold $r^* = 0.0166$ for 50- to 55-year-old women in the NHS validation cohort

Accuracy measure	**Estimate**	**95% CI**
Positive predictive value (PPV)	84/3,461 = 0.024	(0.019, 0.030)
Negative predictive value (NPV)	13,456/13,624 = 0.988	(0.986, 0.990)
Probability of correct classification (PCC)	(13,456+ 84)/ 17,085 = 0.793	(0.786, 0.799)
Probability of misclassification (PMC)	(3,377+168) / 17,085 = 0.208	(0.201, 0.214)
Sensitivity	84/252 = 0.33	(0.28, 0.40)
Specificity	13,456/16,833= 0.80	(0.79, 0.81)

95% confidence intervals were calculated assuming binomial variation and conditional on the denominators.

had a risk greater than 0.0166 (sensitivity = 0.333). Of the 16,833 women without breast cancer, 13,456 had risks below the threshold (specificity = 0.799). Of 3,461 women with risks above 0.0166, only 84 developed breast cancer (PPV = 0.024), whereas 13,456 of the 13,624 women with risks below the threshold remained free of breast cancer (NPV = 0.988). The overall misclassification rate was $100 \times PMC = 20.8\%$.

These measures of accuracy are based on the binary outcome indicator O_i rather than on time to breast cancer incidence. We do this because failure times are quite variable, compared to their mean. For example, the coefficient of variation of an exponentially distributed failure time is 1.0, regardless of the mean. Henderson and Keiding (2005) discussed the difficulties of projecting survival times in clinical practice. Korn and Simon (1990) and Korn and Simon (1991) discussed expected losses for models that predict survival times.

6.4.3 Discriminatory accuracy

Discriminatory accuracy measures how well separated the distributions of risk are for cases and non-cases.

Some measures of discriminatory accuracy are based on the receiver operating characteristic (ROC) curve (see e.g., Pepe (2003)), which extends the idea of classification at a single threshold in Section 6.4.2 by varying the threshold. The ROC curve is generated by plotting $1 - G(r^*)$ (or TP) on the ordinate against $1 - K(r^*)$ (FP) on the abscissa, as r^* varies from 0 to 1. If risks in cases are higher than risks in non-cases, the ROC curve will fall above the line of equality; thus the ROC curve provides an indication of how different the distribution G of absolute risk in cases is from the distribution K of risk in non-cases. Figure 6.4 plots the ROC curve for the NHS validation data for women in various age groups.

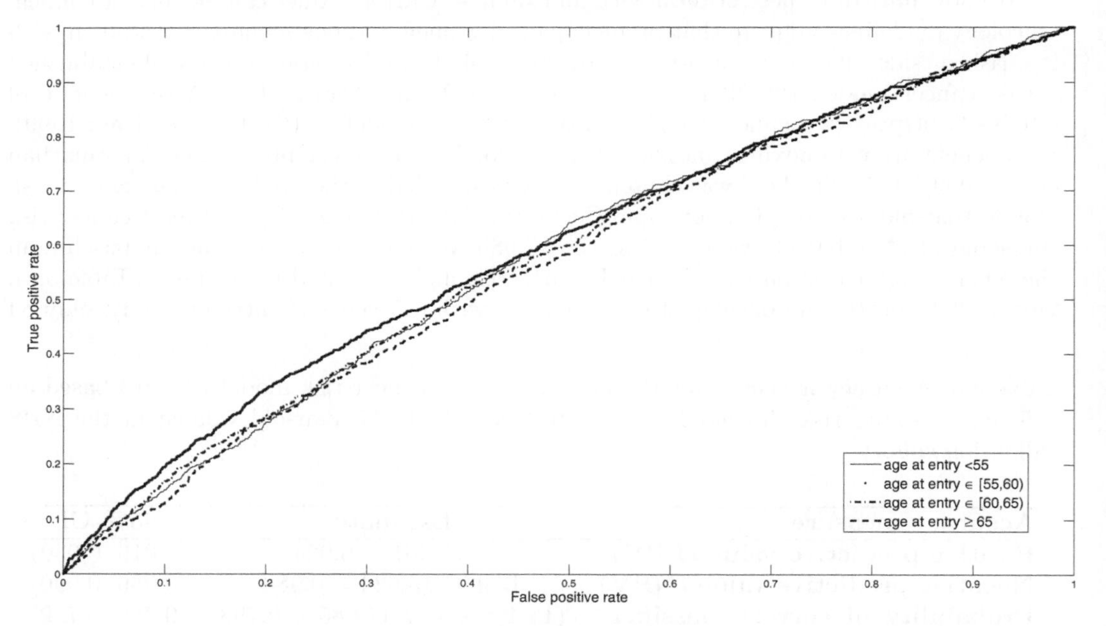

Figure 6.4: ROC curve for absolute breast cancer risk estimates from the BC2013 model in the NHS validation cohort for various age groups.

Pepe (2003) described key properties of the ROC curve. It is unchanged by any monotone increasing transformation of the risks R. The slope for the ROC curve at risk threshold r^* equals the likelihood ratio, namely the ratio of risk densities, $g(r^*)/k(r^*)$ for cases and non-cases. By assigning costs to misclassifications of cases and non-cases in a screening program, Pepe (2003) wrote the expected costs in terms of ROC and derived similar optimal thresholds as described in Section 6.6.

A popular summary measure of the ROC is the area under the ROC curve (AUC or $AUCROC$), which is equivalent to the probability that a randomly selected case will have a risk that is greater than that of a randomly selected non-case. AUC can be computed as

$$AUC = \int_0^1 \{1 - G(u)\}dK(u), \tag{6.20}$$

and can be estimated from the risks r_i^K of l non-cases and the risks r_j^G of m cases as

$$\widehat{AUC} = (lm)^{-1} \sum_{i=1}^{l} \sum_{j=1}^{m} \{I(r_j^G > r_i^K) + 0.5I(r_j^G = r_i^K)\}. \tag{6.21}$$

The non-parametric estimate in Equation (6.21) can also be viewed as $\widehat{AUC} = U/ml$, where U is the MannWhitneyWilcoxon test statistic (Mann and Whitney, 1947), that tests the null hypothesis that two samples come from the same population against an alternative hypothesis that one population (the cases) has larger values. If risk of disease increases with R, values of AUC range from 0.5 if $G(r) = K(r)$ for all r to 1.0 if the support of G lies entirely above the support of K (perfect discrimination). If $AUC = 1.0$, there is a risk r^* that equals or exceeds all risks in non-cases and is less than all risks in cases.

While the ROC curve and the AUC can be estimated from cohort data, they are effectively retrospective measures that compare the risks in cases and non-cases. Thus the ROC can also be estimated from case-control study data, as in Equation (6.21).

An important issue concerns how much of the discriminatory accuracy is attributable to time-related factors, such as variation in age in the population or variation in the risk projection intervals, and how much of the discriminatory accuracy is attributable to risk factors $\mathbf{Z}$. For example, the Framingham model for cardiovascular events (Wilson et al., 1998) includes age and age-squared as covariates in the risk model, whose time scale is time since counseling. High AUC estimates near 0.8 associated with this model derive in part from the strong dependence of cardiovascular risk on age. Cancer risk also increases strongly with age, and age has often been used as the time scale for modeling cancer risk. One approach to estimate the discriminatory accuracy contributed by $\mathbf{Z}$ and not age is to stratify cases and non-cases into 5-year age intervals (Chen et al., 2006a) and compute an estimate of AUC within each age stratum. An average over these stratum-specific AUC estimates indicates the discriminatory accuracy contributed by $\mathbf{Z}$, not by age variation.

In the NHS validation of the breast cancer risk model the age-specific ROC curves plotted in Figure 6.4 do not differ appreciably, and the corresponding AUC values were also similar, with values 0.581, 0.595, 0.578, and 0.567 for the age groups < 55, $[55, 60)$, $[60, 65)$ and ≥ 65 years, respectively. These AUC values indicate modest discriminatory accuracy from the factors in BC2013, apart from age.

6.4.4 Extensions of accuracy measures to functions of time and allowance for censoring

Especially when the time scale is time on study with projection interval $(0, \tau]$, it may be useful to define the previous criteria as functions of τ, as reviewed in Gerds et al. (2008). The earlier literature in this area concerned *pure risk*, not absolute risk. Graf et al. (1999) described how expected loss, such as the Brier criterion, could be estimated and plotted as function of τ with right censored data, provided censoring was independent of survival time. Schoop et al. (2008) relaxed this assumption to conditional independence given covariates and allowed the projection interval to advance with time. Heagerty et al. (2000) developed the concepts of *sensitivity*, *specificity* and the ROC curve as a function of time. Heagerty and Zheng (2005) extended this work to include covariates and to define a "case" either as incident at a given time t or as having occurred at or before time t (cumulative case). Moskowitz and Pepe (2004) showed how to estimate NPV and PPV as a function of time on study. Uno et al. (2007) provided estimates of PMC, *sensitivity*, *specificity*, NPV and PPV by minimizing PMC for a "working model" of the probability of failure by time t, provided censoring was conditionally independent of failure time given covariates. Cai et al. (2010) showed how to recalibrate a parametric working model non-parametrically for pure cumulative risk to time t in the presence of censoring.

Recent literature extended many of these ideas to *absolute risk*. Li et al. (2011) showed how to recalibrate a working model for absolute risk non-parametrically. Saha and Heagerty (2010) extended the notions of incident and cumulative cases to include type of failure and thereby defined cause-specific *sensitivity* (TP), *specificity* (1-FP) and associated ROC curves and AUC as functions of follow-up time τ, both for incident and for cumulative case definitions. Saha and Heagerty (2010) provided non-parametric estimates of these quantities. Zheng et al. (2012) used semi-parametric models to allow for covariates and censoring to estimate TP, FP, the ROC curve, PPV and NPV at a fixed time τ.

6.5 Criteria for applications of risk models for screening or high-risk interventions

Rose (1992) outlined two approaches to preventive intervention in a population. The "general population strategy" is to intervene on the entire population. This strategy has the greatest potential for preventive effect, but it can only be used when the intervention is so safe that everyone can receive it with negligible risk. For example, if an information campaign to reduce salt intake could lower systolic blood pressure in the general population by 2 mm Hg on average, that would prevent more heart attacks than a campaign to identify and treat only those with very high blood pressure. A second strategy is to focus on high risk subjects. Such a "high risk" strategy might be useful if the intervention had serious side effects. Then one should only intervene on individuals with high enough risk of the main health outcome that the benefits of risk reduction outweigh the risks from adverse intervention effects (see Sections 6.6.2 and 10.5). Another motivation might be economic, if there are not enough preventive resources to intervene on all members of the population. Then allocating the intervention to those at highest risk will prevent more disease than random allocation of the intervention, provided the risk assessment is not too expensive (Gail, 2009a). The following criteria are useful for implementing the "high risk" prevention strategy.

6.5.1 Proportion of cases followed and proportion needed to follow

Suppose that the risk model R can be applied to an entire population to assign a disease risk r to each person. The model-based risks are then ranked, and a proportion of those individuals at highest risk of developing disease is followed up. Depending on the specific application, follow-up could consist of a diagnostic test, screening, or a preventive intervention. For example, the risk of breast cancer could be computed based on a risk model, and then a proportion of those with highest risk would receive more intensive screening with mammography or ultrasound to detect disease early and treat it more effectively.

Pfeiffer and Gail (2011) and Pfeiffer (2013) proposed and studied two criteria to assess the usefulness of models that predict risk of disease incidence for screening and prevention, or the usefulness of prognostic models for management following disease diagnosis. The first criterion, the *proportion of cases followed*, $PCF(p)$, is the proportion of cases who are included in the proportion p of individuals in the population at highest risk, given by

$$PCF(p) = 1 - G \circ F^{-1}(1-p) = 1 - G(\phi_{1-p}), \tag{6.22}$$

where $G \circ F(x) = G\{F(x)\}$ is the composition of G with F and $\phi_{1-q} = F^{-1}(1-q)$ denotes the $(1-p)^{th}$ quantile of F. As before, G and F are the distributions of risk in cases and in the population, respectively. This criterion has been used by others, e.g., Pharoah et al. (2002), but the statistical properties of its estimate had not been described. The second criterion is the *proportion needed to follow-up*, $PNF(q)$, namely the proportion of the general population at highest risk that one needs to follow in order that a proportion q of cases will be followed, defined as

$$PNF(q) = 1 - F \circ G^{-1}(1-q) = 1 - F(\gamma_{1-q}), \tag{6.23}$$

where $\gamma_{1-q} = G^{-1}(1-q)$ denotes the $(1-q)^{th}$ quantile of the distribution of risk in cases, G. If risk is concentrated in a small proportion of the population at highest risk, then $PCF(p)$ will be high, even for small p and $PNF(q)$ will be small, even for large q. These quantities are useful for assessing the potential usefulness of a screening program. For example, if $PCF(0.10) = 0.20$, only 20% of those destined to develop disease will be screened in a program focused on the top 10% of the population at highest risk. Likewise $PNF(0.5) = 0.40$ means that 40% of the population at highest risk needs to be screened to cover 50% of future cases.

To lessen the dependency of $PCF(p)$ and $PNF(q)$ on the given thresholds p and q, Pfeiffer (2013) defined the integrated PCF and the integrated PNF as

$$iPCF(p^*) = \int_{p^*}^{1} PCF(p)dW(p) \text{ and } iPNF(q^*) = \int_{q^*}^{1} PNF(q)dW(q), \tag{6.24}$$

where W is a probability measure on the unit interval. For $dW(p) = dp$,

$$iPCF(p^*) = 1 - p^* - \frac{1}{1-p^*} P\{R^G \leq R^F | R^F \in (0, \phi_{1-p^*})\}, \tag{6.25}$$

and

$$iPNF(q^*) = 1 - q^* - \frac{1}{1-q^*} P\{R^F \leq R^G | R^G \in (0, \gamma_{1-q^*})\}, \tag{6.26}$$

where R^F and R^G are random risks from F and G. For the special case of $p^* = q^* = 0$, $iPCF(0) = 1 - P(R^G \leq R^F) = P(R^F < R^G)$. Thus, $iPCF(0)$ is the probability that a randomly selected case has a higher risk than a randomly selected member of the general population. This measure is more appropriate for population interventions than the AUC, namely the probability that a randomly selected case has a higher projected risk than a randomly selected non-case, $AUC = P(R^G > R^K)$, because at the time of intervention one does not know the eventual case status of members of the population. Equations (6.25) and (6.26) resemble expressions for the partial area under the ROC curve (McClish, 1989). The quantities $iPCF(p^*)$ and $iPNF(q*)$ focus on the high risk portion of the population to be screened. While the AUC compares ranks of the estimated risks in the cases to those in non-cases, $iPCF(0)$ compares risk in cases to risks in the whole population, which is a mixture of cases and non-cases. However, for a rare disease, $K \approx F$, and the values of the AUC and $iPCF(0)$ will be close. Figure 6.5 shows a PCF curve when the population distribution of risk F is a beta distribution with parameters $\alpha = 1.5$, $\beta = 28.5$, corresponding to event probability $\mu \equiv P(Y = 1) = 0.05$. The area under this curve is $iPCF1(0) = 0.71$. The corresponding AUC value is 0.72.

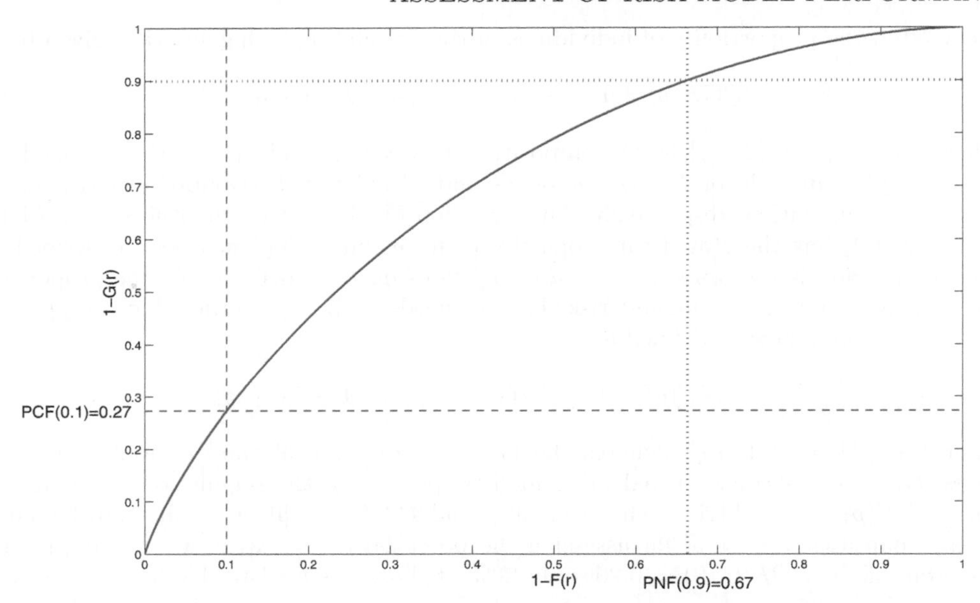

Figure 6.5: PCF curve when the distribution F of risk is a Beta distribution with parameters $\alpha = 1.5$, $\beta = 28.5$, corresponding to mean $\mu = 0.05$ and $iPCF(0) = 0.71$.

Pfeiffer and Gail (2011) and Pfeiffer (2013) developed estimates of PCF, PNF, $iPCF$ and $iPNF$ for three types of sampled data and derived their asymptotic distributions. First, Pfeiffer and Gail (2011) considered a random sample of risk estimates $r_i^F, i = 1, \ldots, n$ from the cohort and assumed that the risk model was well calibrated. Second, Pfeiffer (2013) considered case-control data with random samples of risks in cases, $r_i^G \sim G, i = 1, \ldots, m$, and controls, $r_j^K \sim K, j = 1, \ldots, l$, and assumed that the event probability $\mu \equiv P(Y = 1)$ in the population was known from external sources. From this information, Pfeiffer (2013) estimated PCF, PNF, $iPCF$ and $iPNF$ non-parametrically. Third, Pfeiffer (2013) studied the corresponding estimates when a random sample of risks and the associated binary outcomes $(r_i^F, O_i), i = 1, \ldots, n$ were available from the population. The second and third scenarios do not require well calibrated risk models for unbiased estimation of $PCF, PNF, iPCF$ and $iPNF$. We expand on these comments in the following paragraphs.

6.5.1.1 Estimation of PCF and PNF

Estimation using observed risks in a population

If the risk model R is well calibrated, that is $P(O = 1|r) = r$, then $\mu \equiv P(O = 1) = E(R) = \int_0^1 rdF(r)$, and the distribution G of risk in cases can be derived from the population distribution F as shown in Equation (6.14). In this setting,

$$PCF(p) = 1 - G(\phi_{1-p}) = 1 - \frac{1}{\mu} \int_0^{\phi_{1-p}} tdF(t) = 1 - L(1-p), \qquad (6.27)$$

where L is the Lorenz curve of F (Lorenz, 1905). Likewise, $PNF(q) = 1 - F(\gamma_{1-q}) = 1 - L^{-1}(1-q)$, where L^{-1} denotes the inverse of the Lorenz curve (Goldie, 1977).

Thus if the risk model is well calibrated, PCF and PNF can be estimated nonparametrically based on empirical estimates of L and L^{-1} from a random sample $r_1^F, \ldots, r_n^F$ of risks. Let $r_{(1)}^F \leq \ldots \leq r_{(n)}^F$ denote the order statistics of the estimated risks, and let $[x]$ be the largest integer less than or equal to x. Let $S_i = \sum_{k=1}^i r_{(k)}$. An estimate of the Lorenz curve and thus PCF is $\widehat{PCF} = 1 - L_n(1-q) = 1 - S_{[n(1-q)]}/S_n$. Using Goldie's (Goldie, 1977) result for the inverse function of the Lorenz curve, L_n^{-1}, for a fixed value of $1-p$, the PNF is estimated as $\widehat{PNF} = 1 - L_n^{-1}(1-p) = i/n, \quad S_i/S_n < 1-p \leq S_{i+1}/S_n, i = 0, \ldots, n$.

If the model is well calibrated, $iPCF$ and $iPNF$ are functionals of the integrated Lorenz curve and its integrated inverse. A popular summary measure of the Lorenz curve, the Gini index (Gini, 1912) defined as $Gini = 1 - 2\int_0^1 L(p)dp$ is related to $iPCF(0)$ through $Gini = 2iPCF(0) - 1$. A non-parametric estimate of $iPCF$ is thus obtained by interpolation as $\widehat{iPCF}(p^*) = 1 - p^* - \sum_{i=1}^{[(1-p^*)n]}([(1-p^*)n] - i + 1)r_{(i)}/nS_n$. Similarly, we estimate $iPNF$ as $\widehat{iPNF}(q^*) = 1 - q^* - \sum_{i=1}^{k^*} ir_{(i+1)}/nS_n$, where k^* satisfies $\quad S_{k^*}/S_n < q^* \leq S_{k^*+1}/S_n$.

Estimation using risks in a case-control sample when $\mu = P(O = 1)$ is known

From random samples $r_i^G \sim G, i = 1, \ldots, m$, of cases and $r_j^K \sim K, j = 1, \ldots, l$, of non-cases we obtained the empirical distribution functions $G_m(r^*)$ and $K_l(r^*)$. Assuming that the event probability $\mu = P(O = 1)$ in that population is known, we estimated the distribution of risk in the general population as $\hat{F}(r^*) = \mu G_m(r^*) + (1-\mu)K_l(r^*)$. Plugging G_m, K_l, $\hat{F}$, and $\hat{\phi}_{1-p} = \hat{F}^{-1}(1-p)$ and $\hat{\gamma}_{1-q} = G_m^{-1}(1-q)$ into (6.22), (6.23), and (6.24) yields estimates $\widehat{PCF}$, $\widehat{PNF}(q)$, $\widehat{iPCF}(p^*)$ and $\widehat{iPNF}(1-q^*)$.

Estimation using risks and outcomes in a population

Here we observe i.i.d. samples $(r_i^F, O_i), i = 1, \ldots, n$ of risks and the corresponding event outcomes in a population. For a model that predicts disease incidence, these data would be risk estimates at baseline and observed outcomes at the end of the follow-up period, and for a model that predicts prevalence of a disease, the risks and outcomes could be based on a cross-sectional sample.

Pfeiffer (2013) estimated PCF and PNF by plugging estimates of F, G and the corresponding quantiles ϕ and γ into the expressions (6.22) and (6.23), respectively. Estimates of $iPCF$ and $iPNF$ were obtained in a similar way. The distribution of risk in the general population, F, was estimated from Equation (6.2), and G was estimated from Equation (6.13).

Variance calculations

Pfeiffer (2013) derived the asymptotic properties and variances for the estimates of PCF, PNF, $iPCF$ and $iPNF$ for the three types of data described above using a Taylor linearization approach, that yields variance estimates of a statistic $\hat{T}$ through a first order approximation of $\hat{T}$, such that $\text{var}(\hat{T}) \approx \text{var}\{\sum_1^n \Delta_i(\hat{T})\}$, as described in more detail in Section 4.6.1. Again, $\Delta_i(\hat{T})$ denotes the influence function operator for the influence of observation i on $\hat{T}$ (Graubard and Fears, 2005; Shah, 2002; Deville, 1999; Hampel, 1974; Reid and Crepeau, 1985). For estimates based on (r_i^F, O_i) observed in a cohort, Pfeiffer (2013) used bivariate influence functions (Pires and Branco, 2002).

Estimates for the NHS validation data

Table 6.4 shows estimates $\widehat{PCF}_R$ and $\widehat{PNF}_R$ from the NHS validation cohort, based on risks R only, under the assumption that the risk model BC2013 is well calibrated; it also shows estimates $\widehat{PCF}_{(R,O)}$ and $\widehat{PNF}_{(R,O)}$ based on (R, O) without the calibration assumption. Estimates $\widehat{PCF}_{(R,O)}$, which are unbiased, were lower than $\widehat{PCF}_R$ for $p = 0.10$ and $p = 0.20$. The width of the 95% confidence intervals was appreciably larger for $\widehat{PCF}_{(R,O)}$, which shows how much efficiency is gained by assuming that the model is well calibrated. If the assumption is violated, however, $\widehat{PCF}_R$ can be biased. For PNF with $q = 0.90$, a fraction $\hat{q}_{(R,Y)} = 0.901$ of cases was found in the $100 \times \widehat{PNF}_{(R,O)} = 76.9\%$ of the population with the highest risk; this is evidence that $\widehat{PNF}_{(R,O)}$ is unbiased. In contrast, a fraction $\hat{q}_R = 0.945$ of cases was found in the $100 \times \widehat{PNF}_R = 84.1\%$ of the population with highest risk when $q = 0.90$. Thus 94.5% of cases instead of the desired 90% had risks in the highest 84.1% of the population, reflecting a lack of model calibration and consequent bias in $\widehat{PNF}_R$ (Table 6.4).

The AUC value for this example was 0.616, very close to the integrated PCF, $\widehat{iPCF}(0) = 0.614$, as expected for a rare outcome.

Table 6.4: Estimates of PCF and PNF from the NHS validation cohort based on 5-year BC2013 risk projections for 50- to 55-year-old women

	Estimate based on cohort data	
	Assume well-calibrated model, use data R only	**No assumption on calibration, use data (R, O)**
% screened (100 × p)		
10%	$\widehat{PCF}_R = 0.168$ 95%CI: (0.167, 0.169)	$\widehat{PCF}_{(R,O)} = 0.178$ 95%CI: (0.127, 0.229)
20%	$\widehat{PCF}_R = 0.299$ 95%CI: (0.298, 0.301)	$\widehat{PCF}_{(R,O)} = 0.328$ 95%CI: (0.261, 0.395)
% cases to be captured (100 × q) in screen		
90%	$\widehat{PNF}_R = 0.841$ 95%CI: (0.840, 0.842)	$\widehat{PNF}_{(R,O)} = 0.769$ 95%CI: (0.649, 0.890)
80%	$\widehat{PNF}_R = 0.588$ 95%CI: (0.706, 0.709)	$\widehat{PNF}_{(R,O)} = 0.533$ 95%CI: (0.533, 0.777)

95% bootstrap confidence intervals (CIs) are shown.

6.6 Model assessment based on expected costs or expected utility specialized for a particular application

Minus the sample mean square error of prediction (Brier statistic) and the sample mean logarithmic score (minus half the binomial deviance) converge to expectations of general criteria called "proper scores" (Gneiting and Raftery, 2007)). A risk model that yields a higher mean value of a proper score is preferred to one with a smaller mean value. If possible, however, it is desirable to choose criteria that *meet the special requirements of a particular application*, rather than choose a general proper score. If it is possible to assign "costs", which are also called "losses", to various outcomes that are specialized for a particular problem, then optimal risk thresholds for decision can be determined that minimize the expected cost or loss. A figure of merit for a given risk model is its expected cost for that optimal threshold. In comparing two risk models, the preferred model is the one with smaller expected cost. In the following sections we elaborate on these ideas. Rather than specifying costs or losses, some investigators equivalently specify "utilities". An optimal risk threshold can be determined from utilities, and with this threshold, a preferred risk model is the one that yields the larger expected utility.

6.6.1 Two health states and two intervention options

Many important problems in clinical epidemiology and clinical practice can be represented in terms of two health states and two intervention options. In screening for disease, a person either has screen-detectable disease or not, and an intervention choice is whether or not to apply a screening test to that person, perhaps based on an estimate of the probability that the person is diseased. In predicting whether a man will have a myocardial infarction in the next ten years, the man either will or will not be so diagnosed, and an intervention might be whether or not to recommend taking statins to prevent cardiovascular events, perhaps based on the risk of such events. Such considerations could also apply after disease diagnosis. For example, a 65-year-old man diagnosed with prostate cancer with a favorable pathology (Gleason score 2) has a chance of dying of prostate cancer of less than 5%, because he is likely to die of other causes first (Albertsen et al., 2005). The outcomes are death from prostate cancer or not, and the intervention choice is whether to treat vigorously with surgery or radiation or to wait for laboratory or other signs of cancer progression before treating.

Problems of this type can be characterized by the data in Table 6.5. A risk estimate r is used to decide on intervention or not, according to some risk threshold, t. The rule is to intervene if $r > t$ and not to intervene if $r \leq t$. The risk r for the screening example is the risk of prevalent disease, but the risks for the other two examples should be absolute risks of the adverse outcome. Costs (or losses) for the various combinations of intervention choice and disease state are shown, but if appropriate utilities are used instead of costs, the results obtained by minimizing costs are analogously obtained by maximizing utilities. Letting π denote the true probability of disease or of an adverse health outcome, $sens(t)$ the sensitivity of the risk model at threshold t, and $spec(t)$ the corresponding specificity, one can express the joint probability of being diseased and having the intervention as $\pi \times sens(t)$. Other joint probabilities are shown in Table 6.5.

Table 6.5: Definitions for a decision problem with two health states and two intervention options[a]

Intervention	**Disease state**	**Costs**	**Risk criterion at threshold t**	**Outcome probability**
Yes	Diseased	C_{TP}	$r > t$	$\pi \times sens(t)$
No	Diseased	C_{FN}	$r \leq t$	$\pi \times \{1 - sens(t)\}$
Yes	Not diseased	C_{FP}	$r > t$	$(1-\pi)\{1 - spec(t)\}$
No	Not diseased	C_{TN}	$r \leq t$	$(1-\pi)spec(t)$

[a]Abbreviations: TP, true positive; FN, false negative; FP, false positive; TN, true negative; C, cost; r, absolute risk; t, threshold; π, probability of disease; *sens*, sensitivity; *spec*, specificity.

Assuming there is a cost, C_{test}, associated with assessing risk, the total expected cost is

$$\begin{aligned}\bar{C}(t) &= \pi \times sens(t)C_{TP} + \pi \times \{1 - sens(t)\}C_{FN} + (1-\pi)\{1 - spec(t)\}C_{FP} \\ &\quad +(1-\pi)spec(t)C_{TN} + C_{test} \\ &= -\pi \times sens(t)B_{case} - (1-\pi)spec(t)B_{non-case} + \pi C_{FN} + (1-\pi)C_{FP} + C_{test},\end{aligned} \tag{6.28}$$

where $B_{case} = C_{FN} - C_{TP} \geq 0$ is the net benefit of intervening on a case (or reduction in cost from intervening on a case) and $B_{non-case} = C_{FP} - C_{TN} \geq 0$ is the net cost from intervening on a non-case. The risk threshold t^* that minimizes $\bar{C}(t)$ is

$$t^* = B_{non-case}/(B_{non-case} + B_{case}) = (1 + B_{case}/B_{non-case}),^{-1} \tag{6.29}$$

and the corresponding minimum expected cost is

$$\begin{aligned}\bar{C}_{\min} &= -\pi \times sens(t^*)(C_{FN} - C_{TP}) + (1-\pi)\{1 - spec(t^*)\}(C_{FP} - C_{TN}) + \pi C_{FN} \\ &+(1-\pi)C_{TN} + C_{test} = -\pi \times sens(t^*)B_{case} - (1-\pi)spec(t^*)B_{non-case} \\ &+\pi C_{FN} + (1-\pi)C_{FP} + C_{test}.\end{aligned} \tag{6.30}$$

A perfect model r has $sens(t) = spec(t) = 1$ and

$$\bar{C}_{\min}^{\text{perfect}} = \pi\, C_{TP} + (1-\pi)C_{TN} + C_{test}. \tag{6.31}$$

If one intervenes on all subjects ($sens(t) = 1$, $spec(t) = 0$), then

$$\bar{C}_{\min}^{\text{all}} = \pi\, C_{TP} + (1-\pi)C_{FP} + C_{test}. \tag{6.32}$$

If one never intervenes ($sens(t) = 0$, $spec(t) = 1$), then

$$\bar{C}_{\min}^{\text{none}} = \pi C_{FN} + (1-\pi)C_{TN} + C_{test}. \tag{6.33}$$

These three quantities can be used as benchmarks for the performance $\bar{C}_{\min}$ of an imperfect risk model (Weinstein et al., 1980; Gail and Pfeiffer, 2005; Gail, 2009b; Baker et al., 2009).

Equation (6.29) is remarkable because the optimal threshold depends only on the costs and not on which risk model is used. Equation (6.29) was first derived by Pauker and Kassirer (1975) by finding the threshold at which the expected loss is the same for the intervention and no intervention options. This important result shows that specifying a threshold is equivalent to specifying the cost ratio $B_{case}/B_{non-case}$, as emphasized and used by Pauker and Kassirer (1975). Metz (1978) showed that this threshold corresponded to the point where the slope of the ROC curve equals $(1-\pi)B_{non-case}/\pi B_{case}$. Gail and Pfeiffer (2005) derived the threshold by differentiating Equation (6.28).

$\bar{C}_{\min}$ in Equation (6.30) decreases with increasing sensitivity and specificity at t^*. Model 1 is preferred to model 2 if

$$\bar{C}_{\min,2} - \bar{C}_{\min,1} = \pi\, B_{case}\{sens_1(t^*) - sens_2(t^*)\} + (1-\pi)B_{non-case}\{spec_1(t^*) - spec_2(t^*)\} > 0. \tag{6.34}$$

Equivalently, model 1 is preferred to model 2 if

$$\{sens_1(t^*) - sens_2(t^*)\} + \{spec_1(t^*) - spec_2(t^*)\}\{(1-\pi)B_{non-case}/\pi\, B_{case}\} > 0. \tag{6.35}$$

If both the sensitivity and specificity of model 1 are greater than that of model 2 at t^*, then model 1 is preferred. If either $sens_1(t^*) > sens_2(t^*)$ and $spec_1(t^*) < spec_2(t^*)$ or $sens_1(t^*) < sens_2(t^*)$ and $spec_1(t^*) > spec_2(t^*)$, then whether or not model 1 is preferred depends on the weight assigned to the difference in specificities, $\{(1-\pi)B_{non-case}/\pi\, B_{case}\}$.

In terms of the previous notation, Vickers and Elkin (2006) defined the "net benefit" at a risk threshold t as

$$NB(t) = \pi \times sens(t) - (1-\pi)\{1 - spec(t)\}\{t/(1-t)\}. \tag{6.36}$$

One can obtain *NB(t)* from Equation (6.28) by discarding terms that do not depend on t, dividing by $-B_{case}$, and recognizing from Equation (6.29) that $t/(1-t) = B_{non-case}/B_{case}$. Baker et al. (2009) showed that discarding those terms is equivalent to subtracting $\bar{C}_{\min}^{\text{none}}$ from $\bar{C}_{\min}$. Vickers and Elkin (2006) recommended a "decision curve", which is a plot of $NB(t)$ against t . By varying t between 0 and 1, one is implicitly examining net benefit for a range of values of implied cost ratios $B_{non-case}/B_{case}$, and one risk model might be preferred to another if its net benefit were larger over a relevant range of values of t. If none receive the intervention, $NB(t) = 0$. If all receive the intervention, $NB(t) = \pi - (1-\pi)t/(1-t)$, which is very nearly linear with slope $-(1-\pi)$ for small t. The decision curve can be compared with these two loci to see whether using the risk model is preferable to intervening on all or intervening on none, without a risk model.

Van Calster and Vickers (2015) studied the effects of miscalibration on the decision curve. Miscalibration always lowers *NB(t)*. Miscalibration can lead to worse decisions than no model if risks are underestimated for true event rates less than π or overestimated for true event rates over π. Baker et al. (2009), who used utilities instead of costs, reviewed several alternative measures of performance based on the equivalents of $\bar{C}(t)$, $\bar{C}_{\min}$, $\bar{C}_{\min}^{\text{perfect}}$, $\bar{C}_{\min}^{\text{all}}$, and $\bar{C}_{\min}^{\text{none}}$. They presented a scaled statistic, the "relative utility" and "relative utility curve". We define the corresponding relative cost curve, *RCC*, as

$$\begin{aligned} RCC(t) &= \{\bar{C}_{\min}^{\text{none}} - \bar{C}(t)\}/\{\bar{C}_{\min}^{\text{none}} - \bar{C}_{\min}^{\text{perfect}}\} \text{ for } t^* \geq \pi \\ &= \{\bar{C}_{\min}^{\text{all}} - \bar{C}(t)\}/\{\bar{C}_{\min}^{\text{all}} - \bar{C}_{\min}^{\text{perfect}}\} \text{ for } t^* < \pi. \end{aligned} \tag{6.37}$$

At the optimal threshold for a given model, $RCC(t^*)$ is given by Equation (6.37) with $\bar{C}_{\min}$ replacing $\bar{C}(t)$. Peirce (1884) calculated $-\pi \times sens(t)B_{case} + (1-\pi)\{1 - spec(t)\}B_{non-case}$ but did not define an optimal threshold. Van Calster et al. (2013) presented a unified treatment of net benefit, relative utility, *AUC* and some other measures, such as the net reclassification index, which is further discussed in Chapter 7.

6.6.2 *More complex outcomes and interventions*

Although the previous formulation for two health states and two intervention actions has many applications and has been well studied, there may be multiple health states to consider, and the intervention choices may be more elaborate.

6.6.2.1 *Example with four intervention choices*

Pauker and Kassirer (1980) considered diagnostic tests, such as renal biopsies, which themselves carry risk. The resulting 4 possible intervention actions included: administer treatment without the diagnostic test, withhold treatment without the diagnostic test, perform the diagnostic test and administer treatment if it is positive, and perform the diagnostic test and withhold treatment if it is negative. For each of these 4 possible actions, the disease was either present or absent, resulting in 8 possible combinations of intervention actions and disease states. By assigning utilities to each of these 8 conditions and allowing for the cost associated with performing the diagnostic test, Pauker and Kassirer (1980) were able to define two risk thresholds for clinical management. We translate their notation for utilities into the previous notation for costs. They first presented a risk threshold for withholding treatment without diagnostic testing versus diagnostic testing. This threshold was

$$t_{test}^* = \frac{P(\text{Test}+|\text{no disease})B_{non-case} + C_{test}}{P(\text{Test}+|\text{no disease})B_{non-case} + P(\text{Test}+|\text{disease})B_{case}}. \tag{6.38}$$

Thus, the disease risk threshold t_{test}^* for performing the diagnostic test increases with the cost of the test C_{test}, and with the cost of treating a non-case, $B_{non-case}$; the threshold decreases with the benefit B_{case} of treating a case and with the diagnostic test's specificity and sensitivity. The second threshold was for the decision to treat without testing versus diagnostic testing. The threshold for treatment without diagnostic testing was

$$t_{treat}^* = \frac{P(\text{Test-}|\text{no disease})B_{non-case} - C_{test}}{P(\text{Test-}|\text{no disease})B_{non-case} + P(\text{Test-}|\text{disease})B_{case}}. \tag{6.39}$$

This threshold decreases with increasing C_{test}, increasing B_{case}, and decreasing test sensitivity; it increases with increasing $B_{non-case}$ and increasing test specificity. Based on these thresholds, one treats without testing if $r > t_{treat}^*$. If $r \leq t_{test}^*$, one does not test or treat. If $t_{test}^* < r \leq t_{treat}^*$, one tests and treats according as the test is positive or negative.

6.6.2.2 *Multiple outcomes in prevention trials*

Sometimes an intervention affects multiple health outcomes. For example, Fisher et al. (1998) studied whether tamoxifen would prevent breast cancer in 13,388 women followed on average for 4 years. Although tamoxifen reduced the risk of invasive breast cancer (relative risk 0.51) compared to placebo, it had other effects (Table 6.6). In particular, it reduced the risk of hip fractures and *in situ* breast cancer, but increased the risk of endometrial cancer, stroke, pulmonary emboli and deep vein thromboses.

Table 6.6: Relative risks (RRs) from tamoxifen treatment for various health outcomes, and absolute numbers of health outcomes expected in 5 years with and without tamoxifen in a population of 10,000 white 40-year-old women with uteri and with a projected breast cancer risk of 2%

Health events	**RR (95% CI)**[a]	**None get tamoxifen**	**All get tamoxifen**	**Prevented by tamoxifen**
Invasive breast cancer	0.51 (0.39–0.66)	200	103	97
Hip fracture	0.55 (0.25–1.15)	2	1	1
Endometrial cancer	2.53 (1.35–4.97)	10	26	–16[b]
Stroke	1.59 (0.93–2.77)	22	35	–13
Pulmonary emboli	3.01 (1.15–9.27)	7	22	–15
Net life-threatening events		241	187	54
In situ breast cancer	0.50 (0.33–0.77)	106	53	53
Deep vein thrombosis	1.60 (0.91–2.86)	24	39	–15
Net serious events		130	92	38

[a]From B. Fisher, J.P. Costantino, D.L. Wickerham, C.K. Redmond, M. Kavanah, W.M. Cronin, V. Vogel, A. Robidoux, N. Dimitrov, J. Atkins, M. Daly, S. Wieand, E. Tan-Chiu, L. Ford, and N. Wolmark. Tamoxifen for prevention of breast cancer: Report of the national surgical adjuvant breast and bowel project p-1 study. *Journal of the National Cancer Institute*, 90(18):1371–1388, 1998.
[b]A negative number means that tamoxifen increases the number of events.

To provide guidance to women as to whether there was a net expected benefit from taking tamoxifen, Gail et al. (1999a) classified the health outcomes as life-threatening or serious (Table 6.6) and estimated the absolute risk of each outcome in the absence and presence of tamoxifen. Suppose a woman with a uterus had a breast cancer risk assessment, and her projected 5-year absolute risk was 2%. She might consider what would happen to 10,000 women just like her over 5 years. On the basis of absolute risk estimates one might expect 241 life-threatening events without tamoxifen and 187 life-threatening events with tamoxifen, a reduction of 54 events (Table 6.6). Likewise, tamoxifen reduces the expected number of serious events in this population by 38. It seems that such a woman should consider the use of tamoxifen.

If one is willing to assign a cost (or loss) c_k to each outcome, $k = 1, 2, \ldots K$, where $k = 1$ corresponds to invasive breast cancer and $K = 7$ to deep vein thrombosis (Table 6.6), one can determine whether there is a net benefit from taking tamoxifen by testing

$$\text{Net Benefit} = \sum_{k=1}^{K} c_k P_{0k} - \sum_{k=1}^{K} c_k P_{1k} = \sum_{k=1}^{K} c_k (P_{0k} - P_{1k}) > 0. \tag{6.40}$$

In this equation, P_{0k} is the probability of the outcome in the absence of tamoxifen and P_{1k}

is the probability in the presence of tamoxifen. The *net benefit* is the expected cost in the absence of tamoxifen minus the expected cost in the presence of tamoxifen. In Gail et al. (1999a), the relative risks RR_k in Table 6.6 were used to compute $P_{1k} = \text{RR}_k P_{0k}$, and the costs were defined as $c_k = 1$ for $k = 1, 2, ..., 5$ (life-threatening events) and as $c_k = 0.5$ for $k = 6, 7$ (serious events). Using these costs, one could classify women according as whether or not the net benefit was positive. Young women with high breast cancer risk had positive net benefits, whereas older women tended to have a negative net benefit because they had higher baseline risks, P_{0k}, for stroke, pulmonary emboli, deep vein thromboses, and endometrial cancer. Cross-classifications on age and breast cancer absolute risk indicated which women had a net benefit for tamoxifen (Gail et al., 1999a) and for raloxifene (Freedman et al., 2011).

Several comments follow. First these calculations ignore the possibility that a woman would develop more than one of these conditions. This approximation is reasonable over short time intervals, like 5 years. This assumption means that one does not need to assign costs to multiple simultaneous outcomes. Moreover, one does not need to know the joint distribution of these various events with and without tamoxifen; marginal estimates like P_{0k} and P_{1k} are sufficient. Second, we have assumed that we can calculate $P_{1k} = \text{RR}_k P_{0k}$, regardless of the characteristics of the woman. Prevention trials of this type rarely provide sufficient information to detect heterogeneity of the intervention effect, but these methods can be extended to allow for it (Janes et al., 2014). Third, not everyone would agree to the costs used. Sensitivity analyses based on varying costs can be used to see if conclusions are robust, as in Gail et al. (1999a). Fourth, the estimates of net benefit in Equation (6.40) are subject to random variation, primarily because the relative risk estimates are variable (Table 6.6). Gail et al. (1999a) showed how to account for such variability by using a parametric bootstrap to resample the numbers of health outcomes and categorized the evidence that the net benefit was positive as strong (probability 0.9 to 1.0) or moderate (probability 0.6 to 0.89). Finally, these analyses only estimated the risks of health outcomes other than breast cancer on the basis of race and age. More precise estimates of P_{0k} based on risk models for other outcomes have the potential to improve the net benefit (Gail, 2012).

6.6.2.3 Expected cost calculations for outcomes following disease diagnosis

Therapeutic decisions after disease diagnosis also depend on the interventions that are available and the costs that might be associated with various interventions and outcomes. The following simple example indicates that the computation of expected loss and the data requirements can be more complex for therapeutic decisions. Suppose a standard cancer chemotherapy is to be compared with a new chemotherapy, and that the two health outcomes of interest are fatal chemotherapy toxicity (k =1) or disease recurrence (k =2). Denote the bivariate outcome $\mathbf{O} = (O_1, O_2) \equiv \{I(\text{event}\, k = 1 \text{ occurs}), I(\text{event}\, k = 2 \text{ occurs})\}$, and let $P_0(\mathbf{O})$ and $P_1(\mathbf{O})$ be the probability mass functions under standard and new chemotherapies respectively. In this setting, joint events like $\mathbf{O} = (1, 1)$ are unfortunately possible. Now consider some possible cost (or loss) functions, $c(\mathbf{O})$. Here c is a scalar positive function of $\mathbf{O}$. A simple loss function might be the additive model $c(\mathbf{O}) = c_1 O_1 + c_2 O_2$, where c_1 and c_2 are costs associated with events $k = 1$ and 2. It turns out that for additive cost functions like this, the decision rule that minimizes expected costs is to treat if the net benefit in Equation (6.40) is positive, where P_{0k} and P_{1k} are the marginal distributions for O_1 and O_2. Such additive cost functions might apply in a setting where the health outcomes were two different mild conditions, such as itching and redness, but in the present example an additive cost function does not seem appropriate. Suppose we assign costs $c_1 =$ 2 and c_2 =1, because fatal toxicity is more devastating than recurrence. The cost can be no greater than 2, because a recurrence hardly adds costs to fatal toxicity. Thus we might use $c(\mathbf{O}) = \max(c_1 O_1, c_2 O_2)$. The decision rule that minimizes expected cost is to give the new treatment if

$$\text{Net Benefit} = \sum_{\mathbf{O}} c(\mathbf{O})\{P_0(\mathbf{O}) - P_1(\mathbf{O})\} > 0. \tag{6.41}$$

In order to compute this net benefit with non-additive costs, we need the joint distributions $P_0(\mathbf{O})$and $P_1(\mathbf{O})$, not merely the marginal distributions used in Equation (6.40). Thus randomized trials that yield estimates of $P_0(\mathbf{O})$ and $P_1(\mathbf{O})$ should report not only marginal outcomes but joint outcomes (which is rarely done but is feasible with electronic records).

This example is meant only to illustrate that therapeutic decisions can be complex and require elaborate data to estimate net benefit. In fact, to describe realistic costs in the therapeutic setting, one may need to take the timing of health outcomes into account, and there may be several possible outcomes to consider. Formulating realistic outcome possibilities and joint costs is often the main impediment to implementing formal decision methods. Another consideration that applies to the therapeutic setting and more broadly is that minimizing expected cost may not be the best criterion. Some patients may want to adopt the intervention that minimizes the maximum cost that can be encountered, rather than minimizing the expected cost.

Provided one accepts minimizing expected cost (or minimizing maximum cost) as the criterion of choice, one can compare risk models in terms of their associated net benefit in specific applications.

Chapter 7

Comparing the performance of two models

Many of the criteria in Chapter 6 to assess the performance of a single risk model can be used to compare two models. Such criteria include measures of accuracy, such as positive and negative predictive value, misclassification rate, sensitivity, specificity, and additional criteria based on the ROC curve. Other criteria for a single risk model can also be used, such as criteria for quantifying the performance with respect to specific interventions (e.g., PCF or PNF), and criteria based on expected costs, as presented in Chapter 6. All these criteria for single risk models can also be employed to compare the performance of two different models evaluated on the same validation data. In this chapter we illustrate such comparisons. However, we also discuss some more recently proposed criteria for model comparison that have no "single model" analogue. They include risk stratification tables, the net reclassification improvement (NRI), and continuous net reclassification improvement, $cNRI$ (Pencina et al., 2008). These latter criteria were developed to quantify the improvement in a model from adding a novel predictive marker. Examples of serum markers include CA-125 for predicting ovarian cancer incidence, and PSA (prostate-specific antigen) to predict the presence of prevalent prostate cancer and help decide if a biopsy is warranted. There has also been interest in determining how much the performance of risk prediction models could be improved by including information on single nucleotide polymorphisms (SNPs) identified in genome wide association studies (GWAS). Although individual disease-associated SNPs may confer only modest risk for most diseases, the combined effect of all identified disease-associated SNPs, summarized in a "polygenic risk score", might provide substantial information. Unless costly molecular information improves prediction compared to models based on easily obtained risk factors such as clinical or personal characteristics, there may be little value in using the molecular markers. Although assessing the value of adding a new marker to an existing model is an important application of methods for model comparison, these methods can also be used to compare models that use entirely different risk factors.

7.1 Use of external validation data for model comparison

We compare the performance of two models evaluated in the same "test" or "validation" data. These "external validation data" are independent of the data sources used to develop the models. We denote the two models that we wish to compare by R_1 and R_2 and assume the risk estimates for both were calculated using possibly different baseline covariates but the same projection interval for each individual in the validation data set. Thus we observe bivariate risk estimates $(r_i^1, r_i^2), i = 1, \ldots, n$, from models R_1 and R_2. The bivariate distribution of risks can be calculated from the joint distribution of all risk factors used in both models by extending Equation 6.1. However, we are mainly interested in the marginal risk distributions F_1 and F_2 induced by the respective covariate distributions for the risk factors in R_1 and R_2 in the general validation population. As in Chapter 6, G_i and $K_i, i = 1, 2$, denote the distributions of risk in cases and non-cases for models $i = 1, 2$, respectively.

When discussing nested models, we let R_2 denote the "new model" and R_1 denote the original model. For non-nested models, the designation of the subscript is arbitrary. For most of this chapter we assume that the validation data are from a cohort, but we point out when criteria can also be estimated from case-control data. In Section 7.7 we mention problems with trying to compare models using the training data.

7.2 Data example

To illustrate the methods in this chapter, we compared an absolute risk model for invasive breast cancer with potentially modifiable risk factors (BC2013) (Pfeiffer et al., 2013) to the old absolute breast cancer risk model, the National Cancer Institute's publicly available Breast Cancer Risk Assessment Tool (BCRAT at http://www.cancer.gov/bcrisktool), which includes modifications of the original "Gail model" (Gail et al., 1989), as described previously (Costantino et al., 1999; Gail et al., 2007; Matsuno et al., 2011). We used a subset of the 57,906 women in the Nurses' Health Study (NHS) external validation cohort described in Chapter 6. All comparisons were based on 5-year absolute risk estimates from BC2013 and BCRAT for the 17,085 women aged 50–55 years at baseline in the NHS cohort.

The predictors in the new BC2013 model are age and race/ethnicity of a woman, her family history of breast or ovarian cancer, personal history of benign breast disease/breast biopsies, estrogen and progestin menopausal hormone therapy (MHT) use, other MHT use, age at first live birth, menopausal status, age at menopause, alcohol consumption and body mass index (BMI). BCRAT predicts a woman's breast cancer risk based on her age and race/ethnicity, family history of breast cancer, personal history of breast biopsy and diagnosis of atypical hyperplasia, her age at her first live birth of a child and age at menarche. BMI, MHT and alcohol use are not included as predictors in BCRAT, and age at menarche and a diagnosis of atypical hyperplasia are not included in BC2013.

7.3 Comparison of model calibration

First, we applied the criteria presented in Chapter 6 to assess the calibration of each model.

Table 7.1 shows the observed number (O) of cancers, and the expected numbers (E) from both models with corresponding E/O ratios and 95% confidence intervals (CIs), overall and in various subgroups defined by selected covariates. Both models under-predicted the overall observed number of cases ($O = 252$) somewhat. The expected number of events were 231 from BC2013 and 238 from BCRAT; however, neither overall E/O ratio was statistically significantly different from one. Both models statistically significantly ($p < 0.05$) under-predicted the number of events for women with a diagnosis of benign breast disease, and BC2013 also significantly under-predicted the number of events for women with BMI ≥ 35 kg/m^2 and for women with one first degree relative with breast cancer. However, power to detect lack of calibration was limited for cells defined by covariate values that had few cases.

Table 7.2 gives the observed and expected events by deciles of risk for both models. The absolute risks of developing breast cancer were relatively low, reflecting the facts that the validation population was young (aged 50 to 55 years) and the projection interval was only five years long. For BC2013, risk estimates ranged from 0.63% to 4.29%, and for BCRAT from 0.63% to 8.65%. BC2013 overestimated the number of events in the lowest two deciles; for example, in the first decile group, the model predicted 14 events while 6 were observed, with $E/O = 2.31$. For BCRAT, the numbers of women falling into the risk decile groups were less balanced than for BC2013, because BCRAT only yields 108 total covariate patterns, resulting in many tied risk estimates. BCRAT overestimated the number of events in the lowest three deciles with E/O values of $1.20, 1.11$, and 1.66, and slightly under predicted risk in the high-risk deciles. BC2013 under-predicted risk in the high-risk deciles by more than BRCAT.

Letting $G = 10$ correspond to the decile groups, we computed the global test statistic in Equation (6.6), $Q = \sum_{g=1}^{G}(O^g - E^g)^2/E^g$, as $Q = 16.7$ for BC2013 and $Q = 13.4$ for BCRAT. Neither value exceeded the cutoff of $\chi^2_{10} = 18.31$ at the 0.05 level, indicating that both models were adequately calibrated overall.

We also assessed calibration by fitting a logistic regression model to observed outcomes (Equation (6.4)) with $\log\{R_k/(1-R_k)\}, k = 1, 2$ as the independent variable. The regression intercept and slope estimates were $\hat{\nu}_0 = 1.37$ ($p = 0.11$) and $\hat{\nu}_1 = 1.30$ ($p = 0.13$) for BC2013 and $\hat{\nu}_0 = 0.10$ ($p = 0.88$) and $\hat{\nu}_1 = 1.01$ ($p = 0.95$) for BCRAT. The fact that the intercepts are positive but not statistically significantly different from zero is consistent with slight underestimation of risk overall in both models. The estimated slope $\hat{\nu}_1 = 1.30$, though not statistically significantly different from 1.0, is consistent with underdispersion of risk estimates for BC2013, namely underestimation of high risks and overestimation of low risks, as in Table 7.2 and Figure 7.1.

Table 7.1: Comparison of observed (O) and expected (E) incident breast cancers and the corresponding 95% confidence intervals (CIs) based on 5-year predictions from BC2013 (Pfeiffer et al., 2013) and BCRAT (http://www.cancer.gov/bcrisktool) in women ages 50–55 in the Nurses' Health Study (NHS) validation cohort

		BC2013		BCRAT	
	O	**E**	**E/O (95% CI)**	**E**	**E/O (95% CI)**
All women	252	231	0.92 (0.72, 1.04)	238	0.94 (0.84, 1.07)
Variable					
Age at menarche					
< 12	59	53	0.90 (0.70, 1.16)	59	1.00 (0.77, 1.29)
$12 - 13$	146	136	0.93 (0.79, 1.09)	140	0.96 (0.81, 1.12)
≥ 14	47	42	0.89 (0.67, 1.19)	40	0.85 (0.64, 1.13)
BMI					
$< 25\ kg/m^2$	144	122	0.85 (0.72, 1.00)	130	0.90 (0.77, 1.06)
25 to $< 30\ kg/m^2$	77	69	0.89 (0.71, 1.12)	70	0.91 (0.73, 1.13)
30 to $< 35\ kg/m^2$	18	27	1.48 (0.93, 2.35)	26	1.43 (0.90, 2.27)
$\geq 35\ kg/m^2$	13	3	0.26 (0.15, 0.44)	12	0.95 (0.55, 1.64)
Benign breast disease					
No	93	105	1.13 (0.92, 1.38)	106	1.14 (0.93, 1.40)
Yes	159	126	0.79 (0.68, 0.93)	132	0.83 (0.71, 0.97)
# of first degree relatives with breast cancer					
0	208	200	0.96 (0.84, 1.10)	193	0.93 (0.81, 1.06)
1	43	30	0.69 (0.51, 0.93)	41	0.97 (0.72, 1.30)
2	1	1	1.18 (0.17, 8.39)	3	3.49 (0.49, 24.78)

These analyses indicate that both models are reasonably well calibrated in the NHS data. Many of the criteria for comparing risk models that we discuss below can be misleading unless the models being compared are well calibrated, namely $P(O = 1|R_i = r) \approx r, i = 1, 2$. We specifically address the implications of lack of calibration when we discuss the various criteria.

Table 7.2: Comparison of observed (O) and expected (E) incident breast cancers in the NHS validation cohort in deciles of risk computed from the BC2013 and BCRAT models

Decile	BC2013					BCRAT				
	Risk interval	**N**	**E**	**O**	**E/O**	**Risk interval**	**N**	**E**	**O**	**E/O**
1	[0.0063, 0.0088]	1707	14	6	2.31	[0.0063, 0, 0.0090]	1995	17	14	1.20
2	(0.0088, 0.0099]	1724	16	13	1.24	(0.0090, 0.0098]	1289	12	11	1.11
3	(0.0099, 0.0108]	1703	18	25	0.71	(0.0098, 0.0106]	2280	23	14	1.66
4	(0.0108, 0.0118]	1705	19	15	1.28	(0.0106, 0.0112]	1305	14	15	0.95
5	(0.0118, 0.0127]	1698	21	28	0.74	(0.0112, 0.0122]	1757	21	29	0.71
6	(0.0127, 0.0138]	1707	23	27	0.84	(0.0122, 0.0133]	1606	20	29	0.71
7	(0.0138, 0.0150]	1711	25	30	0.82	(0.0133, 0.0149]	1759	25	23	1.08
8	(0.0150, 0.0167]	1710	27	25	1.08	(0.0149, 0.0169]	1655	26	36	0.91
9	(0.0167, 0.0192]	1711	30	38	0.80	(0.0169, 0.0210]	1758	33	36	0.91
10	(0.0192, 0.0429]	1709	39	45	0.86	(0.0210, 0.0865]	1681	47	48	0.98

Each decile group contains N women, which can vary because of ties in risk.

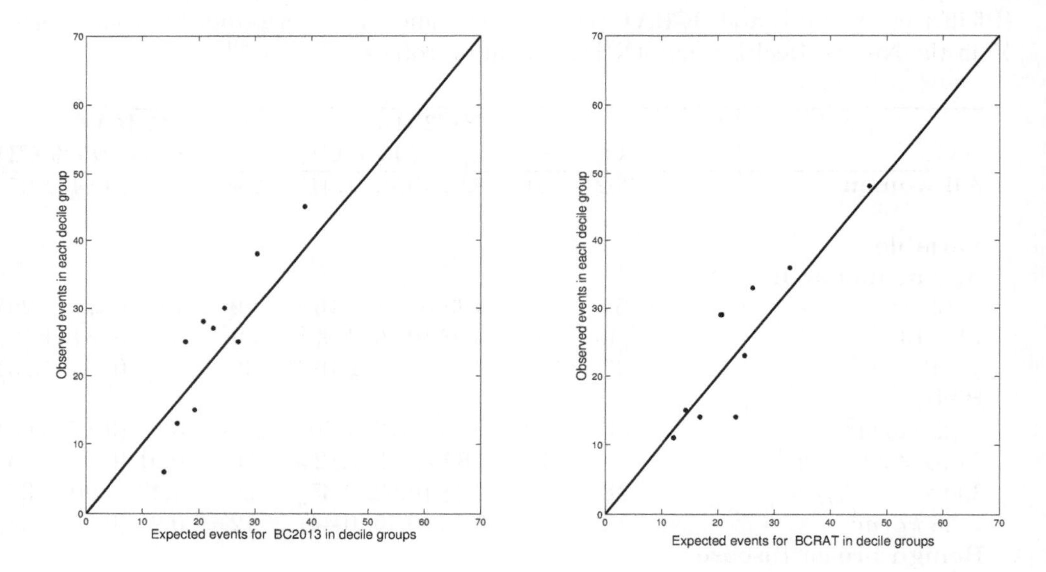

Figure 7.1: Calibration plots for BC2013 and BCRAT for incident breast cancer in the NHS validation cohort.

7.4 Model comparisons based on the difference in separate model-specific estimates of a criterion

The criteria used to characterize the performance of a single model in Chapter 6 can also be used to compare two models by computing the difference of estimates of the criterion from the two models. Each criterion can be estimated from the marginal distributions of risk for the separate models, but the two estimates are correlated because the same individuals in the validation sample contribute to each estimate; the estimated variance of the difference must take this correlation into account.

7.4.1 *Comparisons of predictive accuracy using the Brier and logarithmic scores*

Two widely used measures of predictive accuracy are the Brier and logarithmic scores, as discussed in Section 6.4.1. The mean square error (mean Brier score) was estimated from

$$\widehat{MSE} = n^{-1} \sum_{i=1}^{n} (O_i - r_i)^2 \tag{7.1}$$

as 0.0145017 for BC2013. The corresponding estimate for BCRAT was 0.0145001. To test whether the difference in the two estimates is statistically significant, one can perform a paired t-test on the n paired differences between the summands in Equation (7.1) based on BC2013 and based on BCRAT. The corresponding two-sided p-value was $p = 0.80$.

Similarly, the logarithmic score was estimated from

$$n^{-1} \sum_{i=1}^{n} \{-O_i \log(R_i) - (1 - O_i) \log(1 - R_i)\} \tag{7.2}$$

as 0.0758 for BC2013. The corresponding estimate for BCRAT was 0.0757, and the two-sided p-value based on the paired t-test was $p = 0.85$. Thus, neither model demonstrated statistically significantly better predictive accuracy based on these proper scores.

7.4.2 *Classification accuracy criteria based on single risk threshold*

As mentioned in Section 6.4.2, if there is a single clinical decision threshold, then one can compute various accuracy criteria based on this threshold, separately for the two models. The models will be compared by computing the differences between these estimated criteria. These comparisons depend on predictions $\hat{O}_i$ from model $i = 1, 2$ obtained as

$$\hat{O}_i = \begin{cases} 0 & \text{if } R_i \leq r^* \\ 1 & \text{if } R_i > r^*, \end{cases} \tag{7.3}$$

where r^* is a risk or decision threshold used to predict the actual outcome.

Given the decision rule in Equation (7.3), one can compare two risk prediction models using the summary measures in Section 6.4.2, including sensitivity, specificity, the positive predictive value (PPV), the negative predictive value (NPV) and the probability of correct classification (PCC), or its complement, the probability of misclassification (PMC). These quantities were computed as in Section 6.4.2 separately for models $i = 1, 2$ from the distributions of risk in the population (F_i), in cases (G_i), and in non-cases (K_i).

The American Society for Clinical Oncology concluded that premenopausal women and postmenopausal women with low risk of side effects and a 5-year projected risk $> r^* = 0.0166$ may benefit from chemoprevention (Visvanathan et al., 2009). Using this threshold, we categorized all n women as well as the women who developed breast cancer ("events" or "cases") and women who did not ("non-events" or "non-cases"), as shown in Table 7.3 for both BC2013 and BCRAT. Out of 252 women who developed breast cancer within 5 years of study baseline, only 84 had a BC2013 absolute risk estimate greater than 0.0166 (sensitivity = 0.333). Of the 16,833 women without breast cancer, 13,456 had BC2013 risks at or below that threshold (specificity = 0.799) (Tables 7.3 and 7.4). For BCRAT, only 88 of 252 cases had a risk greater than 0.0166 (sensitivity = 0.349), and of the 16,833 women without breast cancer, 13,285 had BCRAT risks at or below that threshold (specificity = 0.789).

Such computations can be extended to other accuracy measures (Table 7.4). Of 3,461 women with BC2013 risks above 0.0166, only 84 developed breast cancer ($\widehat{PPV}_1 = 84/3461 = 0.024$), whereas 13,456 of the 13,624 women with BC2013 risks at or below

Table 7.3: Categorization of women in the NHS validation cohort (Pfeiffer et al., 2013), ages 50 to 55 years at baseline, who experienced the event ("cases") during 5 years of follow-up and those who did not, based on 5-year absolute breast cancer risk estimates exceeding 1.66% for the BCRAT and BC2013 models

	≤ 1.66%	**> 1.66%**	**Total**
	5-year risk from BC2013		
n	13,624	3,461	17,085
Events	168	84	252
Non-events	13,456	3,377	16,833
Percentage with events(%)	1.23	2.43	1.47
	5-year risk from BCRAT		
n	13,449	3,636	17,085
Events	164	88	252
Non-events	13,285	3,548	16,833
Percentage with events(%)	1.22	2.42	1.47

Table 7.4: Accuracy measures for the absolute breast cancer risk estimates from the BC2013 and BCRAT models based on a 5-year absolute risk threshold $r^* = 0.0166$ for 50- to 55-year-old women in the NHS validation cohort

Measure	**BC2013**	**BCRAT**	
	Estimate (95% CI)	**Estimate (95% CI)**	**Difference (95% CI)**
PPV	0.024 (0.019, 0.030)	0.024 (0.020, 0.030)	-0.0001 (-0.0008, 0.0007)
NPV	0.988(0.986, 0.990)	0.988 (0.986, 0.990)	0.0001 (-0.0009, 0.0012)
PCC	0.793(0.786, 0.799)	0.783 (0.777, 0.789)	-0.0098 (-0.0159, -0.0037)
PMC	0.208(0.201, 0.214)	0.217(0.211, 0.224)	0.0098 (0.0037, 0.0159)
Sens	0.333 (0.28, 0.40)	0.349(0.29, 0.41)	0.0159 (-0.041, 0.073)
Spec	0.799 (0.79, 0.81)	0.789 (0.78, 0.80)	-0.0102 (-0.017, -0.004))

Abbreviations: PPV= Positive predictive value; NPV= Negative predictive value; PCC= Probability of correct classification; PMC= Probability of misclassification; Sens= sensitivity; Spec=specificity.
95% confidence intervals were calculated assuming binomial variation and conditional on the denominators for the estimates. Confidence intervals for the differences were the estimates ±1.96 times the bootstrap estimate of standard error of the difference from $B = 1000$ bootstrap replications.

the threshold remained free of breast cancer ($\widehat{NPV}_1 = 0.988$). The overall misclassification rate was $100 \times \widehat{PMC}_1 = 100(3,377 + 168)/17,085 = 20.8\%$. For BCRAT, of 3,636 women with risks above 0.0166, only 88 developed breast cancer ($\widehat{PPV}_2 = 88/3636 = 0.024$), whereas 13,285 of the 13,449 women with BCRAT risks at or below the threshold remained free of breast cancer ($\widehat{NPV}_2 = 13285/13624 = 0.988$). The overall misclassification rate was $100 \times \widehat{PMC}_2 = 100(3,548 + 164)/17,085 = 21.7\%$.

Thus, both models had the same PPV and NPV. BCRAT had a slightly lower PCC and consequently a higher PMC. Both models had low sensitivity, but it was slightly higher for BCRAT, while specificity only differed by a single percentage point.

These comparisons of accuracy measures are only meaningful if both models are well calibrated. If one of the models systematically over or underestimates risk, then accuracy measures can convey misleading information. For example, a model that consistently overestimates risk would tend to have higher sensitivity and lower specificity. The corresponding biases for PPV, NPV, PCC, and PMC are more complex to evaluate because they depend on the amount by which sensitivity is increased, on the amount by which specificity is decreased, and on $P(O = 1)$.

Let M be one of the criteria $PPV, NPV, PCC, PMC, Sens$ and $Spec$. One can test for a difference between models based on the difference in estimates of M via

$$T_M = \frac{n\{\hat{M}^1 - \hat{M}^2\}^2}{\hat{V}_{M^1-M^2}}, \tag{7.4}$$

where $n^{-1}\hat{V}_{M^1-M^2}$ is the estimated variance of $(\hat{M}^1 - \hat{M}^2)$.

Under the null hypothesis of no difference in the criterion M between the two models, T_M has a χ_1^2 distribution. As the same data are used to obtain $\hat{M}^1$ and $\hat{M}^2$, the measures are not independent and their correlation needs to be accommodated in the variance computation. If one has computed the influence function for each measure, the correlation is accommodated by computing the empirical variance of the difference of the influences. Alternatively, one can bootstrap the differences to estimate $n^{-1}\hat{V}_{M^1-M^2}$.

Based on the statistic in Equation (7.4) with the variances estimated by bootstrap with B=1,000 replications, the two models differed statistically significantly for PCC ($p =$ 0.0027), PMC ($p = 0.0027$) and specificity ($p = 0.0022$). Equivalence of sensitivity and specificity of the two models could also be tested with a McNemar test for correlated proportions (McNemar, 1947). From the McNemar test, there was no statistically significant evidence for a difference in sensitivity for the two models ($p = 0.586$), but the 1% difference in specificity (Table 7.4) was indeed statistically significant($p = 0.002$). These findings are consistent with the confidence intervals for the differences in Table 7.4.

7.4.3 Comparisons based on the receiver operating characteristic (ROC) curve

The receiver operating characteristic curve describes the pairs (sensitivity, 1-specificity) for all choices of thresholds (Section 6.4.3). It is common practice to compare the discriminatory ability of two risk prediction models through a summary measure of the ROC curve, such as the area under the curve (AUC) or partial area under the curve ($pAUC$). One computes the ROC summary measure for each model and the difference (e.g., ΔAUC or $\Delta pAUC$), with confidence intervals. The $pAUC$ is designed to exclude regions of unacceptably poor specificity (Pepe, 2003). Because the ROC depends only on the distribution of risks in cases and non-cases, it can be computed from case-control data as well as from cohort data. Likewise, functionals of the ROC, such as AUC and ΔAUC can be computed from case-control or cohort data.

One can derive confidence intervals and standard errors for ΔAUC and $\Delta pAUC$ from the bootstrap distribution of the estimated differences. For cohort data, one resamples the cohort with replacement. For case-control data, one resamples cases and controls separately with replacement. To test significance, one can use e.g., a Wald statistic, computed by dividing the observed difference by its standard error and comparing it's value to the standard normal distribution to report a p-value. Non-parametric methods for comparing two $pAUC$s were given by Wieand et al. (1989) and by Zhang et al. (2002).

In the NHS data example, $\widehat{AUC}$ (with bootstrap standard errors based on 1000 bootstrap repetitions in parentheses) was $\widehat{AUC}_1 = 0.617(0.0167)$ for BC2013 and $\widehat{AUC}_2 =$ 0.623(0.0173) for BCRAT, resulting in $\widehat{\Delta AUC} = \widehat{AUC}_1 - \widehat{AUC}_2 = -0.006(0.0159)$ with a bootstrap 95%CI= $(-0.0282, 0.0355)$ and a bootstrap p-value = 0.968 for the null hypothesis $H_0 : \Delta AUC = 0$. There is thus no statistically significant evidence that BC2013 has better or worse discriminatory ability than BRCAT in these validation data.

The nonparametric estimate of the ROC curve depends only on the ranks of the risks in the combined sample of cases and non-cases. Thus, monotone transformations of the risks do not affect the ROC curve or functionals of it. In particular the AUC is not affected by miscalibration that is induced by a monotone transformation of the true risks. Moreover, transforming the risk estimates using any monotone transformation, including re-calibration based on the Cox regression intercepts and slopes, does not impact the AUC comparison. Note, however, that $sens(r^*)$ and $spec(r^*)$ are not functionals of the ROC curve alone because they depend on r^*, which is not identifiable from the ROC curve. Likewise $pAUC$ depends on p.

Unlike functionals of the ROC curve, like AUC, which can be estimated from case-control data, the quantities PPV, NPV, PCC and PMC can only be estimated from cohort data, unless $P(O = 1)$ is known from other sources, and they are sensitive to miscalibration.

7.4.4 Integrated discrimination improvement (IDI) and mean risk difference

The mean risk difference (Pepe et al., 2014) for a given risk model can be estimated as the mean risk in cases less the mean risk in non-cases (also called the "Yates slope" (Yates, 1982)). Thus, the mean risk difference can be estimated from case-control data as well as from cohort data. Pencina et al. (2008) proposed the integrated discrimination improvement (IDI), which is equivalent to the difference in mean risk differences between two models, as a criterion for comparing models. Recall that $sens(r^*) = P(R > r^*|O = 1)$ and $1 - spec(r^*) = P(R > r^*|O = 0)$. Pencina et al. (2008) defined the integrated sensitivity and integrated specificity as

$$IS = \int_0^1 P(R > r^*|O = 1)dr^* = \int_0^1 1 - G(r^*)dr^* = E(R|O = 1)$$

and

$$IP = \int_0^1 \{1 - P(R > r^*|O = 0)\}dr^* = \int_0^1 1 - K(r^*)dr^* = E(R|O = 0).$$

Recall that G and K denote the distribution of risk in cases and non-cases, respectively, as defined in Equations (6.11) and (6.12). Using the above expressions, Pencina et al. (2008) defined the integrated discrimination improvement (IDI) as

$$IDI = (IS_2 - IS_1) - (IP_2 - IP_1).$$

The IDI can be estimated from cohort data by computing the mean difference of the predicted probabilities in the cases and non-cases separately,

$$\widehat{IDI} = \frac{\sum_{i=1}^n (r_i^1 - r_i^2)O_i}{\sum_{i=1}^n O_i} - \frac{\sum_{i=1}^n (r_i^1 - r_i^2)(1 - O_i)}{\sum_{i=1}^n (1 - O_i)}.$$

For case-control data these expressions are replaced by means of $r^1 - r^2$ in cases and controls respectively. However, one difficulty in interpreting the IDI is that in low risk populations it tends to be very small. For example, in the NHS validation cohort breast cancer data, the mean risk from BC2013 less that from BCRAT in the 252 cases was -0.0011, and in the 16,833 controls it was -0.0004, resulting in $\widehat{IDI} = -0.0007$.

One can test the null hypothesis $H_0 : IDI = 0$ with the statistic

$$T = \frac{\widehat{IDI}}{\{(\widehat{se}_e)^2 + (\widehat{se}_{ne})^2\}^{1/2}},$$

where $\widehat{se}_e$ is the estimated standard error of paired differences of risk predictions from the new and old models across all case subjects and $\widehat{se}_{ne}$ is the corresponding estimate for subjects without events. With case-control sampling, the mean risk difference among cases is independent of that among controls, and T has an asymptotic standard normal distribution. The same asymptotic distribution holds for T in cohort data, as follows from an analysis of the four summations in the equation that defines $\widehat{IDI}$. For our breast cancer model example, $T = -1.89$ with an asymptotic two-sided p-value $p = 0.0588$ and no rejection of the null hypothesis.

Hilden and Gerds (2014) noted that IDI can yield misleading results, even when estimated with independent test data, because a miscalibrated model can appear superior to the correct model. Their simulated examples showed that IDI analyses are particularly sensitive to miscalibration, and they suggested not to rely on the IDI for model comparisons.

7.4.5 Comparing two risk models based on PCF, PNF, iPCF, or iPNF

In Section 6.5 we presented criteria for assessing usefulness of a model for implementing a "high risk" prevention strategy. One criterion was the proportion of cases who are included in the proportion p of individuals in the population at highest risk, $PCF(p)$. A second criterion was the proportion needed to follow, $PNF(q)$, namely the proportion of the general population at highest risk that one needs to follow in order that a proportion q of cases will be followed. We also considered integrated versions of these criteria, $iPCF$ and $iPNF$. We showed how to estimate these four criteria from various observational study designs, including cohort and case-control data, and, under the additional assumption of a well calibrated model, from only the model-based risk estimates in a cohort.

Pfeiffer and Gail (2011) and Pfeiffer (2013) also proposed test statistics to compare two risk models, both of which were applied to the same validation population. To test whether, for fixed p, $PCF^1 = PCF^2$, or for a fixed q, $PNF^1 = PNF^2$, or $iPCF^1 = iPCF^2$, or $iPNF^1 = iPNF^2$, using correlated risk estimates (r^1, r^2), one can use the test statistics

$$T_{PCF}(p) = \frac{n\{\widehat{PCF^1}(p) - \widehat{PCF^2}(p)\}^2}{\hat{V}_{PCF}} \text{ and } T_{PNF}(q) = \frac{n\{\widehat{PNF^1}(q) - \widehat{PNF^2}(q)\}^2}{\hat{V}_{PNF}}, \quad (7.5)$$

or

$$T_{iPCF}(p) = \frac{n\{\widehat{iPCF^1} - \widehat{iPCF^2}\}^2}{\hat{V}_{iPCF}} \text{ and } T_{iPNF} = \frac{n\{\widehat{iPNF^1} - \widehat{iPNF^2}\}^2}{\hat{V}_{iPNF}}, \quad (7.6)$$

where $\hat{V}/n$ are consistent estimates of the variance of the difference of the estimates.

Asymptotically all test statistics in (7.5) and (7.6) have a central χ_1^2 distribution under H_0. Under the alternative, the non-centrality parameters for the test statistics are $\delta_{PCF} = n(PCF^1 - PCF^2)^2/V_{PCF}$, $\delta_{PNF} = n(PNF^1 - PNF^2)^2/V_{PNF}$, $\delta_{iPCF} = n(iPCF^1 - iPCF^2)^2/V_{iPCF}$, and $\delta_{iPNF} = n(iPNF^1 - iPNF^2)^2/V_{iPNF}$, respectively. The variances for the test statistics can be computed based on the respective influence functions ψ^{R_1} and ψ^{R_2} for models 1 and 2 as $V = Var(\psi^{R_1} - \psi^{R_2})$, or alternatively, by using a bootstrap variance estimate.

Estimates of PCF, PNF, and $iPCF$ are shown for BC2013 and BCRAT in Table 7.5. If one screens the $100 \times p = 10\%$ of the population at highest risk, one would detect $\widehat{PCF} = 17.9\%$ of cases with BC2013, and 19.0% of cases with BCRAT. To detect $100 \times q = 90\%$ of cases, one would need to screen 77.2% of the population at highest risk with BC2013 and 80.8% with BCRAT. The integrated PCF curve was $iPCF = 0.618$ for BCRAT and $iPCF = 0.615$ for BC2013, values very slightly less than the corresponding AUC values.

For none of the criteria in Table 7.5 did we observe a statistically significant ($p < 0.05$) difference in performance between the two models, based on tests in (7.5) and (7.6).

Table 7.5: Estimates of $iPCF$, PCF, and PNF based on (R, O) data from the NHS validation cohort, where R is the 5-year risk projection for 50- to 55-year-old women from BC2013 and BCRAT, and where O is the observed case status

	Estimate for	
	BC2013	**BCRAT**
	$\widehat{iPCF}_{(R,O)} = 0.615(0.017)$	$\widehat{iPCF}_{(R,O)} = 0.618(0.017)$
% screened (100 × p)		
10%	$\widehat{PCF}_{(R,O)} = 0.179(0.025)$	$\widehat{PCF}_{(R,O)} = 0.190(0.026)$
20%	$\widehat{PCF}_{(R,O)} = 0.325(0.038)$	$\widehat{PCF}_{(R,O)} = 0.333(0.035)$
% cases to be captured (100 × q) in screen		
90%	$\widehat{PNF}_{(R,O)} = 0.772(0.017)$	$\widehat{PNF}_{(R,O)} = 0.808(0.038)$
80%	$\widehat{PNF}_{(R,O)} = 0.654(0.027)$	$\widehat{PNF}_{(R,O)} = 0.627(0.044)$

Standard errors (in parentheses) were based on 1000 bootstrap repetitions.

7.4.6 Comparisons based on expected loss or expected benefit

Most of the previous criteria for comparing risk models are general and can be applied without specifying details of the decision problem or intervention that would be affected by information from a risk model. For example, measures of accuracy, such as AUC or PPV can be applied quite generally. Measures such as PCF and PNF are also quite general, although one frequently has an idea of what constitutes an acceptable PCF or PNF. In this section, we discuss criteria for comparing risk models that are based on the expected losses for a specific intervention. Information from the better risk model reduces the expected loss (or increases the expected utility) more than information from the inferior risk model.

As an example, suppose we want to help women aged 50–59 decide whether to take tamoxifen to prevent breast cancer. From data in Fisher et al. (1998) and Gail et al. (1999a), the expected rates per 10^5 women-years in the absence of tamoxifen are 246.6 for invasive breast cancer, 101.6 for hip fracture, 81.4 for endometrial cancer, 110.0 for stroke and 50.0 for pulmonary embolism. In the presence of tamoxifen, these rates are 125.8, 55.9, 326.4, 174.9, and 150.5, respectively. The aggregated non-breast cancer rates are 343.0 and 707.7 in the absence and presence of tamoxifen respectively. These rates of life-threatening events can be used to compute losses (costs), defined as the expected number of life-threatening events. These costs are presented in Table 7.6, a cross-classification of costs by use of tamoxifen (designated by $r>t$, namely a risk r exceeding the threshold for administration of tamoxifen, t) and by whether breast cancer would occur ($O = 1$) or not ($O = 0$). The administration of tamoxifen in a person destined to develop breast cancer is assumed to cut the risk by the factor 0.51 (Fisher et al., 1998).

From this table the net benefit of giving tamoxifen to a case (O =1) is B_{case} = 100,343 − 51,707.7 = 48,635.8, and the net cost from giving tamoxifen to a non-case is $B_{non-case}$ =707.7-343=364.7. From Equation (6.29), the optimal threshold is t^* =364.7/(364.7+48,635.8)=744.3 per 10^5(see Gail (2009b)), or $t^* = 5 \times 744.3 \times 10^{-5}$ = 0.03722, expressed as a 5-year risk. For a risk model R, the expected loss at this threshold is given by Equation (6.30), where π is the probability of breast cancer, $C_{FN} = 100,343$,

Table 7.6: Costs (expected number of life-threatening events per 100,000) cross-classified by the presence or absence of breast cancer and on whether tamoxifen is given

Decision whether to give tamoxifen based on risk threshold, t	**Breast cancer status if no tamoxifen**	
	O = 1	**O = 0**
r > t	51,000+707.7=51,707.7	707.7
r ≤ t	100,000+343=100,343	343

and $C_{FP} = 707.7$. Using data from the NHS on risk estimates r_i and observed breast cancer outcomes, O_i for the ith cohort member, $i = 1, 2, \ldots, n$, we can estimate the expected loss with this risk model for decisions as

$$\hat{\hat{C}}_{\min} = n^{-1}\sum_{i=1}^{n}\{I(r_i > t^*, O_i = 1) \times 51{,}707.7 + I(r_i > t^*, O_i = 0) \times 707.7 + I(r_i \leq t^*, O_i = 1) \times 100{,}343 + I(r_i \leq t^*, O_i = 0) \times 343\} \tag{7.7}$$

From this formula we calculated $\hat{\hat{C}}_{\min} = 1818.17$ for BC2013 and $\hat{\hat{C}}_{\min} = 1808.90$ for BCRAT. Thus, in 100,000 women like the 50- to 55-year-old women in NHS, one would expect 9.27 fewer life-threatening events from using BCRAT to decide which women should receive tamoxifen, compared to using BC2013. To test whether this difference in expected loss is statistically significant, one can perform a paired t-test on the n differences computed by subtracting the summand in Equation (7.7) computed with risk model BCRAT from the summand computed with risk model BC2013 on the same woman. In this example, the two-sided p-value was 0.8459, indicating no significant difference between the two models. Note that the expected losses are expressed in terms of expected life-threatening events in one year in a population of 100,000 women in their fifties, but the risk thresholds in Equation (7.7) can be expressed in units of 5-year or 1-year risk without changing the result, so long as the risk projections are changed accordingly.

This example illustrates how two risk models can be compared in terms of expected risk when the costs can be specified for a specific decision problem. Often the costs are hard to specify, in which case the optimal risk threshold for intervention is not precisely known. This led Vickers and Elkin (2006) to define the "decision curve." The decision curve plots the "net benefit" in Equation (6.36) against the corresponding threshold, t, expressed as percent, namely $100 \times t$. The net benefit can be estimated from a cohort study such as the NHS by

$$\widehat{NB}(t) = n^{-1}\sum_{i=1}^{n}[I(r_i > t, O_i = 1) - \{t/(1-t)\}I(r_i > t, O_i = 0)]. \tag{7.8}$$

Again we express t as a 5-year absolute risk of breast cancer. For each fixed t, the one can test for a difference in net benefits with a paired t-test on the n differences computed by subtracting the summand in Equation (7.8) computed with risk model BCRAT from the summand computed with risk model BC2013 on the same woman. For example, for $t = 0.0166$, a threshold on the drug label for the use of tamoxifen to prevent breast cancer, the estimated net benefits were 0.0016452 for BCRAT and 0.0015801 for BC2013. The difference in net benefits, 0.000065, was not statistically significant, however (p= 0.8801). Figure 7.2 shows the estimated net benefit plots for BCRAT (dashed line) and BC2013 (solid line). The two curves are virtually identical. $\widehat{NB}(t)$ can be regarded as a stochastic

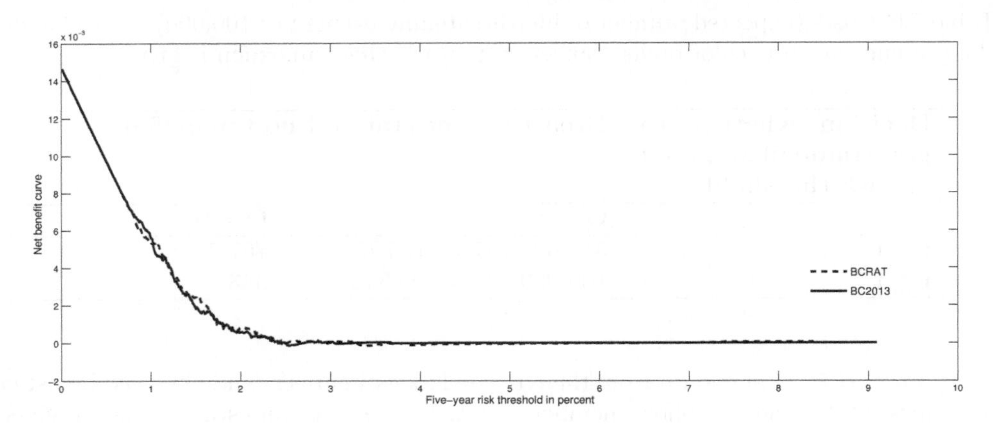

Figure 7.2: Net benefit plots for BCRAT and BC2013 for 50- to 55-year-old women from the independent NHS validation cohort.

process in t whose covariance is easily calculated from Equation (7.8). This approach can be used to put simultaneous confidence intervals on each decision curve and on their difference.

7.5 Joint distributions of risk

The joint risks computed from the two models (R_1, R_2) have empirical joint distributions $\hat{F}(r_1, r_2)$ in the general validation population, $\hat{G}(r_1, r_2)$ in cases, and $\hat{K}(r_1, r_2)$ in non-cases. The criteria in Section 7.4 can be estimated from the margins of these distributions, but to compute covariances of criteria estimates for the two models, the joint distributions are needed. It can be instructive to examine correlations between R_1 and R_2 (or transformations of them like logit(R) or $\log\{-\log(1-R)\}$). Such correlations say nothing about calibration, but if R_1 and R_2 are highly correlated, the models probably have similar AUC values. After calibration, the two highly correlated models also probably yield similar predictions. On the other hand, if the correlations are low, it is possible that the predictive performance of either model can be improved by combining predictors from the two models. Figure 7.3 shows a scatterplot of 5-year BCRAT risk versus 5-year BC2013 risk for women aged 50–55 years from the NHS cohort. Although the agreement is good for the bulk of the observations, some larger risks from BCRAT correspond to women with a strong family history and are higher than those from BC2013. The Pearson correlations were 0.633 for the risks R in Figure 7.3, 0.677 for logit(R), and 0.677 for $\log\{-\log(1-R)\}$. These high correlations are consistent with the close agreement of the AUC values estimated for these two models.

7.6 Risk stratification tables and reclassification indices

The criteria for model comparisons in Section 7.4 could be estimated separately from the data for each risk model, namely from the margins of $\hat{F}(r_1, r_2)$, $\hat{G}(r_1, r_2)$, and $\hat{K}(r_1, r_2)$. We now consider some criteria that can only be estimated from the joint risks at the individual level. These criteria do not have a "single model analogue."

Cook et al. (2006) and Cook (2007) proposed criteria based on risk stratification tables. To construct a risk stratification table, one first defines risk categories that are clinically relevant, such as [0,1%), [1%,1.66%], (1.66%,2.5%), and $\geq$ 2.5% for 5-year absolute breast cancer risk (Table 7.7). These categories were partly based on the risk threshold 1.66% recommended by the American Society for Clinical Oncology (ASCO) (Visvanathan et al., 2009).

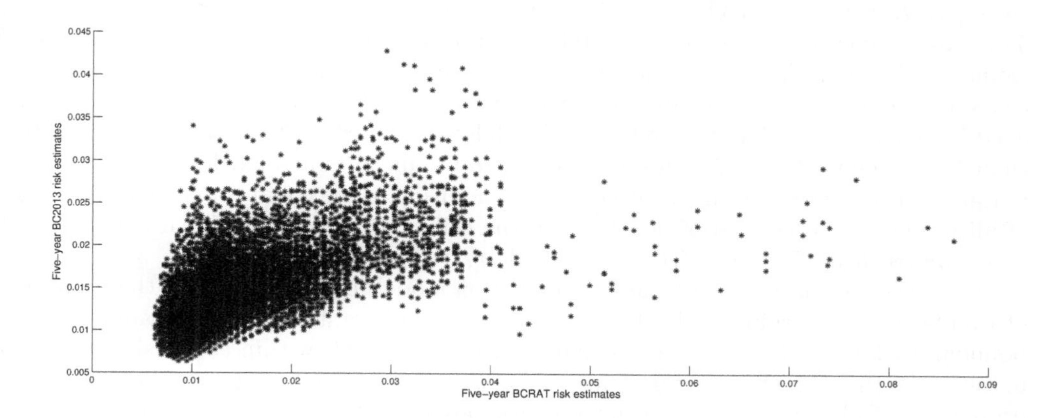

Figure 7.3: Scatterplot of 5-year absolute risk estimates from BCRAT and BC2013 for 50- to 55-year-old women in the NHS validation cohort data.

Table 7.7: Risk stratification based on 5-year absolute breast cancer risk estimates from the BCRAT and BC2013 (Pfeiffer et al., 2013) models for women in the NHS validation cohort (Pfeiffer et al., 2013), ages 50- to 55-years at baseline

5-year risk from BCRAT		**5-year risk from BC2013**				
		0 to < 1%	1 to ≤1.66%	> 1.66 to <2.5%	≥2.5%	Total
0 to < 1%	n	2,291	1,675	114	2	4,082
	Events[a]	13	16	1	0	30
	Non-events	2,278	1,659	113	2	4,052
	Prop. Events (%)	0.57	0.96	0.88	0.00	0.73
1% to ≤1.66%	n	1387	6632	1299	49	9367
	Events	10	100	24	0	134
	Non-events	1,377	6,532	1,275	49	9,233
	Prop. Events (%)	0.72	1.51	1.85	0.00	1.43
> 1.66% to <2.5%	n	9	1,522	1,120	78	2,729
	Events	0	27	38	0	65
	Non-events	9	1,495	1,082	78	2,664
	Prop. Events (%)	0.00	1.77	3.39	0.00	2.38
≥2.5%	n	1	107	598	201	907
	Events	0	2	13	8	23
	Non-events	1	105	585	193	884
	Prop. Events (%)	0.00	1.87	2.17	3.98	2.54
Total	n	3,688	9,936	3,131	330	17,085
	Events	23	145	76	8	252
	Non-events	3,665	9,791	3,055	322	16,833
	Prop. Events (%)	0.62	1.46	2.43	2.42	1.47

[a]Events correspond to women who developed breast cancer (cases) and non-events to those who did not (non-cases). "Prop. Events (%)" is the percentage of cases in each cell.

Each interior cell in the risk stratification table contains the number of women with joint risks (R_1, R_2) from BCRAT and BC2013 that fall into the cross-classified risk categories. The cross-tabulations are done separately for all n women in the validation population, for women with events (cases), and for women without events (non-cases). The percentages of cases in each interior cell are labeled "Prop. Events(%)". For example, of the 17,085 women aged 50 to 55 years at baseline in the NHS validation cohort, 2,291 had joint risks each less than 1%, of whom 13 (0.57%) were cases. The rows and columns labeled "Total" show the marginal proportions of women with events, in addition to the count totals. The proportions of all women, of cases, and of non-cases in the cells and margins of this table can be also be computed from $\hat{F}(r_1, r_2)$, $\hat{G}(r_1, r_2)$, and $\hat{K}(r_1, r_2)$ respectively.

To assess the calibration of the risk prediction models one can compare the proportions of events in the margins of Table 7.7 with the corresponding row and column category boundaries. For BCRAT, the proportions of observed events within each risk category are in the far-right "Total" column. They agree well with the row category boundaries; the proportion of observed events within the risk category of 0% to less than 1% was 0.73%, which falls inside the risk category. Similarly, the proportions of events for the risk category of 1% to 1.66%, 1.67% to 2.5%, and greater or equal to 2.5% were 1.43%, 2.38% and 2.54%, indicating that BCRAT is well calibrated in this validation dataset. The new BC2013 model shows some evidence of lack of calibration. The observed proportions of events listed in the last row of Table 7.7 are 0.62%, 1.46%, 2.43 %, and 2.42%. While the first three values fell well within the category boundaries, the mean BC2013 risk in the largest risk category is lower than 2.5%, reflecting that true risk among those at highest risk is underestimated by the BC2013 model. Equations (6.6) and (6.7) provide formal tests of calibration based on the observed and expected events in these marginal categories.

Janes et al. (2008) warn that the interior cells of the table may give misleading information on calibration. For example, if model 2 contains factors not in model 1 and model 2 has high risks in some cells because of those factors, then model 1 may appear to be mis-calibrated in those cells, which constitute a subpopulation, even though model 1 is well calibrated in the entire population and satisfies the definition of good calibration with respect to its risk factors, $P(O = 1|r_1) = r_1$.

BCRAT and BC2013 in Table 7.7 are not nested models. Suppose instead of BC2013, we considered a model 2 that was identical to BCRAT except that it had an additional marker. Then BCRAT (model 1) would be nested in model 2. Although the performance of model 2, reflected in the bottom totals of the risk stratification table are of primary interest, one might want to investigate the performance of model 2 in a subset of the population with intermediate risk from model 1. For example if the marker was expensive, one might only want to use it if it were informative in the segment of the population for which model 1 gave non-definitive intermediate risk estimates. Looking at the distributions of women and events within rows of the risk stratification table could be useful in this context.

Risk stratification tables were originally proposed for use with cohort data (Cook et al., 2006; Cook, 2007). However, some authors cross-classify case-control data instead. Although the joint distributions of risks amoung cases and among non-cases are valid in such tables, corresponding to $\hat{G}(r_1, r_2)$, and $\hat{K}(r_1, r_2)$, the population totals obtained by adding cases to controls do not reflect the general population and are usually greatly enriched in cases. In particular, tests of calibration from risk stratification of case-control data are misleading.

We turn next to criteria for comparing two models that depend on joint risks (R_1, R_2), either as shown in risk stratification tables or as continuous versions based on $\hat{F}(r_1, r_2)$, $\hat{G}(r_1, r_2)$, and $\hat{K}(r_1, r_2)$.

7.6.1 Net reclassification improvement (NRI)

To improve upon the ΔAUC, Pencina et al. (2008) proposed a novel measure for dichotomous outcomes, the net reclassification improvement (NRI), to quantify the improvement in risk prediction offered by including new information, such as a new marker into a risk model. While the NRI has been immensely popular in the medical literature, several authors (e.g., Kerr et al., 2014; Pepe et al., 2015, 2014) have pointed out limitations and pitfalls of this measure that we also address in this section.

Assume that risks predicted from two models are cross-classified based on some clinically meaningful risk thresholds as in a risk stratification table. Let events be those with the outcome of interest (cases, $O = 1$) and non-events be those without the outcome of interest (controls, $O = 0$), and define "upward movement" (*up*) as a change into higher risk category based on the second (new) model and "downward movement" (*down*) as a change to a lower risk category. Pencina et al. (2008) defined the NRI (see also Kerr et al. (2014)) as

$$\begin{aligned} NRI =& NRI_e + NRI_{ne} \\ &\equiv \{P(up|O=1) - P(down|O=1)\} + \{P(down|O=0) - P(up|O=0)\} \end{aligned} \tag{7.9}$$

where

$$P(up|O=i) = \frac{\#\text{ in group }(O=i)\text{ moving up}}{\sum_{i=1}^{N} I(O=i)}, i = 0, 1,$$

and where $P(down|O = i)$ is defined similarly. The NRI can be interpreted as the net change in the proportion of subjects assigned to a more appropriate risk category under the new model (Kerr et al., 2014). The quantities NRI_e and NRI_{ne} are, respectively, the net change in the proportion of cases assigned to a higher risk category and the net change in the proportion of non-cases assigned to a lower risk category by the new model, R_2. From Equation (7.9) it is easy to see that the maximum value of the NRI is 2. Thus, although the NRI combines four proportions, it cannot be interpreted as a proportion itself. The NRI is frequently misinterpreted as "the proportion of patients reclassified to a more appropriate risk category" (Kerr et al., 2014; Pepe et al., 2014). The proportion of patients reclassified to a more appropriate risk category is instead given by $P(up, O = 1) + P(down, O = 0)$.

For our data example, we calculate the NRI with BCRAT regarded as the old (model 1) and BC2013 as the new model 2. Based on the risk thresholds in Table 7.7, the $NRI_e = (16+1+0+24+0)/252 - (10+0+27+0+0+2+13)/252 = -0.0437$ and $NRI_{ne} = (1377+9+1495+1+105+585)/16833 - (1659+113+2+1275+49+78)/16833 = 0.0235$; thus $NRI = -0.0201$.

If there are only two risk categories in the risk stratification table, $NRI_e = sens(R_2) - sens(R_1) = \Delta sens$, and $NRI_{ne} = spec(R_2) - spec(R_1) = \Delta spec$. These values quantify how much model R_2 improves risk predictions for cases and controls respectively.

Kerr et al. (2014) considered a "population-weighted net reclassification index", $NRI(\rho) = \rho NRI_e + (1-\rho) NRI_{ne}$, where ρ denotes the prevalence of the outcome in the population. However, the authors do not recommend using $NRI(\rho)$ or NRI, as information is lost when NRI_e and NRI_{ne} are combined into a single number.

Assuming independence between risks in cases and non-cases, we can test the null hypothesis H_0: $NRI = 0$ based on properties of the multinomial distribution with the test statistic

$$T = \frac{\widehat{NRI}}{\left\{ \frac{\hat{P}(up|O=1)+\hat{P}(down|O=1)}{\sum_i O_i} + \frac{\hat{P}(down|O=0)+\hat{P}(down|O=0)}{\sum_i (1-O_i)} \right\}^{1/2}},$$

which has an asymptotic normal distribution. For our example, $T = -0.0201/0.0386 = -0.521$ which corresponds to two-sided p = 0.602; thus, we do not reject the null hypothesis of no net reclassification improvement.

The NRI is sensitive to model mis-calibration. To illustrate this point we use an example presented in Gail (2009b). Suppose that a well-calibrated baseline risk model R_1 has risks distributed uniformly on the interval [0, 0.1] in control subjects and on the interval [0, 0.2] in cases and that there is only one risk threshold at risk 0.2. Then, the sensitivity is 0 and the specificity is 1.0. Suppose a new poorly calibrated model R_2 adds 0.05 to all risk estimates, thus shifting the apparent risk distributions to be uniform on the interval [0.05, 0.15] in control subjects and on the interval [0.05, 0.25] in cases and yielding a new average risk in the entire population that is 0.05 above the true average risk. The new "sensitivity" is then 5(0.25 - 0.20) = 0.25 and the "specificity" remains 1.0. Thus, the NRI=(0.25 - 0) + (1.0 - 1.0) = 0.25 is large, even though R_2 is badly calibrated and is no more discriminating than R_1. Indeed, the AUC is 0.75 for both models and thus $\Delta AUC = 0$.

The NRI has also been criticized because the risk categories may not be appropriate for clinical decisions and because the NRI weights each type of classification change equally, without regard to clinical consequences (Vickers et al., 2009). For example a change in risk estimate among intermediate risk categories or among low risk categories might have less impact on patient management than a change from intermediate to high risk categories. Weighting to take costs of mis-classifications into account has been recommended instead.

7.6.2 Extensions of NRI

To allow for varying costs in the two-category setting, Pencina et al. (2011) defined a weighted NRI, namely $wNRI$. Let s_1 be the savings from identifying a case as high risk and s_2 the savings from identifying a non-cases as low risk. The quantity s_1 captures the adverse events that are avoided by labeling a person destined to have an event as high risk, and s_2 captures the savings (adverse events, money) from allowing a non-case to avoid unnecessary treatment. The "weighted net reclassification index" ($wNRI$) is the average savings per person, computed as $wNRI = s_1 NRI_e + s_2 NRI_{ne} = s_1 \Delta sens + s_2 \Delta spec$. Setting $B_{case} = s_1$ and $B_{non-case} = s_2$, we note that $wNRI$ is not equivalent to the reduction in expected losses from using model 2 (see Equation (6.35)) for the fixed threshold used to define the risk stratification table, because $wNRI$ does not take the prevalence of disease into account.

A limitation of the definition of the NRI, and reclassification tables in general, is that in many fields of application there are no clinically well established or relevant risk thresholds. To address this issue, Pencina et al. (2011) proposed a category-free extension of the NRI, the continuous NRI, or $cNRI$, given by

$$cNRI = P(R_2 > R_1 | O = 1) - P(R_2 > R_1 | O = 0). \tag{7.10}$$

$cNRI$ is estimated by simply computing the mean of the indicator function $I(r_i^2 > r_i^1), i = 1, \ldots, n$ for cases and noncases separately. For BCRAT and BC2013, $cNRI = 0.454 - 0.468 = -0.014$.

The $cNRI$, like the NRI, does not take the costs of misclassification into account. Also, it is based on within person differences in risk estimates that may not reflect performance at the population (marginal) level (Kerr et al., 2014).

Recent work shows that even when evaluated on independent validation data, $cNRI$, like IDI, can lead to false positive results. In simulations in which un-informative markers were added to a base model 1 in training data and the models were then compared in independent validation data, the $cNRI$ and IDI often yielded statistically significant results in favor of the new model 2 with markers that contained no information (Pepe et al., 2014; Hilden and Gerds, 2014).

7.7 Concluding remarks

We have discussed methods for comparing models based on independent validation data. Some authors attempt to perform such comparisons on the same training data used to estimate the models. This typically leads to over-optimistic assessments of each model and unreliable comparisons. Moreover, standard asymptotic normal distribution theory does not apply in many cases, because parameter estimates are at the boundary (Vickers et al., 2011; Demler et al., 2012; Pepe et al., 2013). For example, a standard test like the Delong test (Delong et al., 1988) for comparing two AUC values is conservative and has low power when assessed on the training data.

When it is possible to define costs for a specific decision problem, the expected loss specific to that problem is an attractive measure of model performance and can be used to compare models. The more general criteria in Section 7.4 can also be used and have the advantage of familiarity from other applications. For example, risk modelers have a general sense of whether an AUC value is promising for a given application, based on other experience with the AUC. Some of these criteria, like the IDI are very sensitive to mis-calibration, whereas others, like the AUC, are robust to mis-calibration induced by monotonic transformations.

Although risk stratification tables are a valuable descriptive device and can be used with nested models to examine the risk distribution in the enhanced model within strata defined by risk in the base model, serious issues have been raised regarding the interpretability, sensitivity to miscalibration, and consequent likelihood of yielding false positive findings for the NRI and $cNRI$. Pepe and Janes (2013) discuss this and other aspects of comparing risk models.

It is good practice to assess model calibration carefully before comparing models using any of the criteria in this chapter.

Chapter 8

Building and updating relative risk models

8.1 Introductory remarks

Absolute risk estimates based on cause-specific models rely on survival analysis methods that were first widely applied for estimating pure risks following disease diagnosis. In Chapter 4 we discussed how standard inference for the Cox proportional hazards model (Cox, 1972) could be used to estimate relative risks for cause-specific hazards as well as cumulative and instantaneous contributions to the cause-specific hazards. Thus, a vast literature on survival regression modeling also applies to modeling cause-specific hazards and absolute risk estimation based on cause-specific hazard modeling. Excellent discussions of topics such as how to code covariates, flexible representations of dose-response for quantitative covariates (e.g., splines), handling missing values and model checking by examining residuals and other tests of goodness-of-fit, are found in classic books on survival and risk modeling, including Andersen et al. (1993), Harrell (2001), Kalbfleisch and Prentice (2002), Steyerberg (2009), Therneau and Grambsch (2000), and van Houwelingen and Putter (2012). We do not attempt to discuss these topics comprehensively, but we briefly touch on three important issues for modeling absolute risk: covariate selection, missing covariate data, and updating previously well-established risk models by adding new covariates.

8.2 Selection of covariates

An important aspect of regression modeling is selecting covariates for the model. The criteria for and approach to covariate selection can depend on the intended use of the model and the scientific information available on potential risk factors from previous studies. One possible goal is to obtain unbiased estimates and valid inference on previously established risk factors. Another related but distinct goal is prediction, and in our particular applications, predicting the probability of disease (risk prediction).

If previous studies have identified the risk factors, there may be little need for covariate selection, although some modeling may be needed to identify a good coding for the variables and perhaps to identify interactions. For example, in developing the breast cancer risk models BCRAT and BC2013, the investigators had access to a large literature on breast cancer epidemiology that had established a set of risk factors such as family history, reproductive history, biopsy history, alcohol consumption and hormone replacement therapy use. In this context, classical methods applied to a previously defined set of risk factors would be expected to yield valid parameter estimates and inference. Such estimates could be used either to assess the strength of the associations with outcome or for the construction of risk prediction models. Within this well-defined regression framework, one can also draw on previous studies to improve the precision of parameter estimates (see Section 8.4).

When the investigator examines many possible regression models defined by the selection of various subsets of variables in the training data and then estimates the parameters of the selected model from these data, classical methods of inference on those parameters are misleading. For example, Pötscher (1991) and Leeb (2005) have shown that the asymptotic distributions of the post-model-selection parameter estimates are typically non-normal and depend on the unknown parameters in a complex fashion. Even a small amount of modeling, such as the choice of the number of polynomial terms needed for regression on a continuous covariate, can lead to distorted operating characteristics based on classical theory (Efron, 2014). There is a growing literature on valid inference after model selection. For example, Efron (2014), Wasserman and Roeder (2009), and Meinshausen et al. (2009) proposed resampling approaches or data splitting. Lockhart et al. (2014) derived the exact asymptotic null distribution of a statistic for testing significance of variables that enter the LASSO model (Tibshirani, 1996). Berk et al. (2013) proposed an approach for post-selection inference ("PoSI") for the linear model that is valid over all possible selected models and does not assume that a linear model is correct. Our primary concern, however, is not with inference on model parameters but with predicting the disease outcome for a new individual, based on that person's covariates.

Selecting a regression model by finding a subset of covariates that appear to perform well in the training data also has implications for prediction, and, in particular, for predicting the risk of disease for a new individual based on his or her covariates and the selected risk prediction model. Selecting too many predictors often leads to "over-fitting", whereby the model appears to perform well in the training data but not in independent validation samples. In the context of logistic risk prediction, models that are over-fitted tend to overestimate risks among those in the highest decile of predicted risk and underestimate risk among those in the lowest decile of predicted risk. Methods to shrink the parameter estimates toward zero are sometimes used to ameliorate over-fitting (Harrell, 2001; Steyerberg, 2009; Van Houwelingen and Le Cessie, 1990; van Houwelingen, 2001, 2000; Copas, 1987).

The problem of over-fitting can be extreme when there are a very large number of covariates from which to choose, such as in genome-wide association studies to detect single nucleotide polymorphisms (SNPs) associated with disease. A SNP might be selected only if its chi-square statistic exceeds a Bonferroni-corrected quantile of the chi-square distribution ("hard thresholding"). The estimated log odds ratios associated with selected SNPs are biased away from zero, a phenomenon called the "winner's curse" (Zöllner and Pritchard, 2007). Without bias correction, the winner's curse can contribute to over-fitting. With a well-defined selection criterion, such as hard thresholding, and assuming the various SNPs are statistically independent, one can correct for such bias by relying on a likelihood that is conditioned on the selection condition (Zöllner and Pritchard, 2007). In general, however, the various risk factors might be correlated, as in the case of RNA expression arrays, and the precise selection algorithm may be difficult to describe, making such bias correction difficult or impossible.

As described in Section 6.4, one important measure of the performance of a risk model R is its expected mean square error, $MSE = E(O_i - R_i)^2 = E\{Var(O_i)|\pi_i\} + E(R_i - \pi_i)^2 = E\pi_i(1-\pi_i)+E\{(bias)^2\}$ in future samples. As discussed in Chapters 1 and 7 of (Hastie et al., 2009), as one increases the complexity of a risk model, for example by adding additional risk factors, one tends to decrease the bias in the predictor but increase its variance. Thus, in future data, a complex model R may have little bias but large variance, leading to large MSE. Similar comments apply to another measure of performance, the expected entropy, $E\{-O_i \log(R_i) - (1 - O_i)\log(1 - R_i)\}$ in future samples.

An approach used to avoid over-fitting is to penalize the complexity of the risk model. If there are a modest number of models to be examined that are nested within a global model, and if the sample size n is larger than the number of parameters in the global model, one can apply a complexity penalty as follows. One selects the model with the smallest Akaike Information Criterion, $AIC = -2\log(\hat{L}) + 2p$, where p is the number of parameters (risk factor degrees of freedom) in the model and $\hat{L}$ is the maximized likelihood. Here the complexity penalty is $2p$. Alternatively one can select a model that minimizes the Bayes Information Criterion, $BIC = -2\log(\hat{L}) + p\log(n)$. Unlike the AIC criterion, the

BIC criterion leads to correct model selection as n goes to infinity faster than the number of covariates, if the true model is included in the model space. However BIC leads to more parsimonious models than AIC, and in samples of practical size the BIC procedure may lead to models that are too simple and have large bias.

If the number of covariates p exceeds n, there are multiple solutions that maximize the likelihood, and one needs to impose constraints based on considerations external to the available data, to obtain a model (Chapter 7 in Hastie et al. (2009)). These constraints may concern the smoothness of the regression functions or other conditions on sets of parameters. If the number of risk factors thought to be truly associated with disease is small, compared to p ("sparsity"), or if it is thought to be unlikely that parameters have large effects, such conditions can be reflected in a penalty that when added to the log likelihood yields models with parameter estimates shrunk toward 0. The widely used LASSO procedure (Albert, 1982; Tibshirani, 1996) finds $\boldsymbol{\beta}$ that minimizes $-2\log\{L(\boldsymbol{\beta})\} + J_\lambda(\boldsymbol{\beta}) = -2\log\{L(\boldsymbol{\beta})\} + \lambda\sum_{i=1}^{p}|\beta_i|$. The LASSO penalty is based on an L-1 norm. The penalty for ridge regression $J_\lambda(\boldsymbol{\beta}) = \lambda\sum_{i=1}^{p}\beta_i^2$ is based on the L-2 norm. Penalties for the elastic net (a combination of the L1 and L2 penalties) and other procedures are described in books on data mining (Hastie et al., 2009; Giraud, 2015). These methods have been applied not only to linear regression, but to generalized linear models (Friedman et al., 2010), including logistic regression (Steyerberg et al., 2000), and more recently to regression for survival data. For the Cox proportional hazards model, penalized partial likelihood methods have been proposed based on the LASSO (technical report cited in Tibshirani (1996)) and on the smoothly clipped absolute deviation method (Fan and Li, 2001, 2002). Zhang and Lu (2007) proposed an adaptive LASSO method based on a penalized partial likelihood with adaptively weighted L-1 penalties on regression coefficients. Unlike the LASSO and smoothly clipped absolute deviation methods, which apply the same penalty to all the coefficients, the adaptive LASSO penalty has the form $\lambda\sum_{i=1}^{p}|\beta_i|\tau_i$, with small weights τ_i chosen for large coefficients and large weights for small coefficients. The adaptive LASSO has the "oracle property". A penalized estimator has the oracle property if it is asymptotically equivalent to the "oracle" estimate that one would obtain if one knew *a priori* the truly outcome-associated variables and used unpenalized regression on them. The LASSO estimator does not have oracle properties (Fan and Li, 2001). However, even penalized algorithms that enjoy the (asymptotic) oracle property can result in misleading estimates and inference on individual covariate effects when applied to finite samples of real data and may not outperform non-oracle procedures. Penalties based on L-2 norms have also been described for the Cox model (Verweij and Van Houwelingen, 1994; van Houwelingen et al., 2006).

The quantity λ in penalized regression is sometimes called a "tuning parameter" and needs to be specified in order to obtain regression estimates. As discussed in Chapter 7 of Hastie et al. (2009), if one had a huge amount of data, one could divide it into training data (A) and test data (B) and further divide A into estimation data (A1) and selection data (A2). For each value of λ, one estimates the regression model from A1, giving rise to a large number of regression models indexed by λ. Then one selects the regression model (i.e., the value of λ) that provides the best predictions in the independent A2 data. Usually one re-estimates the final model by using the previously selected λ but fitting the corresponding model to all the training data, A. Finally, one obtains an unbiased estimate of the predictive performance of the final model (e.g., the MSE of prediction) by applying the final model to the test data, B. This paradigm avoids the over-optimistic assessment of performance that is obtained by applying the selected model to the training data.

If there are insufficient training data to permit separate estimation (A1) and selection (A2) phases, one can instead use cross-validation to choose λ (see, e.g., Tibshirani (1996)). With five-fold cross validation, one randomly divides all the training data into five equal portions. For a fixed λ, one begins by estimating the model indexed by λ on the first four portions and using the remaining portion to estimate the prediction error (e.g., MSE). One repeats this process four more times by successively using different portions to estimate the model and estimate the prediction error. The average of these five estimates of prediction error is the criterion used to characterize the performance of the model with that value of λ. This entire procedure is repeated for many values of λ, and the λ value with the smallest predicted error is selected. A final model is obtained by re-estimating the model with the selected λ using all the training data. Finally, to obtain an unbiased estimate of the prediction error for the final model, one applies the final model to the test data, B. This paradigm can also be applied to procedures like stepwise regression, where the "tuning parameter" corresponds to the significance level chosen to retain covariates. For procedures like all subset selection, λ indexes each of the 2^p possible models.

In the previous two paragraphs, we have assumed that there are independent test data B that were held in reserve and never used in estimating the models or selecting the best model. The test data were only used to estimate the prediction error of the selected model. An advantage of this approach is that valid estimates of prediction error are obtained no matter how complex (and possibly ill-defined) the procedures for selecting covariates and estimating the model are. If there are insufficient training data to permit this approach, and if the selection and estimation procedures are well defined, as for example in LASSO, cross-validation can also be used to estimate prediction error using all the data. We use the LASSO as an example. One might randomly divide all the training plus test data into five parts. One further divides the first four portions into five parts and proceeds as in the previous paragraph to estimate and select what appears to be the best model. Then one estimates its prediction error with the left-out portion. Repeating this process five times, one has five selected LASSO models and their estimated prediction errors. The average of these five prediction errors indicates how well the process of fitting the LASSO (with estimation of λ by an internal cross-validation step) will perform when applied to all the training and test data to obtain the final model. Better estimates of prediction error may be obtained by using leave-one-out-at-a-time cross-validation rather than five-fold cross-validation on the entire data set (Molinaro et al., 2005). A serious error that is sometimes made is to omit the model selection step in the cross-validation (or bootstrap as in Hastie et al. (2009)) evaluation (Dupuy and Simon, 2007). For example, suppose the LASSO procedure is applied to all the training plus test data and yields a small set of covariates to be included in the model and a given optimal value of λ. If one holds this value of λ and the selected set of covariates fixed but only allows the regression parameters to vary in the double cross-validation procedure above, one will seriously underestimate the prediction error.

In Chapter 6 we stressed the importance of independent validation data to assess the performance of a previously developed risk model. Such independent validation can provide an even more rigorous assessment than the test data (B) described above, because independent validation data may also reveal whether a model developed in one population applies to another population. When covariate selection is an important aspect of model development, and especially when the training data are used to discover useful covariates among many possible covariates, some form of test data (B) or re-sampling techniques are needed to obtain a realistic assessment of the model's prediction error in the same population that gave rise to the model, and further testing in independent validation is highly desirable.

8.3 Missing data

In any real data set, some values on some variables are missing for some subjects. Molenberghs et al. (2015) provide a general overview of classifications of types of missing data and approaches to handling them. Here we concentrate on approaches that have been developed to account for missing covariates in the Cox model, because these approaches apply, with little modification, to estimation of absolute risk under the cause-specific hazard model.

Kalbfleisch and Prentice (2002) reviewed early work for the Cox model and provided a useful framework for thinking about the literature.

8.3.1 *Types of missing data*

Rubin (1976) introduced the following hierarchy of missing data mechanisms, which we specialize for survival data. Let $\mathbf{Z} = (\mathbf{Z}^{\mathrm{m}}, \mathbf{Z}^{\mathrm{c}})$ be the vector of covariates, of which $\mathbf{Z}^{\mathrm{c}}$ is always observed and $\mathbf{Z}^{\mathrm{m}}$ may or may not be missing on an individual. Let $\mathbf{V}$ be a p $\times$ 1 vector of indicators that take value 1 if the corresponding component of $\mathbf{Z}^{\mathrm{m}}$ is observed and 0 otherwise. In addition to $\mathbf{Z}^{\mathrm{c}}$, we also always observe $X = min(T, C)$ and $\delta = I(T \leq C)$. Here T is a survival time and C is a censoring time that is conditionally independent of T given $\mathbf{Z}$. In the competing risk framework, T is the time to the first of the competing events, and δ is 0 if censored and otherwise is $1, 2, \ldots, M$ according as the observed event is of type k. The data are *missing completely at random* (MCAR) if $\mathbf{V}$ is independent of $\mathbf{Z}, X$, and δ. Although the MCAR assumption cannot be verified empirically, it can be refuted empirically if the distribution of $(\mathbf{Z}^{\mathrm{c}}, X, \delta)$ varies across patterns of missingness $\mathbf{V}$. The data are *missing at random* (MAR) if $\mathbf{V}$ is conditionally independent of $\mathbf{Z}^{\mathrm{m}}$ given $(\mathbf{Z}^{\mathrm{c}}, X, \delta)$. A stronger assumption sometimes used in the survival literature is that $\mathbf{V}$ is conditionally independent of $\mathbf{Z}^{\mathrm{m}}$ given $\mathbf{Z}^{\mathrm{c}}$. The MAR assumption cannot be verified statistically, but is sometimes justified based on substantive considerations or when the missingness is by design. If the missingness is neither MCAR nor MAR, it is *not missing at random* (NMAR), which is also called *informative missingness.* Whereas various analytical approaches are applicable for MCAR and MAR data, NMAR data require an unverifiable explicit model for the conditional distribution $(\mathbf{V}|\mathbf{Z}^{\mathrm{m}}, \mathbf{Z}^{\mathrm{c}}, X, \delta)$. Such models can be used to explore the sensitivity of analyses to the MCAR or MAR assumptions or to the baseline NMAR model.

8.3.2 *Approaches to handling missing data*

If missing data are MCAR from a cohort, then those cohort members with complete data are a random subsample of the cohort and can be analyzed using standard methods for cohorts. Assume first a strong MAR assumption that $\mathbf{V}$ is conditionally independent of $\mathbf{Z}^{\mathrm{m}}$ given $\mathbf{Z}^{\mathrm{c}}$. Then those members of a risk set with complete data on $\mathbf{Z}^{\mathrm{m}}$ constitute a random subsample of the risk set, and their contribution to the partial likelihood can be used in a "complete case" analysis (Kalbfleisch and Prentice, 2002). Instead, Zhou and Pepe (1995) estimated the expectation of $\exp(\mathbf{Z}'\boldsymbol{\beta})$ for each risk set non-parametrically from the members of the risk set with always observed covariates $\mathbf{Z}^{\mathrm{c}}$, and maximized the estimated partial likelihood. Lin and Ying (1993) proposed an estimated set of score equations with the conditional "expectations" from the partial likelihood score equations replaced by estimated "expectations" from the members of risk sets with complete data. See also Martinussen et al. (2016).

A weaker MAR assumption is that $\mathbf{V}$ is conditionally independent of $\mathbf{Z}^{\mathrm{m}}$ given $(\mathbf{Z}^{\mathrm{c}}, X, \delta)$. Several investigators have considered this less stringent MAR assumption. Paik and Tsai (1997) extended the approach of (Lin and Ying, 1993). Chen and Little (1999) developed a non-parametric maximum likelihood procedure, NPML, but required two notable assumptions, namely a model for the joint distribution of the observed and missing covariates and the assumption that C is conditionally independent of T given $\mathbf{Z}^{\mathrm{c}}$, rather than the weaker usual assumption that C is conditionally independent of T given $\mathbf{Z}$.

A second approach based on inverse weighting assumes that $\tilde{V} = I(V_i = 1, i = 1, \ldots, p)$, an indicator that is one if an individual has any missing covariates and zero otherwise, is conditionally independent of $\mathbf{Z}^{\mathrm{m}}$ given $(\mathbf{Z}^{\mathrm{c}}, X, \delta)$. Letting $\pi = P(\tilde{V} = 1|X, \delta, \mathbf{Z}^{\mathrm{c}})$, one can multiply contributions to the partial likelihood score from individuals with measured $\mathbf{Z}$ by π^{-1}, but this simple inverse weighting can be quite inefficient. Wang and Chen (2001) developed a more efficient augmented inverse weighting method that requires a parametric model for the expectation $E(\mathbf{Z}^m|X, \delta, \mathbf{Z}^c)$ as well as the model for π. This method is "doubly robust" in that consistent estimates are obtained if either the model for π or for $E(\mathbf{Z}^m|X, \delta, \mathbf{Z}^c)$ is correct, and the method is valid if C is conditionally independent of T given $\mathbf{Z}$. Qi et al. (2005) showed that efficiency could be gained by estimating π non-parametrically, and surprisingly that this approach was asymptotically as efficient as augmentation, which they also implemented by kernel estimation of $E(\mathbf{Z}^m|X, \delta, \mathbf{Z}^c)$. Their methods are valid if C is conditionally independent of T given $\mathbf{Z}$ and also do not make parametric assumptions on $E(\mathbf{Z}^m|X, \delta, \mathbf{Z}^c)$, but their kernel augmentation method might be impractical for multivariate $\mathbf{Z}^m$. Further extensions of weighting methods allow for non-monotone missingness (Xu et al., 2009) and weights that perform better when some values of π are very small (Luo et al., 2009).

A third general approach is to impute missing covariates. Let $\mathbf{Z}^{mm}$ be the missing components of $\mathbf{Z}^m$ and $\mathbf{Z}^{mo}$ be the observed components of $\mathbf{Z}^m$. One can impute values for $\mathbf{Z}^{mm}$ by drawing from the predictive distribution $[\mathbf{Z}^{mm}|\mathbf{Z}^{mo}, \mathbf{Z}^c, X, \delta]$. The practical problem is how to specify the joint distribution $[\mathbf{V}, \mathbf{Z}^m, \mathbf{Z}^c, X, \delta]$ from which to estimate the required predictive distribution (see Fitzmaurice et al. (2015) and Kenward and Carpenter (2007)). Under the MAR assumption, $[\mathbf{V}, \mathbf{Z}^m, \mathbf{Z}^c, X, \delta] = [\mathbf{Z}^m, \mathbf{Z}^c, X, \delta][\mathbf{V}|\mathbf{Z}^c, X, \delta]$. It is important to include X and δ as well as the observed covariates in the predictive distribution (Sterne et al., 2009). Once a complete data set has been imputed in a single set of imputations as above, the analysis of the "complete" data can proceed with standard methods, as in Chapter 4. To account for the added uncertainty from the imputed data, however, one repeats the entire process multiple times to obtain $m \geq 2$ imputed datasets and m sets of estimates. The variance of the estimate, such as the 10-year absolute risk for a fixed set of covariates, can be computed from the expected variance of the estimate given the imputed complete data plus the variance of the expected estimate given the imputed data, as discussed in Rubin (1987). The latter term accounts for the uncertainty induced by imputation. These methods, though very attractive computationally, depend on the validity of the predictive distributions.

8.4 Updating risk models with new risk factors

When novel risk factors become available from new data, it is desirable to combine their information with information from existing prediction models, to improve predictions and risk stratification. New molecular markers are often measured in relatively small case-control or cohort studies that provide little new information on well established risk factors. For example, when data on new risk factors such as mammographic density, single nucleotide polymorphisms (SNPs) or circulating hormone measures become available, it would be desirable to also utilize available information on the well established effects of many reproductive risk factors to develop new models that predict breast cancer risk.

In this section, we discuss various methods in the literature for building logistic regression models based on individual-level data that include a new predictor, while using parameter estimates from an existing logistic model with "standard" factors. Some authors refer to this approach as "model updating". For rare diseases, the odds ratios from logistic modeling of cohort or case-control data approximate the relative hazards needed in cause-specific hazard models of absolute risk. Thus we can take advantage of the literature on updating logistic models to update cause-specific hazard models of absolute risk. In particular we can use the approach in Chapter 5 that combines relative risks with external composite hazard rates to estimate the cause-specific hazard function

$$\hat{\lambda}_1(t; \mathbf{z}^1) = \hat{\lambda}_{01}(t) rr(\hat{\boldsymbol{\beta}}_1' \mathbf{z}^1) = \{1 - \widehat{AR}(t)\} \lambda_1^*(t) rr(\hat{\boldsymbol{\beta}}_1' \mathbf{z}^1), \tag{8.1}$$

where rr denotes the relative risk and $\mathbf{z}^1$ denotes risk factors for the cause-specific hazard for which absolute risk is being calculated, λ_1. In what follows we omit any super- and subscripts and use $rr(\mathbf{Z})$ to denote the relative risk term that depends on covariates $\mathbf{Z}$.

As in Grill et al. (2016), we consider several approaches to updating the relative risk part of a model. We let $\mathbf{X} = (X_1, \ldots, X_p)'$ denote a vector of p established covariates, and Z a covariate that we term "new marker". We first let Z be a single marker, but later extend methods to multivariate markers. We assume that the true relative risk model (or relative odds model for logistic regression with rare outcome) in the population is given by

$$rr(\mathbf{X}, Z) = rr\{\boldsymbol{\beta}'_{\mathbf{X}}(\mathbf{X} - \mathbf{X}_0), \beta_Z(Z - Z_0)\} = \exp\{\boldsymbol{\beta}'_{\mathbf{X}}(\mathbf{X} - \mathbf{X}_0) + \beta_Z(Z - Z_0)\}, \quad (8.2)$$

where $\boldsymbol{\beta}_{\mathbf{X}} = (\beta_1, \ldots, \beta_p)'$ are the log-relative risks for $\mathbf{X}$, β_Z is the log relative risk for Z, and $\mathbf{X}_0$ and Z_0 are referent covariate levels.

We assume that the original relative risk model we wish to update only included factors $\mathbf{X}$,

$$rr(\mathbf{X}) = \exp\{\boldsymbol{\gamma}'(\mathbf{X} - \mathbf{X}_0)\}. \quad (8.3)$$

The methods presented here can be extended to other relative risk functions.

8.4.1 Estimating an updated relative risk model, $rr(\mathbf{X}, Z)$, from case-control data

We assume that a new case-control study is available that has information on $\mathbf{X}$ and on the marker, Z. Our goal is to update the relative risk model with information on Z, while also utilizing information available from model $rr(\mathbf{X})$ in (8.3). Letting D denote the binary disease outcome, where $D = 1$ denotes diseased and $D = 0$ denotes non-diseased individuals, we wish to obtain the estimate

$$R_{\mathbf{X},Z} = \hat{P}\{D = 1|Z, \mathbf{X}, rr(\mathbf{X})\} \quad (8.4)$$

from the new dataset. We then approximate the joint relative risk given $\mathbf{X}$ and Z by the odds ratio from model (8.4) to obtain the updated relative risk model,

$$\hat{rr}(\mathbf{X}, Z) = \frac{\hat{P}\{D = 1|Z, \mathbf{X}, rr(\mathbf{X})\} / \hat{P}\{D = 0|Z, \mathbf{X}, rr(\mathbf{X})\}}{\hat{P}\{D = 1|Z_0, \mathbf{X}_0, rr(\mathbf{X}_0)\} / \hat{P}\{D = 0|Z_0, \mathbf{X}_0, rr(\mathbf{X}_0)\}} = \frac{R_{\mathbf{X},Z}/(1 - R_{\mathbf{X},Z})}{R_{\mathbf{X}_0,Z_0}/(1 - R_{\mathbf{X}_0,Z_0})}. \quad (8.5)$$

Note, however, that in general if $P(D = 1|\mathbf{X}, Z)$ is logistic then $P(D = 1|\mathbf{X})$ cannot be logistic, because from Bayes theorem,

$$P(D|Z, \mathbf{X}) = P(D|\mathbf{X}) \frac{P(Z|D, \mathbf{X})}{\sum_D P(D|\mathbf{X}) P(Z|D, \mathbf{X})} = P(D|\mathbf{X}) f(Z|D, \mathbf{X}), \quad (8.6)$$

where $f(Z|D, \mathbf{X}) = P(Z|D, \mathbf{X}) / \sum_D P(D|\mathbf{X}) P(Z|D, \mathbf{X})$. Only when the outcome is rare and $\mathbf{X}$ and Z are independent can both models, $P(D = 1|\mathbf{X})$ and $R_{\mathbf{X},Z}$, be logistic as discussed further in Section 8.4.3.

We now summarize several approaches for combining information from an existing relative risk model $rr(\mathbf{X})$ with information on the new marker Z to estimate a model $rr(\mathbf{X}, Z)$ based on case-control observations $(D, \mathbf{X}, Z)$. One of the approaches assumes independence between Z and $\mathbf{X}$ in the source population, while the others allow for dependence between Z and $\mathbf{X}$.

8.4.2 Estimating $rr(\mathbf{X}, Z)$ from new data only

A simple approach is to completely ignore information from the old model $rr(\mathbf{X})$ and to fit a logistic regression model

$$R_{\mathbf{X},Z} = P(D = 1|Z, \mathbf{X}) = \frac{\exp(\mu + \boldsymbol{\beta}'_X \mathbf{X} + \beta_Z Z)}{1 + \exp(\mu + \boldsymbol{\beta}'_X \mathbf{X} + \beta_Z Z)}. \quad (8.7)$$

Then

$$rr(\mathbf{X}, Z) = \exp\{\hat{\boldsymbol{\beta}}'_{\mathbf{X}}(\mathbf{X} - \mathbf{X}_0) + \hat{\beta}_Z(Z - Z_0)\}.$$

While this is not model "updating", we study this approach, called "logistic-new", in simulations (Section 8.4.7) to quantify the gain in predictive performance and efficiency when including information on $rr(\mathbf{X})$.

8.4.3 Incorporating information on $rr(\mathbf{X})$ into $rr(\mathbf{X}, Z)$ via likelihood ratio (LR) updating

Several authors have proposed updating risk models using the likelihood ratio (LR) of $[Z|D, \mathbf{X}]$, for example (Janssens et al., 2005; Ankerst et al., 2008, 2012). We first outline this approach and then discuss various methods for estimation.

From Equation (8.6),

$$\log\left(\textit{posterior odds}\right) = \log\left\{\frac{P(D=1|Z,\mathbf{X})}{P(D=0|Z,\mathbf{X})}\right\} = \log\left\{\frac{P(D=1|\mathbf{X})}{P(D=0|\mathbf{X})}\right\} + \log\left\{\frac{f\,(Z|D=1,\mathbf{X})}{f\,(Z|D=0,\mathbf{X})}\right\}$$
$$= \log\left(\textit{prior odds}\right) + \log\{LR_D\,(Z|\mathbf{X})\}, \quad (8.8)$$

where

$$\mathrm{LR}_D(Z|\mathbf{X}) = \frac{f(Z|D=1,\mathbf{X})}{f(Z|D=0,\mathbf{X})} = \frac{P(Z|D=1,\mathbf{X})}{P(Z|D=0,\mathbf{X})} \quad (8.9)$$

is the likelihood ratio for the new marker Z with respect to outcome D conditional on covariates $\mathbf{X}$. If we assume that

$$R_{\mathbf{X}} = \hat{P}\,(D=1|\mathbf{X}) = \frac{\exp(\gamma_0)rr(\mathbf{X})}{1+\exp(\gamma_0)rr(\mathbf{X})}, \quad (8.10)$$

then an estimate of the $\log(\textit{posterior odds})$ is

$$\log\left(\widehat{\textit{posterior odds}}\right) = \gamma_0 + \log\{rr(\mathbf{X})\} + \log\left\{\widehat{\mathrm{LR}_D}\,(Z|\mathbf{X})\right\}. \quad (8.11)$$

However, this relationship is only approximate, because usually $R_{\mathbf{X}}$ only approximates $P(D=1|\mathbf{X})$.

Expression (8.11) can be applied to any functional form of the model $rr(\mathbf{X})$. When $rr(\mathbf{X}) = \exp(\boldsymbol{\gamma}'_1\mathbf{X})$, then Equation (8.11) reduces to

$$\log\left(\widehat{\textit{posterior odds}}\right) = \gamma_0 + \boldsymbol{\gamma}'_1\mathbf{X} + \log\left\{\widehat{\mathrm{LR}_D}\,(Z|\mathbf{X})\right\}. \quad (8.12)$$

Under the rare disease assumption, the posterior odds can be used as an approximation to $P(D=1|\mathbf{X}, Z)$, and a similar approximation holds at the reference covariate levels for $P(D=1|\mathbf{X}_0, Z_0)$. By exponentiating the log posterior odds, we obtain the estimated relative risk

$$\hat{rr}(\mathbf{X}, Z) = P(D=1|\mathbf{X}, Z)/P(D=1|\mathbf{X}_0, Z_0) = rr(\mathbf{X})\mathrm{LR}_D\,(Z|\mathbf{X})\exp(c_0), \quad (8.13)$$

where $c_0 = -\log\{P(Z_0|D=1,\mathbf{X}_0)/P(Z_0|D=0,\mathbf{X}_0)\}$. If $rr(\mathbf{X}) = \exp(\boldsymbol{\gamma}'_1\mathbf{X})$, this simplifies to

$$\hat{rr}(\mathbf{X}, Z) = \mathrm{LR}_D\,(Z|\mathbf{X})\exp(c_0 + \boldsymbol{\gamma}'_1\mathbf{X}). \quad (8.14)$$

The variance of $\hat{rr}(\mathbf{X}, Z)$ can be calculated from the covariance matrices of the component models $Var(\boldsymbol{\gamma}, \widehat{\mathrm{LR}_D}) = diag(Var(\boldsymbol{\gamma}), Var(\widehat{\mathrm{LR}_D}))$, using the delta method, which could be implemented e.g., via the *deltamethod* function in the *R* package *msm* (see Ankerst et al. (2012)) or via a parametric bootstrap.

We now summarize and extend several approaches for estimating the LR_D in Equation (8.11).

8.4.3.1 Joint estimation of $\text{LR}_D(Z|\mathbf{X})$

If $P(Z|\mathbf{X})$ is a distribution within the exponential family, i.e., $P(Z|\mathbf{X}) = \exp(\zeta Z)h(z)c(\zeta)$, where h and c are known functions, $\zeta = \mathbf{X}'\boldsymbol{\beta}_{\mathbf{X}}$, and the disease is rare, then $P(Z|\mathbf{X}, D)$ also is in the exponential family. This result is immediate for controls ($D = 0$), because unmatched controls are representative of the general population for a rare disease,

$$P(Z|D = 0, \mathbf{X}) \approx P(Z|\mathbf{X}). \tag{8.15}$$

For cases, Equation (8.4) can be approximated by an exponential function for a rare disease, and

$$\begin{aligned} P(Z|\, D = 1, \mathbf{X}) &= \frac{\exp(\mu + \beta_z Z + \boldsymbol{\beta}'_{\mathbf{X}}\mathbf{X})P(Z|\, \mathbf{X})}{\int \exp(\mu + \beta_z Z + \boldsymbol{\beta}'_{\mathbf{X}}\mathbf{X})\, dF(Z|\mathbf{X})} = \frac{\exp(\beta_z Z)\exp(\zeta Z)h(z)c(\zeta)}{\int \exp(\beta_z Z)\exp(\zeta Z)h(z)c(\zeta)dZ} \\ &= \exp\{(\zeta + \beta_Z)Z\}h(z)c(\zeta + \beta_Z), \end{aligned} \tag{8.16}$$

which is in the exponential family with $\tilde{\zeta} = \zeta + \beta_Z$ and an appropriately adjusted normalizing constant c.

Special cases of interest in the exponential family are the logistic and normal distributions. When logit $\{P(Z = 1|\mathbf{X})\} = \alpha_0 + \boldsymbol{\alpha}'_1\mathbf{X}$ in the general population, then in the cases, logit $\{P(Z = 1|D = 1, \mathbf{X})\} = \alpha^* + \boldsymbol{\alpha}'_1\mathbf{X}$, with a new intercept α^* and otherwise the same coefficients as in the logistic model for the controls, $D = 0$. The different intercept terms in the models for cases and controls can be accommodated by fitting a single logistic model, logit $\{P(Z = 1|D, \mathbf{X})\} = \alpha_0 + \alpha_2 D + \boldsymbol{\alpha}'_1\mathbf{X}$, that also includes D as a predictor in addition to $\mathbf{X}$, to the combined case-control data. The LR_D model (8.9) for a binary marker Z is then given by

$$\text{LR}_D(Z|\mathbf{X}) = \frac{\{1 + \exp(-\alpha_0 - \boldsymbol{\alpha}'_1\mathbf{X})\}^Z \{1 + \exp(\alpha_0 + \boldsymbol{\alpha}'_1\mathbf{X})\}^{1-Z}}{\{1 + \exp(-\alpha_0 - \alpha_2 - \boldsymbol{\alpha}'_1\mathbf{X})\}^Z \{1 + \exp(\alpha_0 + \alpha_2 + \boldsymbol{\alpha}'_1\mathbf{X})\}^{1-Z}}. \tag{8.17}$$

Similarly, for a marker Z that follows a normal distribution, $Z|\mathbf{X} \sim N(\alpha_0 + \boldsymbol{\alpha}'_1\mathbf{X}, \sigma^2)$, under the rare disease assumption $Z|(\mathbf{X}, D) \sim N(\alpha_0 + \alpha_2 D + \boldsymbol{\alpha}'_1\mathbf{X}, \sigma^2)$, where the mean of Z has different intercept parameters for $D = 0$ and $D = 1$. The joint log-LR model for a normally distributed marker Z is

$$\log\{\text{LR}_D(Z|\mathbf{X})\} = \alpha_2(Z - \alpha_0 - \boldsymbol{\alpha}'_1\mathbf{X} - \alpha_2/2)/\sigma^2. \tag{8.18}$$

8.4.3.2 Estimating $\text{LR}_D(Z|\mathbf{X})$ *based on fitting separate models for cases* ($D = 1$) *and non-cases* ($D = 0$)

For $P(Z|\mathbf{X})$ in the exponential family, and assuming rare disease, we can separately estimate the numerator and the denominator of $\text{LR}_D(Z|\mathbf{X})$ in Equation (8.9) by fitting different models to cases ($D = 1$) and to controls ($D = 0$). If Z is a binary marker, $P(Z|D, \mathbf{X})$ can be estimated using separate logistic regression models for cases and controls, yielding

$$\text{LR}_D(Z|\mathbf{X}) = \frac{\{1 + \exp(-\alpha_{00} - \boldsymbol{\alpha}'_{10}\mathbf{X})\}^Z \{1 + \exp(\alpha_{00} + \boldsymbol{\alpha}'_{10}\mathbf{X})\}^{1-Z}}{\{1 + \exp(-\alpha_{01} - \boldsymbol{\alpha}'_{11}\mathbf{X})\}^Z \{1 + \exp(\alpha_{01} + \boldsymbol{\alpha}'_{11}\mathbf{X})\}^{1-Z}}, \tag{8.19}$$

where $\boldsymbol{\alpha}_{1D} = \left(\alpha^D_{11}, \ldots, \alpha^D_{1p}\right)', D = 0, 1$, indicates parameters in the models for controls and cases, respectively. For a normally distributed marker, $Z|(\mathbf{X}, D) \sim N(\boldsymbol{\alpha}'_D\mathbf{X}, \sigma^2_D)$, fitting separate linear models to cases and controls yields

$$\log\{\text{LR}_D(Z|\mathbf{X})\} = \log(\sigma_0/\sigma_1) - (Z - \alpha_{01} - \boldsymbol{\alpha}'_{11}\mathbf{X})^2/(2\sigma^2_1) + (Z - \alpha_{00} - \boldsymbol{\alpha}'_{10}\mathbf{X})^2/(2\sigma^2_0). \tag{8.20}$$

In contrast to Equation (8.18), which corresponds to linear discriminant analysis, estimating the LR_D separately in cases and controls also allows the variances to differ between the two groups, and thus corresponds to quadratic discriminant analysis, see, e.g., Chapter 6 of Anderson (1984).

8.4.3.3 LR updating assuming independence of Z and $\mathbf{X}$ (independence Bayes)

A special case of the LR approach defined above, described, e.g., in Hand and Yu (2001), is to assume that the new marker Z is independent of $\mathbf{X}$ in cases and non-cases, and therefore

$$\mathrm{LR}_D\,(Z|\mathbf{X}) = \frac{P(Z|D=1,\mathbf{X})}{P(Z|D=0,\mathbf{X})} = \frac{P(Z|D=1)}{P(Z|D=0)} = \mathrm{LR}_D\,(Z)\,. \tag{8.21}$$

When case-control data are used for updating, and the outcome is rare, then if $\mathbf{X}$ is independent of Z in the general population, $\mathbf{X}$ and Z are also independent in cases and controls, as shown, e.g., in Gail et al. (2008). Thus, for a rare disease, the assumption of independence of $\mathbf{X}$ and Z in the general population implies independence conditional on D.

When the outcome is rare, Z is in the exponential family and $\mathbf{X}$ and Z are independent, then $P(D|\mathbf{X}) \approx \int_Z \exp(\mu_{\mathbf{X}} + \boldsymbol{\beta}'_{\mathbf{X}}\mathbf{X} + \beta_Z Z)dF(Z|\mathbf{X}) = \exp(\mu + \boldsymbol{\beta}'_{\mathbf{X}}\mathbf{X})$ and

$$\log\{\mathrm{LR}_D(Z)\} = \log\left\{\frac{\exp\{(\zeta+\beta_Z)Z\}h(z)c(\zeta+\beta_Z)}{\exp\{\zeta Z\}h(z)c(\zeta)}\right\} = \beta^* + \beta_Z Z. \tag{8.22}$$

Thus the coefficients for $\mathbf{X}$ and Z in $\hat{rr}(\mathbf{X}, Z)$ in Equation (8.14) are approximately unbiased.

8.4.3.4 LR updating with multiple markers

The methods presented above for a single marker can be extended to two or more markers, $\mathbf{Z}$. For example, to compute the LR for two markers $\mathbf{Z} = (Z_1, Z_2)$, we use that

$$\begin{aligned}\log\{\mathrm{LR}_D(Z_1,Z_2|\mathbf{X})\} &= \log\left\{\frac{P(Z_2|D=1,Z_1,\mathbf{X})P(Z_1|D=1,\mathbf{X})}{P(Z_2|D=0,Z_1,\mathbf{X})P(Z_1|D=0,\mathbf{X})}\right\}\\ &= \log\left\{\frac{P(Z_2|D=1,Z_1,\mathbf{X})}{P(Z_2|D=0,Z_1,\mathbf{X})}\right\} \qquad (8.23)\\ &+ \log\left\{\frac{P(Z_1|D=1,\mathbf{X})}{P(Z_1|D=0,\mathbf{X})}\right\} = \log\{\mathrm{LR}_D(Z_2|Z_1,\mathbf{X})\} + \log\{\mathrm{LR}_D(Z_1|\mathbf{X})\}. \qquad (8.24)\end{aligned}$$

To estimate $\log\{\mathrm{LR}_D(Z_2|Z_1,\mathbf{X})\}$ one simply includes the marker Z_1 along with the predictors $\mathbf{X}$.

8.4.4 Joint estimation, logistic model with offset

The linear dependency of $\log\{\mathrm{LR}_D(Z)\}$ on Z in Equation (8.22) was also noted by Albert (1982), who proposed to include the prior odds with parameters from the original risk model as an offset term in a logistic regression model that included Z as the predictor to obtain $R_{Z,\mathbf{X}}$. In our setting, this corresponds to estimating two new parameters (δ_0, δ_1) based on the model

$$\begin{aligned}R_{\mathbf{X},Z} = \hat{P}\,(D=1|Z,\mathbf{X},rr(\mathbf{X})) &= \frac{\exp[\log\{rr(\mathbf{X})\} + \hat{\delta}_0 + \hat{\delta}_1 Z]}{1+\exp[\log\{rr(\mathbf{X})\} + \hat{\delta}_0 + \hat{\delta}_1 Z]}\\ &= \frac{\exp(\boldsymbol{\gamma}'_1(\mathbf{X}-\mathbf{X}_0) + \hat{\delta}_0 + \hat{\delta}_1 Z)}{1+\exp(\boldsymbol{\gamma}'_1(\mathbf{X}-\mathbf{X}_0) + \hat{\delta}_0 + \hat{\delta}_1 Z)}.\end{aligned} \tag{8.25}$$

The updated relative risk model is thus

$$rr(\mathbf{X}, Z) = \exp\{\boldsymbol{\gamma}'_1(\mathbf{X}-\mathbf{X}_0) + \hat{\delta}_1(Z - Z_0)\}. \tag{8.26}$$

8.4.5 Independence Bayes with shrinkage

Spiegelhalter and Knill-Jones (1984) generalized (8.21) to allow for dependence between $\mathbf{X}$ and Z by fitting one additional shrinkage parameter θ that multiplies $\log\{\mathrm{LR}_D(Z)\}$ in (8.8). Spiegelhalter and Knill-Jones (1984) first estimated the $\mathrm{LR}_D(Z)$ based on the new data and then estimated θ by fitting

$$\log(\textit{posterior odds}) = \gamma_{01} + \boldsymbol{\gamma}_1'\mathbf{X} + \theta\log\{\mathrm{LR}_D(Z)\} = \gamma_{01} + \boldsymbol{\gamma}_1'\mathbf{X} + \theta\log\{\mathrm{LR}_D(Z)\}\,. \quad (8.27)$$

If θ is estimated to be zero, the new marker does not add any information to the model, and when $\theta = 1$, Z is independent of $\mathbf{X}$. We refer to model (8.27) as "LR-shrink" in the numerical studies and compare the two-step estimation approach to a single step approach that directly maximizes (8.27) as a function of θ and all parameters in LR_D.

8.4.6 Updating using constrained maximum likelihood estimation (CML)

Chatterjee et al. (2016) considered building regression models based on individual-level data from an "internal" study while utilizing information on parameters for a reduced model estimated from an "external" big-data source, see also Qin (2000). They identified a set of general constraints that link internal and external models and used them to propose a semi-parametric maximum likelihood estimate for the new model that is equivalent to a form of empirical likelihood (Han and Lawless, 2016).

Following Chatterjee et al. (2016), let $U(D|X;\boldsymbol{\gamma}) = \partial\log g_{\boldsymbol{\gamma}}(D|\mathbf{X})/\partial\boldsymbol{\gamma}$ denote the score function associated with the "external" reduced model $rr(\mathbf{X})$ in (8.10). The population parameter value $\boldsymbol{\gamma}$ for this model satisfies the equation

$$E\{U(D|\mathbf{X},\boldsymbol{\gamma})\} = \int U(D|\mathbf{X},\boldsymbol{\gamma})P(D|\mathbf{X})P(\mathbf{X})dDd\mathbf{X} = 0, \quad (8.28)$$

where $P(D,\mathbf{X}) = P(D|\mathbf{X})P(\mathbf{X})$ is the true underlying joint distribution of $(D,\mathbf{X})$. When the model (8.10) is misspecified, then $R_{\mathbf{X}} = P(D=1|\mathbf{X}) \neq \hat{P}(D=1|\mathbf{X})$, but the above equation still holds true under mild conditions. Under the assumption that $f_\beta(D|Z,\mathbf{X})$ is correctly specified, we can write $P(D|\mathbf{X}) = \int f_{\beta_0}(D|Z,\mathbf{X})P(Z|\mathbf{X})dZ$, with β_0 the true value of β. Thus, the constraint imposed by Equation (8.28) can be rewritten, after changing the order of integration, as

$$\int_{Z,\mathbf{X}}\int_D U(D|\mathbf{X},\boldsymbol{\gamma})f_{\beta_0}(D|Z,\mathbf{X})dF(\mathbf{X},Z) = 0.$$

The above equation converts the external information to a set of constraints, which is used in the analysis of internal data to improve efficiency of parameter estimates. The dimension of the constraint space is the number of parameters by which the external model has been summarized.

If the internal sample is a case-control sample and $p_1 = 1 - p_0$ is the disease probability in the source population, the likelihood is

$$L_{\beta,F} = \left\{\prod_{i=1}^{n_0+n_1} f_\beta(D_i|Z_i,\mathbf{X}_i)dF(\mathbf{X}_i,Z_i)\right\}p_0^{-n_0}p_1^{-n_1}$$

where n_1 and n_0 denote the number of cases and control sampled. The goal is to maximize $\log(L_{\beta,F}) + \lambda^T\int_{Z,\mathbf{X}}\int_D U(D|\mathbf{X},\boldsymbol{\gamma})f_\beta(D|Z,\mathbf{X})dF(\mathbf{X},Z)$, where λ is a vector of Lagrange multipliers, and $dF(\mathbf{X},Z)$ has mass only at the unique observed data points among $(\mathbf{X}_i,Z_i), i = 1,\ldots,n_0+n_1$; see Chatterjee et al. (2016) for details.

The method does not require parametric assumptions for $F(\mathbf{X}, Z)$ and produces consistent estimates of parameters of the updated model, assuming that one correctly specifies the risk distribution $[D|\mathbf{X}, Z]$ for the internal study, irrespective of whether the external risk model is correctly specified. The method applies to any type of regression model, including logistic regression, and does not require a rare disease assumption. The authors showed that the empirical-likelihood approach allows tractable computation of CML irrespective of the dimensions of the risk-factors. The point masses for $\hat{F}(\mathbf{X}, Z)$ can be estimated using either the internal sample or an external reference sample.

Table 8.1 summarizes all these methods and the number of parameters that are estimated for each.

Table 8.1: Summary of updating methods

Method	log (**posterior odds**)	**Assumes independence of X** and **Z**	**Number of parameters estimated for**	
			Z binary	**Z continuous**
Logistic-new	$\mu + \boldsymbol{\beta}_{\mathbf{X}}^T\mathbf{X} + \beta_z Z$	No	p+2	p+2
LR-joint	$\boldsymbol{\gamma}_1^T\mathbf{X} + \log(LR_{dep})$	No	p+2	p+3
LR-separate	$\boldsymbol{\gamma}_1^T\mathbf{X} + \log(LR_{dep})$	No	2(p+1)	2(p+1)+2
LR-ind	$\boldsymbol{\gamma}_1^T\mathbf{X} + \log(LR_{ind})$	Yes	2	4
LR-offset	$\boldsymbol{\gamma}_1^T\mathbf{X} + \delta_0 + \delta_1 Z$	Yes	2	2
LR-shrink	$\boldsymbol{\gamma}_1^T\mathbf{X} + \theta\log(LR_{ind})$	No	3	5
CML		No	p+2	p+2

p: number of risk factors in $\mathbf{X}$
The prior odds from original risk model based only on standard covariates $\mathbf{X} = (X_1, ...X_p)^T$ is $\exp(\boldsymbol{\gamma}_1^T\mathbf{X})$. The quantities $LR_{ind} \equiv P(Z|D=1)/P(Z|D=0)$, and $LR_{dep} \equiv P(Z|D=1, \mathbf{X})/P(Z|D=0, \mathbf{X})$, which is estimated separately (LR-separate) or jointly (LR-joint). Note that only the "Logistic-new" method and CML estimate the parameters in Equation (8.2) corresponding to the correct model.

8.4.7 Simulations

We present selected simulations from Grill et al. (2016) that assess bias and variability in $\hat{P}(D|\mathbf{X}, Z)$ from logistic models updated using the methods in Table 8.1.

To obtain realistic correlations between predictors, we simulated data based on variables from the Viral Resistance to Antiviral Therapy of Chronic Hepatitis C (ViraHepC) study. This study was conducted from 2002-2006 to investigate differences between African Americans and Caucasians in response to antiviral therapy for hepatitis virus C (HCV) (Conjeevaram et al., 2006). The outcome was sustained virological response ($D = 1$ if present and $D = 0$ otherwise). We considered the following covariates $\mathbf{X}$: race (white, non-white), sex (male, female), Ishak fibrosis score that assesses liver fibrosis stages ranging from normal to cirrhosis (regrouped into four categories) and AST/ALT enzyme ratio (in quartiles).

The original model $R_{\mathbf{X}}$ was obtained by including the covariates $\mathbf{X}$ in a logistic regression model.

We then updated the risk models by adding two new markers, interferon lambda 4 (IFNL4) genotype in two categories ($\Delta G/\Delta G$ or $\Delta G/TT$ corresponding to $Z_1 = 0$, and TT/TT corresponding to $Z_1 = 1$), and continuous levels of pre-treatment HCV-RNA ($\log_{10}$(IU/ml); Z_2) to obtain the updated risk prediction model, $R_{\mathbf{X},Z_1,Z_2}$. The marginal distributions of $\mathbf{X}$ and (Z_1, Z_2) are shown in Table 8.2 for the 350 patients with complete predictor information, together with the log odds ratio estimates from the baseline model that included only $\mathbf{X}$, and from the model that included $\mathbf{X}$, Z_1 and Z_2. The variable Z_1 was more common in Caucasians. The variable Z_2 was negatively correlated with AST/ALT ratio (Spearman ρ =-0.23), but only weakly correlated with other baseline covariates (data not shown).

To generate data, we used the estimates of $\beta_{\mathbf{X}}, \beta_{Z_1}$ and β_{Z_2} from the last column of Table 8.2. We first sampled covariate vectors $(\mathbf{X}, Z_1, Z_2)$ with replacement from the 350 study subjects to obtain covariate data for n patients. We then used these covariate vectors to generate outcomes D from a logistic regression model,

$$P(D=1|\mathbf{X}, Z_1, Z_2) = \frac{\exp\{\beta_0 + \boldsymbol{\beta}'_{\mathbf{X}}\mathbf{X} + \beta_{Z_1}Z_1 + \beta_{Z_2}Z_2\}}{1+\exp\{\beta_0 + \boldsymbol{\beta}'_{\mathbf{X}}\mathbf{X} + \beta_{Z_1}Z_1 + \beta_{Z_2}Z_2\}}, \tag{8.29}$$

with $\beta_0 = 0.8$, corresponding to an outcome prevalence of $P(D=1) = 0.1$.

Table 8.2: Distribution of the predictors of sustained virologic response ($D = 1$) and estimated predictor effects in the $n = 350$ ViraHepC participants from whom predictors were sampled for simulations

Variable	**Categories**	**Distribution**	**Baseline model, covariates X** $\boldsymbol{\beta}$ **(std err)**	**Model with covariates X, IFNL4 genotype (Z₁) & HCV-RNA (Z₂)** $\boldsymbol{\beta}$ **(std err)**
Race	Caucasian	52.7%	Ref	Ref
	Non-white	48.3%	−0.85 (0.241)	−0.62 (0.261)
Sex	Male	65.4%	Ref	Ref
	Female	34.6%	0.73 (0.262)	0.68 (0.269))
Ishak fibrosis	0	10.6%	−0.29 (0.156)	−0.33 (0.161)
score	1–2	52.9%		
(ordinal)	3–4	29.7%		
	5–6	6.9%		
AST/ALT ratio (ordinal)	per quartile		−0.39 (0.117)	−0.32 (0.121)
IFNL4	$\Delta G/(\Delta G$ or $TT)$	72.0%	–	Ref
	TT/TT	28.0%	–	0.93 (0.282)
log_{10}HCV-RNA level (median, IQR^a)	–	$6.5(5.6, 6.8)$	–	−0.41 (0.162)
*AUC**			0.701	0.738

[a]IQR - Interquartile range (25th percentile - 75th percentile); * AUC based on c-statistics from SAS PROC logistic. Log odds ratios β (with standard errors) are shown for the baseline model and for the model updated with genetic and viral load information. Parameter estimates from the baseline model were used as the values $\boldsymbol{\gamma}$ in Equation (8.12). Quartile cutoffs for AST/ALT ratio: 0.3165 (min.), 0.6307 (25%), 0.7705 (50%), 0.9302 (75%), 2.275 (max.).

After generating D for each set of covariates from model (8.29), we created three disjoint sets, A, B and C. Dataset A with $n_A = 1,000,000$ samples that only included predictors $\mathbf{X}$ was used to fit model $R_{\mathbf{X}}$ in (8.10). Dataset B, comprised of $n_{cases} = n_{controls} = 250$ cases and controls, with information on $(D, \mathbf{X}, Z)$ was used to estimate $R_{Z,\mathbf{X}}$ based on all methods presented in Table 8.1. To compute the $LR_D(\mathbf{Z}|\mathbf{X})$ for two markers, we used Equation (8.23).

As our prediction is based on a logistic model, we needed to ensure that the intercept term in $R_{\mathbf{X},Z}$ yielded the correct population prevalence or incidence of the outcome. We thus modified models (8.7), (8.25) and (8.27) to match the true disease prevalence $P(D = 1)$, which is assumed known without error from external data, by solving the following equation for μ^*:

$$P(D=1) - \int_Z \int_{\mathbf{X}} \frac{\exp(\mu^* + \hat{g}(\mathbf{X}, Z))}{1 + \exp(\mu^* + \hat{g}(\mathbf{X}, Z))} d\hat{F}(\mathbf{X}, Z) = 0. \tag{8.30}$$

For model (8.7), $\hat{g}(\mathbf{X}, Z) = \hat{\boldsymbol{\beta}}_X' \mathbf{X} + \hat{\beta}_Z Z$, and for model (8.25), $\hat{g}(\mathbf{X}, Z) = \boldsymbol{\gamma}_1' \mathbf{X} + \hat{\delta}_1 Z$. To adjust the intercept for LR-shrink in (8.27), we first included an additional intercept θ_0 in the model to absorb the case-control sampling ratio and γ_{01},

$$\log(\textit{posterior odds}) = \boldsymbol{\gamma}_1' \mathbf{X} + \theta_0 + \theta_1 \log\{\mathrm{LR}_D(Z)\}, \tag{8.31}$$

and after obtaining $\hat{\theta}_1$, solved (8.30) for $\hat{g}(\mathbf{X}, Z) = \boldsymbol{\gamma}_1' \mathbf{X} + \hat{\theta}_1 \log\{\mathrm{LR}_D(Z)\}$. For a rare disease, the empirical distribution function in the controls in the case-control study provides an estimate $\hat{F}(\mathbf{X}, Z)$, if the controls constitute a random sample from the general population. Here we estimated the empirical distribution of $\mathbf{X}$, $\hat{F}(\mathbf{X})$, from dataset A, and the empirical distribution $\hat{F}_{control}(Z|\mathbf{X})$ from the controls in dataset B, to obtain $\hat{F}(Z, \mathbf{X}) = \hat{F}_{control}(Z|\mathbf{X})\hat{F}_A(\mathbf{X})$.

We used data from a third independent dataset, C, a random sample of size n_C = 100,000, to evaluate the predictive performance of the models updated using the various methods. Letting $r_i = \hat{R}_{\mathbf{X}_i, Z_i}$ be the estimated risk and π_i be the corresponding true risk in the simulation model, we assessed the bias of r_i with the ratio of expected to observed cases, $E/O = \sum r_i / \sum O_i$ overall and in subgroups in the third independent dataset, C. To be consistent with notation in Chapter 6, we use O_i instead of D_i to denote the observed outcomes here. For each setting we present means over 1,000 simulations. The variability of the prediction was assessed by first taking the mean of the predicted probabilities $\sum r_i/n$ in each simulation and then computing the standard deviation of the means over the simulation runs with the same setting. We also present results for the area under the receiver operating characteristic (*ROC*) curve (*AUC*), the mean squared bias, $Bias2 = n^{-1}\sum(r_i - \pi_i)^2$, and the estimated mean Brier score (Brier, 1950), $\widehat{MSE} = n^{-1}\sum(O_i - r_i)^2$. See Chapter 6.

Table 8.3 shows the performance of a model $R_{\mathbf{X}, Z_1, Z_2}$ that was updated with the binary genotype, Z_1, and continuous HCV-RNA levels, Z_2. Logistic-new, LR-indep, LR-offset, LR-separate and LR-shrink overestimated risk on the entire population by 8 to 13% (see E/O ratios). Models updated using LR-indep underestimated risks for the IFNL4 $\Delta G/\Delta G$ or $\Delta G/TT$ genotype by 6% and overestimated them for the TT/TT genotype group by 29%, while models updated using LR-separate overestimated in these genotype groups by 4% and 10% respectively. The *AUC* values ranged from 0.740 for CML and LR-joint to 0.729 for LR-separate, which also had a much larger mean squared bias (*Bias*2) overall and in subgroups than the other methods (Table 8.3).

The limited variation of the Brier scores and the *AUC* values across the different methods indicates that the mean Brier score (or mean square error), which is the sum of the squared bias and the Bernoulli variation of the outcome, was dominated by Bernoulli variability. The *AUC* is generally not sensitive to bias, as it is a function of the ranks of the predicted probabilities. However, the standard errors for the *AUC* were noticeably larger for logistic-new and LR-separate than for the other methods, and the standard error of the $\widehat{MSE}$ was large for LR-ind and LR-separate. There were noticeable differences in the mean squared bias (*Bias*2) among the various methods, with the lowest values seen for LR-joint and CML, as expected from the E/O ratios.

8.4.8 Summary

The two procedures LR-joint and CML exhibited little bias overall or in subgroups defined by genotypes of IFNL4, as reflected in E/O ratios near 1.0 and small *Bias*2. Other updating procedures exhibited more bias and larger MSE, especially LR-indep. Other performance

Table 8.3: Performance of various updating procedures for two markers, IFNL4 and HCV-RNA

Method	Overall					In subgroups based on IFNL4 genotype							
						$\Delta G/\Delta G$ or ΔG/TT				TT/TT			
	E/O (se)	**sd(Ē)**	**AUC (se)**	**Bias2 (se)**	**MSE (se)**	**E/O (se)**	**sd(Ē)**	**Bias2**	**MSE**	**E/O (se)**	**sd(Ē)**	**Bias2**	**MSE**
Logistic-new	1.089 (0.002)	0.0053	0.736 (0.000141)	0.0009 (0.000021)	0.085 (0.000030)	1.095 (0.003)	0.0058	0.0005	0.060	1.084 (0.004)	0.0222	0.0021	0.149
LR-joint	1.005 (0.001)	0.0030	0.740 (0.000102)	0.0003 (0.000010)	0.085 (0.000024)	0.992 (0.002)	0.0047	0.0001	0.060	1.016 (0.003)	0.0182	0.0008	0.148
LR-separate	1.078 (0.002)	0.0051	0.729 (0.000171)	0.0066 (0.000094)	0.091 (0.000097)	1.046 (0.003)	0.0053	0.0041	0.064	1.107 (0.003)	0.0206	0.0133	0.160
LR-ind	1.126 (0.002)	0.0052	0.736 (0.000098)	0.0059 (0.000092)	0.090 (0.000095)	0.944 (0.002)	0.0048	0.0039	0.064	1.287 (0.004)	0.0214	0.0112	0.158
LR-offset	1.084 (0.002)	0.0050	0.738 (0.000111)	0.0008 (0.000018)	0.085 (0.000027)	1.092 (0.003)	0.0059	0.0005	0.060	1.077 (0.004)	0.0217	0.0017	0.149
LR-shrink	1.089 (0.002)	0.0053	0.735 (0.000108)	0.0016 (0.000041)	0.086 (0.000046)	1.106 (0.003)	0.0061	0.0013	0.061	1.075 (0.004)	0.0218	0.0025	0.150
CML	1.006 (0.001)	0.0031	0.740 (0.000104)	0.0003 (0.000011)	0.085 (0.000024)	1.004 (0.002)	0.0048	0.0002	0.060	1.008 (0.003)	0.0176	0.0008	0.148

Shown are the ratio E/O of expected number of events(E) to observed number of events (O) (with standard error), the standard deviation of the mean predicted values, $\bar{E}$, and the mean values of AUC, squared bias (Bias2) and the mean square error (MSE or expected Brier score), with their standard errors from simulations based on ViraHepC data. The internal case-control sample had $n_{cases} = 250$ cases and $n_{controls} = 250$ controls. The population disease incidence was $P(D) = 0.1$.

measures such as AUC, which is not affected by bias that preserves rankings, and the expected Brier score, which is dominated by the binomial component of variance, were similar for the various procedures. On the basis of these data, and other results in Grill et al. (2016), we recommend CML or LR-joint for updating.

Some of these methods assume that the distributions of covariates in the data that gave rise to the original model based on $\mathbf{X}$ and in the new internal data that include $\mathbf{X}$ and the novel markers Z are the same. Simulations in Grill et al. (2016) revealed bias in estimates from CML and LR-joint when this assumption was violated. Thus this assumption should be assessed, to the extent possible with data on $\mathbf{X}$, before assuming that the updated model is valid. A more conclusive test would be to study the performance of the updated model in independent validation data (Chapter 6).

This literature pertains to estimates of risk $R_{\mathbf{X},Z} = P(D = 1|\mathbf{X}, Z)$ from logistic models. Further research is needed to apply these methods directly to the absolute risk models in Chapter 4. However, the good performance of LR-joint and CML for estimating $R_{\mathbf{X},Z}$ in these studies also implies good estimation of relative risks, as in Equation (8.5). These relative risks and their associated attributable risks, can be used, as in Chapter 5, to estimate absolute risk with a cause-specific hazard model by incorporating registry data.

Chapter 9

Risk estimates based on genetic variants and family studies

9.1 Introduction

In this chapter we discuss models for estimating absolute risk, pure cumulative risk, and relative risk from family-based studies, such as kin-cohort studies (Struewing et al., 1997; Wacholder et al., 1998) and studies of families ascertained because they have several diseased members ("multiplex pedigrees"). Key considerations include whether the model allows for residual familial correlations apart from those attributable to the genes that are explicitly included in the model (compare Sections 9.2 and 9.3), and how the family was ascertained, which determines the likelihood equations Section(9.4). Section 9.5 compares several genetically based models and an empirical model, the Breast Cancer Risk Assessment Tool (BCRAT) for projecting breast cancer risk (Tables 1.1, 9.1, 9.2 and 9.3). Some of these models, such as BCRAT project absolute breast cancer risk, whereas others project pure breast cancer risk that treats competing risks as random censoring (Chapter 2). The emphasis is on breast cancer models because there is a vast literature on this topic, because various family-based designs have been used to study breast cancer risk, and because both strongly associated mutations and weakly associated genetic markers (SNPs) have been identified for breast cancer. However, the statistical approaches we discuss also apply to other diseases.

Continuous traits, such as height, tend to be normally distributed in the population, reflecting, in part, the variations at many genetic loci, each acting independently and having a modest effect on the trait (Fisher, 1918). Risks of cancer and other diseases are also influenced by such "*polygenic*" effects. Some mutations, however, confer high risks of cancer. For example, women with mutations in the BRCA1 or BRCA2 genes have high risk of breast and ovarian cancer. Mutations that confer high risk are called "*highly penetrant.*" These highly penetrant mutations tend to be rare. Mutations in BRCA1 and BRCA2 occur in less than 1% of the U.S. population. It is therefore hard to study risks conferred by these mutations in population-based cohort or case-control studies. For example, in order to estimate the lifetime risk of developing breast cancer from a highly penetrant (lifetime risk 0.92) dominant mutation with allele frequency 0.0033, as estimated in Claus et al. (1991), with confidence interval of width 0.10, one would need to recruit, genotype and follow 17,301 women (Gail et al., 1999c). Likewise, if the lifetime breast cancer risk is known in the general population, case-control data can be used to estimate the risk in mutation carriers, but the most efficient version of this design would require genotyping 15,506 control women and 1,524 women with breast cancer (Gail et al., 1999c). Thus there is a strong incentive to study populations that are enriched in mutation carriers, such as families with several affected members, in order to reduce the recruitment and genotyping burden. Care must be taken, however, in generalizing the findings from such studies to the general population.

Genetic models are needed to estimate risk from a specific mutation from family-based studies. To analyze such data correctly, one must also take the mode of ascertainment of the family into account. Moreover, other polygenic or environmental factors apart from the gene under study may induce familial aggregation of disease that is not accounted for by the gene under study ("residual familial risk"). For example, mutations in BRAC1 or BRCA2 account for only about 22% of the familial aggregation of breast cancer (Ghoussaini and Pharoah, 2009). Unless the genetic model allows for such residual familial risk, biased risk estimates can be obtained.

We begin our discussion with simple Mendelian models that assume that the only factor that modifies risk, apart from age, is the genotype at a single locus or gene. Then we discuss methods and models that allow for residual familial correlation and analytic methods that take ascertainment and residual correlation into account to estimate risk.

9.2 Mendelian models: the autosomal dominant model for pure breast cancer risk

The simplest genetic models, Mendelian models, assume that a mutation at a single genetic locus (gene) is the only factor that affects pure risk, apart from age. To allow for stratifying factors such as gender or race, separate models might be fitted in each stratum. Under such Mendelian models, it is possible to calculate the joint genotypes of all members of a family, and hence the joint probabilities that each family member carries one or two mutant alleles. Because carrying the mutation is assumed to be the sole determinant of risk, apart from age, it is possible to estimate the genotype-specific risk from family data.

One of the most widely used Mendelian models for cancer risk is the autosomal dominant model. Under an autosomal dominant model, a person with one mutant allele has the same risk as a person with two mutant alleles at the same locus. Even before the BRCA1 and BRCA2 genes had been identified, Claus et al. (1991) estimated the cumulative risk of breast cancer in carriers and in non-carriers of a putative autosomal dominant mutation by using data on the history of breast cancer in the mother and sisters of women with breast cancer (cases) and of women without breast cancer (controls). The cases and controls in this study, the Cancer and Steroid Hormone Study (CASH), were sampled from the general population, rather than from highly affected families. These cases and controls are called probands. For each person in a family, we observe $Y_i = (\delta_i, X_i)$, where $\delta_i = 1$ if the disease of interest (breast cancer) is observed and 0 otherwise, and where $X_i = \min(T_i, C_i)$ is the minimum of age at end of follow-up C_i, which might result from death from competing causes, or age at disease incidence, T_i. The family information on disease outcome is $\mathbf{Y} = (Y_0, Y_1, ..., Y_K)^T = (Y_0, \mathbf{Y}_K^T)^T$, where $i = 0$ denotes the proband and $i = 1, 2, ..., K$ the relatives of the proband. The vector of genotypes is $\mathbf{G} = (G_0, \mathbf{G}_K^T)^T$, but none of these were measured in the study of Claus et al. (1991). Each family contributed the following factor to the likelihood:

$$P(\mathbf{Y}_K|Y_0) = \frac{\sum_{\mathbf{G}} P(\mathbf{G}) \prod_{i=0}^{K} P(Y_i|G_i)}{\sum_{G_0} P(G_0)(Y_0|G_0)}. \tag{9.1}$$

The summations are over the possible genotypes, which were unmeasured, and the likelihood conditions on Y_0, which was determined by design. The genotype probabilities were computed using Mendel's laws and the assumption of Hardy-Weinberg equilibrium. Under this assumption, a randomly selected member of the populations has probabilities p^2, $2p(1-p)$, and $(1-p)^2$ respectively of carrying 2, 1 or 0 copies of a bi-allelic allele (a variant form of a gene or genetic locus) with allele probability p. The product in Equation (9.1) arises from the strong assumption of conditional independence, namely that the breast cancer history for each woman depends only on her genotype and is conditionally independent of the phenotypes of other family members, given her genotype. We will discuss this later. For survival data, Claus et al. (1991) assumed that given G_i,

$$P(Y_i|G_i) = [\gamma_{G_i}\phi\{(X_i - \mu_{G_i})/\sigma_{G_i}\}]^{\delta_i}[1 - \gamma_{G_i}\Phi\{(X_i - \mu_{G_i})/\sigma_{G_i}\}]^{1-\delta_i}\ . \tag{9.2}$$

In expression (9.2), γ_{G_i} is the genotype-specific pure lifetime risk of breast cancer, ϕ and Φ are the density and distribution function for a standard normal variable, and μ_{G_i} and σ_{G_i} are genotype-specific means and standard deviations of the conditional distribution of age-at-disease onset among women with breast cancer. The factor γ_{G_i},which is between 0 and 1, allows for the lifetime probability of breast cancer to be less than one. Nonetheless, Claus et al. (1991) treat competing causes of mortality as independent censoring. Thus expression (9.1) models pure breast cancer risk. Claus et al. (1991) maximized the product over probands of expression (9.1) to estimate a mutant allele frequency of 0.0033 (carrier probability 0.0066) and pure lifetime risks of 92.8% for mutation carriers and 10.0% for non-carriers. Using this model, Claus and her colleagues calculated pure breast cancer risks for women with relatives affected at various ages (Claus et al., 1994). For example, a 49-year-old woman whose mother developed breast cancer at age 25 has a 20-year pure risk of 11.6% of developing breast cancer, whereas, if her mother had been 65 at cancer onset, her 20-year pure risk would be 5.3%.

A linkage study localized a mutation for early-onset breast cancer to chromosome 17q21 in 1990 (Hall et al., 1990), and the corresponding BRCA1 gene was identified by cloning in 1994 (US Patent 5747282), enabling one to measure mutations in it. BRCA2 was localized to chromosome 13q12-13 in 1994 (Wooster et al., 1994) and cloned by 1998 (US Patent 5837492). Subsequent studies measured the prevalence of mutations in these genes and the genotype-specific risk of breast and other cancers, and confirmed that risk from these mutations followed an autosomal dominant pattern. In Section 9.3 we discuss some of the methods used to estimate breast cancer risk that rely on the ability to measure mutations in these genes.

Only women with an appreciable chance of carrying a mutation, say >10%, were recommended for actual genetic testing for mutations. Assuming autosomal dominance and that breast and ovarian cancers were statistically independent given genotype, and using data on the prevalence of mutant alleles and on genotype-specific pure risks for breast and ovarian cancers, Berry et al. (1997) applied Bayes' Theorem to compute $P(G_0|\mathbf{Y})$, where G_0 is the number of mutated BRCA1 alleles in the woman who is being counseled, and $\mathbf{Y}$ includes information on the times to breast and ovarian cancer for the counselee and her relatives. The probability that a mutation is present is $P(\text{a mutation is present}|\mathbf{Y}) = P(G_0 = 1 \text{ or } 2|\mathbf{Y})$. The algorithms were later modified to yield such calculations separately for BRCA1 and BRCA2. A nice feature of this model is that one can also use information on the BRCA1 and BRCA2 mutation carrier status of one or more relatives, $k*$, if available, to produce an improved estimate, say

$$P(G_0|\mathbf{Y}, G_{k*} = g_{k*}). \tag{9.3}$$

One can also project future risk for the counselee at age a to a subsequent age $a + \tau$, given family disease history to age $a, \mathbf{Y}(a)$ and family genotype information if available as

$$\sum_{G_0} P(G_0|\mathbf{Y}(a), G_{k*} = g_{k*})r(a, a + \tau, G_0), \tag{9.4}$$

where $r(a, a + \tau, G_0)$ is the absolute risk of breast cancer between ages a and $a + \tau$ for a woman who does not have breast cancer at age a and has genotype G_0. An algorithm, BRCAPRO, calculates the expressions (9.3) and (9.4). Although the initial version of BRCAPRO used pure risks instead of $r(a, a + \tau, G_0)$ in Equation

(9.4), the current version gives absolute risks that account for competing mortality (http://bcb.dfci.harvard.edu/bayesmendel/brcapro.php).

One indication that mutations in BRCA1 and BRCA2 do not explain the association between family history and breast cancer risk entirely came from a reanalysis of the CASH study after culling out all the women whose BRCAPRO-estimated chance of carrying a mutation in BRCA1 or BRCA2 was 1% or more (Claus et al., 1998). The odds ratio associated with a family history of breast cancer in a first-degree relative was 2.3 for the entire CASH study and 2.1 after removing those with even this slight chance of carrying a mutation. Thus, much of the familial association remained. This suggested a need for models that allowed for residual familial aggregation in addition to the autosomal dominant component, as described in Section 9.3.

9.3 Models that allow for residual familial aggregation to estimate pure breast cancer risk

9.3.1 Polygenic risk

Suppose that the effects of many single nucleotide polymorphisms (SNPs) act multiplicatively on the relative risk (RR) of disease. Let β_i and $G_i = 0$, 1 or 2 be respectively the log relative risk per minor allele and the number of minor alleles for the ith SNP in a set of M such SNPs. If the relative risk for the ith SNP is $\exp(\beta_i G_i)$, then

$$\log(RR) = \sum_{i=1}^{M} \beta_i G_i. \tag{9.5}$$

If the SNP genotypes are independent ("linkage equilibrium"), then $\log(RR)$ is approximately normally distributed with mean $\mu = \sum_{i=1}^{M} 2\eta_i\beta_i \equiv \sum_{i=1}^{M} \mu_i$ and variance

$$\sigma^2 = \sum_{i=1}^{M} 2\eta_i(1-\eta_i)\beta_i^2 \equiv \sum_{i=1}^{M} \sigma_i^2, \tag{9.6}$$

where η_i is the minor allele frequency for SNP i.

As in Fisher (1918), the correlation in $\log(RR)$ between two first-degree relatives is 1/2, and between two second-degree relatives 1/4. Over short time intervals, risks are proportional to relative risks. This type of structure justifies the assumption of log-normally distributed risks used to assess the potential for disease prevention in polygenic models (Pharoah et al., 2002).

9.3.2 Models with latent genetic effects: BOADICEA and IBIS

One way to correct for residual familial correlation is to allow for a latent genetic effect in addition to the measured mutation (Antoniou et al., 2002, 2004; Tyrer et al., 2005). Antoniou and colleagues incorporated an unmeasured polygenic effect in a model that also included separate nuisance hazards for highly penetrant mutations (Antoniou and Easton, 2003; Antoniou et al., 2004, 2008a). Letting $g = 2$, 1, or 0 index carriers of a BRCA2 mutation, carriers of a BRCA1 mutation, and non-carriers, and letting C denote a polygenic normally distributed component with mean 0 and variance σ^2, Antoniou and colleagues modeled the cohort-, genotype-, and age-specific pure breast cancer hazard as

$$\lambda_{G=g}(t|C) = \lambda_0(t) RR_g(t) \exp\{C\}. \tag{9.7}$$

In this expression, $\lambda_0(t)$ is the cohort-specific breast cancer hazard for women without BRCA1 or BRCA2 mutations, and $RR_1(t)$ and $RR_2(t)$ are relative risks that can vary with age t for BRCA1 and BRCA2 mutation carriers respectively. The average hazard for women without BRCA1 or BRCA2 mutation in the general population, $\lambda_0^*(t)$, is obtained by averaging over C as in Equation (9.10). Antoniou et al. (2008a) estimated relative risks mainly from genotyping population-based cases, not cases ascertained through highly affected families. The model was constrained to fit the observed and age-smoothed composite cohort-specific breast cancer incidence rates in England and Wales. The polygenic variance was estimated as $\hat{\sigma}^2 = 4.83 - 0.06 \times \text{age}$. Calculations were facilitated by approximating the normal distribution of C by the hypergeometric distribution. This model (Antoniou et al., 2008a), BOADICEA, predicts pure breast cancer risk and can incorporate data on BRCA1 and BRCA2 mutation status, if available. BOADICEA is available at http://ccge.medschl.cam.ac.uk/boadicea/model/. A test version that includes certain other mutations in addition to BRCA1 and BRCA2 mutations is also available.

Not only does inclusion of a parameter for residual familial correlation affect estimates of genotype-specific hazard rates and hence estimates of pure risk and of mutation carrier probabilities based on family history, but such correlation parameters are also of intrinsic interest for estimating risk. For example, suppose a 55-year old counselee and her mother both tested negative for mutations of BRCA1 and BRCA2. The mother developed breast cancer at age $t_m = 45$ years; the counselee has no sisters and the family history is limited to first-degree relatives. The conditional density of C_m, the polygenic effect of the mother, given $t_m = 45$, is

$$p_{C_m|T_m}(c_m|t_m) = \frac{\exp(c_m)\exp\{-\Lambda_0(t_m)\exp(c_m)\}\varphi(c_m;0,\sigma^2)}{\int \exp(c)\exp\{-\Lambda_0(t_m)\exp(c)\}\varphi(c;0,\sigma^2)dc}, \tag{9.8}$$

where $\varphi(c_m;\mu,\sigma^2)$ is the normal density with mean μ and variance σ^2 and where $\Lambda_0(t)$ is the integral of the baseline hazard $\lambda_0(t)$ to age t. The conditional distribution of the daughter's polygenic effect, C_d, given C_m is normal with mean $C_m/2$ and variance $0.75\sigma^2$, as follows from the fact (Fisher, 1918) that the correlation between C_d and C_m is 0.5. The conditional density of C_d given t_m is

$$p_{C_d|T_m}(c_d|t_m) = \int \varphi(c_d; c_m/2, 0.75\sigma^2)p_{C_m|T_m}(c_m|t_m)dc_m. \tag{9.9}$$

The unconditional hazard of breast cancer for the daughter at age t_d is (Gail, 2008b)

$$\lambda_0^*(t_d) = \frac{\lambda_0(t_d)\int \exp(c)\exp\{-\Lambda_0(t_d)\exp(c)\}\varphi(c;0,\sigma^2)dc}{\int \exp\{-\Lambda_0(t_d)\exp(c)\}\varphi(c;0,\sigma^2)dc}, \tag{9.10}$$

whereas the corresponding conditional hazard given t_m is

$$\lambda_0^*(t_d|t_m) = \frac{\lambda_0(t_d)\int \exp(c)\exp\{-\Lambda_0(t_d)\exp(c)\}p_{C_d|T_m}(c|t_m)dc}{\int \exp\{-\Lambda_0(t_d)\exp(c)\}p_{C_d|T_m}(c|t_m)dc}. \tag{9.11}$$

To compute the desired familial relative risk (Risch, 1990),

$$FRR = \lambda_0^*(t_d|t_m)/\lambda_0^*(t_d), \tag{9.12}$$

requires repeated numerical integration. However, if breast cancer is rare in non-carriers, $\exp\{-\Lambda_0(t_d)\exp(c)\}$ can be set to unity, and, after additional calculations (Gail, 2008b), it follows that

$$FRR \doteq \exp(\sigma^2/2). \tag{9.13}$$

For a 55-year-old counselee, $\hat{\sigma}^2 = 4.83 - 0.06 \times 55 = 1.53$, and $FRR = 2.15$. Thus, the fact that the mother had breast cancer more than doubles the hazard for the daughter, compared to the general population of non-carriers, even though both the mother and daughter are non-carriers. This is a consequence of residual familial risk, and it is in good agreement with the earlier findings of Claus et al. (1998) on residual familial association after taking BRCA1 and BRCA2 into account.

The IBIS model (Tyrer et al., 2005) predicts pure breast cancer risk (with an option to calculate absolute risk) and includes a latent, common, low-penetrant, autosomal dominant gene, in addition to BRCA1 and BRCA2 mutations, to account for residual familial aggregation. The latent gene is assumed to segregate independently of the BRCA1 and BRCA2 genes. The IBIS model includes reproductive risk factors and features of the medical history, such as results of biopsies and a previous diagnosis of lobular carcinoma *in situ*, in addition to the genetic factors. A program for IBIS can be obtained from http://www.ems-trials.org/riskevaluator/.

9.3.3 Copula models

Suppose $S_G(t) = \exp\{-\int_0^{t_i} \lambda_G(u)du\} = P(T > t)$ is the marginal pure survival distribution for time to breast cancer for a woman randomly selected from the general population of women with genotype G. The corresponding marginal hazard is λ_G. Suppose that a family with $K + 1$ individuals is selected at random from the general population. One way to characterize the joint distribution of times to breast cancer in the family is by combining marginal survival probabilities through a copula distribution (Chatterjee et al., 2006, 2007),

$$P(T_0 > t_0,\ T_1 > t_1, \ldots, T_K > t_K) = C_\theta\{S_{G_0}(t_0), S_{G_1}(t_1), \ldots, S_{G_K}(t_K)\}. \quad (9.14)$$

The copula distribution C_θ with association parameter(s) θ is a joint distribution on $K{+}1$ uniform [0,1] random variables. A key question in using such models is how well they fit the joint distribution on the left side of Equation (9.14). However, making some allowance for residual familial correlation, even if not exactly correct, is often more realistic than assuming no residual familial correlation.

9.4 Estimating genotype-specific absolute risk from family-based designs

9.4.1 General considerations

To understand the literature on genotype-specific risk estimation, one must keep several distinctions in mind. First, we assume that the genotypes of interest can be measured. Thus, we can treat these genotypes as risk factors in statistical analyses. We are not discussing segregation analysis, which genetic epidemiologists have used to estimate risk for hypothesized but unmeasured genes, as in Claus et al. (1991). Second, many publications present *pure, not absolute risk*, because they treat death from competing causes as an independent censoring event and apply standard survival estimation procedures, such as the Kaplan-Meier estimator (Chapter 2). Third, one needs to identify the target population to which the risk estimates apply. One might want to estimate risk for a randomly selected *member of the general population* who has a specific genotype. We may attempt to estimate risk by studying families that have been identified because several members have the disease of interest ("multiplex pedigrees"). Unless special care is taken, such data yield risk estimates that are applicable to members of multiplex families, but are too high for the general population.

Large cohorts of people who are representative of the general population and whose genotypes are known may be followed to determine health outcomes. If the cohorts are large enough (Section 9.1), it will be possible to estimate both pure and absolute genotype-specific risk with standard methods from such cohort studies (Chapters 2, 3, and 4). At present, we consider family-based designs that are more efficient for studying rare genotypes and have been used in the literature.

9.4.2 *Combining relative-risks from family-based case-control studies with population-based incidence rates*

Sometimes relative risks are estimated by comparing the genotypes of cases and controls within a family. For example, suppose families with a diseased sibling and at least one non-diseased sibling are ascertained. Regarding each family as a stratum, and genotyping all the siblings, one can use conditional logistic regression or the Mantel-Haenszel procedure for matched data to estimate the relative odds of disease, comparing mutation carrier genotypes $G = 1 \text{ or } 2$ to non-carriers, $G = 0$. For a rare disease, this relative odds approximates a relative risk, $RR_{fam}(G = g)$. If the mutation is rare, incidence rates from the general population $\lambda^*(t)$ approximately equal rates for non-carriers in the general population, $\lambda_0^*(t)$. Hence one can estimate the genotype- and cause-specific hazard in the general population, $\lambda_g(t)$, by substituting estimates in $\lambda_g(t) = RR_{fam}(G = g)\lambda_0^*(t) \doteq RR_{fam}(G = g)\lambda^*(t)$. To compute absolute risks, one can use formula (3.4) to incorporate the competing hazard of (e.g., non-breast cancer) mortality.

The previous estimate of $\lambda_g(t)$ is only valid if the relative risk $RR_{fam}(G = g)$ from family-based case-control data estimates the same relative risk, $RR(G = g)$, as would be obtained from a random sample of cases and controls from the general population. If there are family-associated factors that influence risk independently of the genotype under study, such as polygenic effects or environmental exposures, then the *population-based relative risks will tend to be smaller* than the relative risks estimated from family data. One way to approximate such unmeasured factors is through a random frailty, b, that is associated with each family. Suppose b is a non-negative random variable with mean 1.0, and suppose that the baseline hazard in a family with frailty b is $b\lambda_0^{fam}(t)$. Assume that hazards are proportional within family such that $RR_{fam}(G = g) \equiv \lambda_g^{fam}(t)/\lambda_0^{fam}(t)$ is a constant independent of t. Note that b differs from $\exp(C)$ in Equation (9.7) because the same b applies to every family member, whereas the variables C in Equation (9.7), though correlated among family members, are not identical. It can be shown (Gail, 2008b) that the marginal hazard in the general population, obtained by averaging over the distribution of b, satisfies $\lambda_g \leq \lambda_g^{fam}(t)$. Moreover, the general population (marginal) relative hazard $RR(G = g) \equiv \lambda_g(t)/\lambda_0(t) \leq RR_{fam}(G = g)$ for $RR_{fam}(G = g) \geq 1.0$. Thus, there is a danger of overestimating the genotype-specific relative risks in the general population by using within-family estimates of relative risk. The kin-cohort design, described next, can be used to estimate relative risks that are closer to the general population relative risks.

9.4.3 *Kin-cohort design*

The kin-cohort design is a population-based study design that also incorporates information from family members. Ideally, one obtains a random sample of cases from cases in the general population and a random sample of controls from non-cases in the general population. These sampled cases and controls are called "probands". The probands agree to be genotyped and to provide disease histories (phenotypes Y_k) for their first-degree relatives (Struewing et al., 1997; Wacholder et al., 1998). The sample can be enriched in case probands, and indeed many studies have used case probands only. This design was used to estimate the pure risk of breast cancer in Ashkenazi women carrying mutations BRCA1 or BRCA2 (Struewing et al., 1997). In the notation of Section 9.2, the contribution to the likelihood from each proband's family (Gail et al., 1999c,b), conditional on the ascertainment event, namely the disease status $Y_0 = (\delta, T)$ of the proband, is

$$P(\mathbf{Y}_K, G_0|Y_0) = P(G_0|Y_0) \sum\nolimits_{\mathbf{G}_K} P(\mathbf{G}_K|G_0) P(\mathbf{Y}_K|\mathbf{G}_K, Y_0). \tag{9.15}$$

The summation is over all joint genotypes of relatives, and $P(\mathbf{G}_K|G_0)$ is defined by Mendel's laws and Hardy-Weinberg equilibrium. If each individual's genotype is the only factor that influences his or her phenotype, then phenotypes are conditionally independent given $\mathbf{G}$, and Equation (9.15) can be simplified because

$$P(\mathbf{Y}_K|\mathbf{G}_K, Y_0) = \prod_{i=1}^{K} P(Y_i|G_i). \tag{9.16}$$

Under this "conditional independence" assumption, likelihood methods for survival data (Gail et al., 1999b) applied to (9.15) can be used to estimate the allele frequency and genotype-specific hazards, $\lambda_g^{fam}(t)$. Under conditional independence, the family-specific and marginal hazards in the general population, λ_g, are equal. Absolute risks can be obtained by applying Equation (3.4).

Several biases can arise in kin-cohort studies. If the tendency to participate as a proband and give blood for genotyping is greater in individuals who have several affected first degree relatives than in individuals whose families have few or no affected relatives, estimates of $\lambda_g^{fam}(t)$ will be too high, not only for mutation carriers but also for non-carriers (Wacholder et al., 1998; Gail et al., 1999b). If the proband mistakenly reports disease in his or her relatives, hazards can be seriously overestimated, and if the proband neglects to report disease that has occurred, hazards will be underestimated (Gail et al., 1999c,b, 2001). If the gene in question increases the risk of death from competing causes, the hazard for the disease of interest will be underestimated (Chatterjee et al., 2003; Gail and Chatterjee, 2004). This problem can be eliminated in principle by modeling the effects of the gene on the competing hazards (Chatterjee et al., 2003). This underestimation is even more severe if the risk of mortality following incidence of the disease of interest is higher in mutation carriers than non-carriers (Gail and Chatterjee, 2004). Asymptotic formulas can be inaccurate, even for seemingly large samples (Gail et al., 1999c,b, 2001), and the "reproducibility" assumption, $P(Y_i|g_i, g_0) = P(Y_i|g_i)$, may not hold (Gail and Chatterjee, 2004; Whittemore, 1997).

Absolute risk in mutation carriers will be overestimated if one does not account for residual familial risk (Chatterjee et al., 2006; Gail et al., 1999b, 2001). The key ingredient in Equation (9.15), $P(\mathbf{Y}_K|\mathbf{G}_\mathrm{K}, Y_0)$, does not simplify to Equation (9.16) in the presence of residual familial risk, because components of $\mathbf{Y}_K$ are correlated with Y_0 and with each other. If all probands are a random sample from the source population, then $(\mathbf{Y}_K, Y_0)$ can be regarded as a random sample from the population. Each of the pairs (Y_i, Y_0) from a given family can also be regarded as randomly sampled, though not independent. Thus for each family, a "composite likelihood"

$$P(G_0)P(Y_0|G_0) \prod_{i=1}^{K} \sum_{G_i} P(Y_i|G_i)P(G_i|G_0) \tag{9.17}$$

can be constructed that yields unbiased estimates of the marginal risk $P(Y_i|G_i)$ (Chatterjee and Wacholder, 2001). This approach reduces, but does not eliminate, the upward bias in pure risk estimates for mutation carriers when case probands are over represented in the kin-cohort sample, as is common. Begg (2002) noted that genotype-specific risks would be overestimated if only case probands are used and if risk varies in the population because of factors other than the gene under study. However, applying copula models to the marginal survival probabilities $S_{g_k}(t) = P(T_k > t|g_k)$ to account for residual familial risk, where T_k

is the time to the disease of interest (e.g., breast cancer) for family member k, Chatterjee et al. (2006) found that even if all probands were cases, unbiased estimates of pure risk were obtained, provided that the correct copula was chosen; the results were sensitive to misspecification of the copula, however. Kin-cohort designs that sampled equal numbers of case and control probands yielded nearly unbiased pure cumulative risk estimates that were much less sensitive to the choice of the copula. Estimates of relative risk were more robust to misspecification of the copula than estimates of cumulative risk, especially if only case probands were sampled. Chatterjee et al. (2006) therefore recommended estimating $RR(G = g)$ with a copula model to allow for residual familial risk. Then following the approach in Chapter 5, one estimates attributable risk $AR(t)$ from known allele frequencies and $RR(G = g)$ and then estimates $\lambda_g(t) = RR(G = g)\lambda^*(t)\{1 - AR(t)\}$, which reduces approximately to $\lambda_g(t) \doteq RR(G = g)\lambda^*(t)$ for rare mutations. Note that a dominant mutation like those in BRCA1 or BRCA2 with carrier prevalence 0.0066 and $RR(G = 1) = RR(G = 2) = 20$ (Claus et al., 1991) would have $AR = 0.0066 \times 19/(0.0066 \times 19 + 1) = 0.11$, justifying the approximation.

Unlike estimates of $RR_{fam}(G = g)$ obtained by comparing cases and controls within a family, the relative risk estimated from the kin-cohort design with allowance for residual familial risk via a composite likelihood or copula modeling, has little upward bias for $RR(G = g)$.

9.4.4 Families with several affected members (multiplex pedigrees)

The kin-cohort design is amenable to analysis because the ascertainment criteria are well understood. Nonetheless, the combination of residual familial risk and case-enriched proband ascertainment complicates the analysis. These challenges are even greater when multiplex pedigrees are recruited from high risk clinics. Often the precise features that led to ascertainment of the family are not known.

Estimation of absolute risk from a pedigree could be based on $P(\mathbf{Y}, \mathbf{G}|A)$ where A is the ascertainment condition, which might depend in a complex way on $\mathbf{Y}$. The quantity $P(\mathbf{Y}, \mathbf{G}|A)$ is termed the "ascertainment corrected joint likelihood" by Kraft and Thomas (2000), who also consider the "prospective likelihood", $P(\mathbf{Y}|\mathbf{G}, A)$, and the "retrospective likelihood", $P(\mathbf{G}|\mathbf{Y}, A) = P(\mathbf{G}|\mathbf{Y})$; the last equality follows from the assumption that A is determined by $\mathbf{Y}$ alone. To avoid the difficulty of defining the ascertainment condition, analysts often use the retrospective likelihood, even though it can be less efficient. Use of $P(\mathbf{G}|\mathbf{Y})$ does not avoid the need to consider residual familial risks, however, because

$$P(\mathbf{G}|\mathbf{Y}) = P(\mathbf{Y}|\mathbf{G})P(\mathbf{G})/\sum_{\mathbf{G}} P(\mathbf{Y}|\mathbf{G})P(\mathbf{G})$$

depends on $P(\mathbf{Y}|\mathbf{G})$, which, conditional on $\mathbf{G}$, may include correlations among familial phenotypes that are induced by residual familial risk. Iversen and Chen (2005) used $P(\mathbf{Y}, \mathbf{G}|A)$ but assumed that A depended only on certain functions of $\mathbf{Y}$, such as the number of affected family members. Using external data, they estimated $P(A)$ empirically, permitting inference from

$$P(\mathbf{Y}, \mathbf{G}|A) \propto P(\mathbf{Y}, \mathbf{G})/P(A).$$

This approach does not avoid the need to consider residual familial risk, however.

These issues are important when estimating the pure risk in carriers of BRCA1 and BRCA2 mutations and in non-carriers. Data from a marker tightly linked to BRCA1 were obtained from the Breast Cancer Linkage Consortium (BCLC), consisting of multiplex families with at least four members with breast cancer diagnosed under age 60 or with ovarian cancer. The retrospective likelihood $P(\mathbf{G}|\mathbf{Y})$ was used, where the likelihood describes the marker pattern, rather than BRCA1 mutations themselves. No attempt was made to model residual familial risk. The estimated pure breast cancer risk to age 70 was 0.85 in BRCA1 mutation carriers (Easton et al., 1995). A similar analysis of data for BRCA2 mutations from BCLC (Ford et al., 1998) yielded an estimate of pure breast cancer risk to age 70 of 0.84 for carriers. In contrast, Antoniou et al. (2003) analyzed data from 22 kin-cohort studies with case-only probands (female breast cancer cases in 16 studies, male breast cancer cases in 2 studies, and ovarian cancer cases in 4 studies). These probands were not selected on the basis of family history, but only on the basis of their personal history of cancer. The combined data from these studies yielded an estimate of pure breast cancer risk to age 70 of 0.65 for BRCA1 mutation carriers and 0.45 for BRCA2 mutation carriers. Because no allowance had been made for residual familial risk, the authors noted that these risk estimates might overestimate risks in the general population, despite the fact that they were considerably lower than estimates from the BCLC. The BOADICEA model, which allows for a polygenic residual familial risk, ascribed pure cumulative risks to age 70 of 0.46 to 0.59 for BRCA1 mutations and of 0.39 to 0.51 for BRCA2 mutations, depending on birth cohort. An earlier kin-cohort study (Struewing et al., 1997) of three founder mutations in BRCA1 and BRCA2 in an Ashkenazi population in the region including Washington, DC reported a cumulative pure risk to age 70 of 0.56, and a population-based kin-cohort study of probands with breast cancer in Australia (Hopper et al., 1999) reported a cumulative pure risk of 0.40.

The differences in cumulative risk estimates to age 70 between the more nearly population-based kin-cohort studies and the studies of multiplex pedigrees, such as 56% versus 85%, can affect clinical management. Risk estimates from multiplex families without adequate adjustment for ascertainment and residual familial risk are too high for women who are found to carry mutations through chance testing or through testing occasioned by the incidence of breast cancer in a single relative, for example. The higher mutation-associated risks from multiplex families are probably useful for advising women in multiplex families, not because all the risk comes from the mutation, but because other risk factors impart additional risk in such families. These arguments imply that a woman in a multiplex family who tests negative for a mutation may still have above average breast cancer risk, by virtue of her strong family history.

9.5 Comparisons of some models for projecting breast cancer risk

Several models are widely used for predicting breast cancer risk in women, as described in Chapter 1. Among these are an empirical model, the Breast Cancer Risk Assessment Tool (BCRAT), and genetically based models (Claus, BRCAPRO, BOADICEA, IBIS) (Amir et al., 2010). The models vary in the risk factors used (Table 9.1), although all the models include age, which is a dominant risk factor over long risk projection intervals. The models labeled Claus, BRCAPRO, BOADICEA and IBIS include detailed family history of breast disease in first- and second-degree relatives, as well as some other family history information not shown. Of these models, only IBIS includes data on reproductive factors and history of breast pathology. BCRAT includes reproductive factors and history of breast pathology, but the only family history that BCRAT uses is number of affected first-degree female relatives (mother or sisters). The CLAUS and BRCAPRO models assume conditional independence given autosomal dominant genotypes, whereas BOADICEA and IBIS allow for residual familial correlation. BCRAT implicitly includes all sources of familial aggregation in the estimates of relative risks associated with having affected first-degree relatives.

These models also differ in other important respects (Gail and Mai, 2010) (Table 9.2). The BCRAT and Claus models are calibrated to age-specific breast cancer incidence rates from the US Surveillance Epidemiology and End Results (SEER) Program of the National Cancer Institute (https://seer.cancer.gov/seerstat/), and the BOADICEA and IBIS models are calibrated to breast cancer incidence rates from England and Wales. BRCAPRO

Table 9.1: Selected risk factors used in some models for projecting breast cancer risk

Factor	BCRAT	CLAUS	BRCAPRO	BOADICEA	IBIS
Reproductive factors					
Age at menarche (w)*	Yes				Yes
Age at first birth (m)	Yes				Yes
Age at menopause (m)					Yes
Hormone replacement (s)					Yes
Personal history of breast pathology					
Previous benign biopsies (m)	Yes				
Atypical Hyperplasia (s)	Yes				Yes
Lobular Carcinoma *in situ* (s)	Ineligible				Yes
Family history of breast cancer					
First degree relatives (s)	Yes	Yes	Yes	Yes	Yes
Second degree relatives (w)		Yes	Yes	Yes	Yes
Age at onset in relatives (m)		Yes	Yes	Yes	Yes
Other factors					
Body mass index (w)					Yes

*The symbols w, m, and s denote, respectively, weak, moderate, and strong risk factors.

uses SEER data for non-carriers and a meta-analysis of cumulative pure risks for mutation carriers. The IBIS and Claus models include ductal carcinoma *in situ* (DCIS) as well as invasive breast cancer, whereas BCRAT, BRCAPRO and BOADICEA project risk for invasive breast cancer only. The Claus, BOADICEA and IBIS models compute pure, not absolute risk (although IBIS has an option to compute absolute risk), in contrast to the BCRAT and BRCAPRO models, which compute absolute risk; pure risks should be higher than corresponding absolute risks (Chapter 3). The Claus model only makes projections for women with at least one affected first-degree relative. BRCAT does not make projections for women with a history of lobular carcinoma *in situ* (LCIS), who have high risk.

To compare risk projections to ages 45 and 80 years from the various models, we considered healthy 35-year-old women with menarche at age 11 and age at first live birth at age 25 (Table 9.3). The women vary with respect to biopsy status and family history. For women with no history of breast cancer in first degree relatives, BCRAT and IBIS gave the highest projections when the woman has had a biopsy, especially in the presence of atypical hyperplasia. A history of LCIS greatly increased risk in the IBIS model. For women with one affected first-degree relative, BCRAT and IBIS projected higher risks than the Claus, BRCAPRO and BOADICEA models, whether or not breast cancer pathology was present. For women with two affected first-degree relatives, BCRAT and IBIS again projected the highest risks (30.0% and 24.2% to age 80 respectively in women without biopsies), especially in the presence of atypical hyperplasia (57.5% and 66.9% respectively), but in the absence of pathology, the risks from the Claus and BOADICEA models were not much lower than those of BCRAT and IBIS. BRCAPRO projected noticeably lower risks (12.6% to age 80), possibly because it fails to account for residual familial correlation. A similar pattern was seen for women with three affected first-degree relatives.

There is considerable variation in projections among the models in Table 9.3. Thus, not all the models are well calibrated (Chapter 6). A number of studies have examined the cal-

Table 9.2: Features of selected models for projecting breast cancer risk

Model [citation]	**Calibrated to**	**Type of breast cancer predicted**	**Type of risk predicted**	**Exclusions**
BCRAT (Costantino et al., 1999)	US SEER	Invasive	Absolute	LCIS
Claus (Claus et al., 1994)	US SEER	Invasive and DCIS	Pure	No affected first-degree relatives
BRCAPRO (Berry et al., 1997; Chen and Parmigiani, 2007)	Meta-analysis for mutation carriers; US SEER for non-carriers	Invasive*	Absolute**	
BOADICEA (Antoniou et al., 2008a)	England and Wales	Invasive	Pure	
IBIS (Tyrer et al., 2005)	England and Wales	Invasive and DCIS	Pure with option for absolute	

Abbreviations: Ductal Carcinoma *in situ* (DCIS); lobular carcinoma *in situ* (LCIS); Surveillance, Epidemiology and End Results Program of the National Cancer Institute (SEER)

*A meta-analysis was used to estimate pure cumulative incidence in mutation carriers. Some *in situ* cases may have been included.

**Original versions projected pure risk, but recent versions adjust for competing risks (see http://bcb.dfci.harvard.edu/BayesMendel/software.php).

Table 9.3: Breast cancer risks in percent to ages 45 and 80 for healthy 35-year-old women who began menstruating at age 11 and had first live births at age 25

Number of affected first-degree relatives*	**Age(s) at breast cancer onset in relative(s)** and/or other characteristics of the patient**	**BCRAT**	**Claus**	**BRCAPRO**	**BOADICEA**	**IBIS**
0	No special features	1.0, 10.7†	N/A	0.9, 11.1	0.8, 8.7	0.9, 9.6
0	1 biopsy	1.7, 14.2	N/A	0.9, 11.1	0.8, 8.7	0.9, 9.6
0	1 biopsy with AH	3.2, 24.2	N/A	0.9, 11.1	0.8, 8.7	3.7, 33.6
0	LCIS	N/A	N/A	0.9, 11.2	0.8, 8.7	7.2, 55.8
1	60 y	1.8, 18.2	0.9, 9.2	0.9, 11.3	1.5, 13.4	1.9, 18.8
1	60 y; LCIS	N/A	0.9, 9.2	0.9, 11.3	1.5, 13.4	14.2, 81.2
1	30 y	1.8, 18.2	2.1, 15.5	1.2, 12.1	2.0, 16.2	2.5, 20.2
1	40 y	1.8, 18.2	1.6, 12.5	1.1, 11.7	1.9, 15.4	2.2, 19.6
1	60 y; 1 biopsy	3.1, 23.8	0.9, 9.2	0.9, 11.3	1.5, 13.4	1.9, 18.8
2	40 y, 60 y	3.2, 30.0	3.6, 22.9	1.3, 12.6	3.2, 21.5	2.7, 24.2
2	40 y, 60 y; 1 biopsy	5.4, 38.0	3.6, 22.9	1.3, 12.6	3.2, 21.5	2.7, 24.2
2	40 y, 60 y; 1 biopsy with AH	9.6, 57.5	3.6, 22.9	1.3, 12.6	3.2, 21.5	10.5, 66.9
3	40 y, 50 y, 60 y	3.2, 30.0	4.6, 28.0	2.5, 16.1	4.8, 28.3	3.4, 27.0
3	30 y, 40 y, 50 y; 1 biopsy	3.2, 30.0	6.5, 37.4	5.2, 24.4	6.6, 33.0	8.4, 34.8
3	40 y, 50 y, 60 y; 1 biopsy	5.4, 38.0	4.6, 28.0	2.5, 16.1	4.8, 28.3	3.4, 27.0
3	40 y, 50 y, 60 y; 1 biopsy with AH	9.6, 57.5	4.6, 28.0	2.5, 16.1	4.8, 28.3	12.7, 71.7

Abbreviations: atypical hyperplasia (AH); lobular carcinoma *in situ* (LCIS); not applicable (N/A).

*For no affected first-degree relatives and for one affected first-degree relative, the pedigree includes the mother and the proband. For two affected first-degree relatives, the pedigree includes the mother, sister, and the proband. For three affected first-degree relatives, the pedigree includes the mother, two sisters, and the proband. These pedigree structures are held constant as other risk factors, including ages at breast cancer onset, vary in the table.

**The mother has the oldest age at onset in all scenarios with affected relatives.

†Left number is risk to age 45 in percent; right number is risk to age 80 in percent. Data taken from M. H. Gail and P. L. Mai. Comparing breast cancer risk assessment models. *Journal of the National Cancer Institute*, 102(10):665–668, 2010.

ibration of BCRAT in general populations (Gail and Mai, 2010), such as the Nurses Health Study (Rockhill et al., 2001). Most (e.g., (Rockhill et al., 2001; Costantino et al., 1999)), but not all (Schonfeld et al., 2010), have found BCRAT to be well calibrated in such populations (Gail and Mai, 2010). The web site for BCRAT, http://www.cancer.gov/bcrisktool/, mentions that BCRAT is not appropriate for women with a previous history of radiation treatment to the chest for Hodgkin's lymphoma, for women with a previous history of invasive breast cancer or DCIS or LCIS, for recent immigrants from regions of Asia where breast cancer risk is low, and for women with known mutations in BRCA1 or BRCA2 genes. Although there is evidence that BCRAT is well calibrated for women with a family history of breast cancer (Bondy et al., 1994) and in women with above average risk recruited to a breast cancer prevention trial (Costantino et al., 1999), there is a need for more studies to evaluate the calibration of the various models in high risk clinic populations or in women with strong family histories. Results from a study based on 64 breast cancer cases in a high risk clinic population (Amir et al., 2003) and from a study based on 83 breast cancer cases in women with at least two family members with breast or ovarian cancer (Quante et al., 2012) suggest that the IBIS model, with its higher risk estimates, was better calibrated than the BCRAT, Claus, and BRCAPRO models, but larger calibration studies are needed for such high risk populations. A recent release of IBIS (Version 7 at http://www.ems-trials.org/riskevaluator/) gives somewhat higher risk estimates than in Table 9.3.

9.6 Discussion

We concentrated on methods for estimating risk associated with highly penetrant mutations from family-based designs, such as the kin-cohort design or studies of multiplex pedigrees. If residual familial risk is not allowed for, one tends to overestimate the absolute (and pure) risk associated with a measured mutation in the general population. Measures of residual familial risk also allow one to make better risk predictions by using not only the information on mutation status but also the residual predictive information in the family history, as illustrated in Section 9.3. Ignoring unmeasured polygenic effects leads to underestimation of family-specific genetic relative risks (Kraft and Thomas, 2000; Pfeiffer et al., 2001), but family-specific estimates of genetic relative risk lead to overestimation of relative risk and absolute risk in the general population for carriers of the measured mutation.

Because highly penetrant mutations account for only a small portion of the total familial aggregation of risk, one would expect that a model such as BOADICEA or IBIS, that also account for residual correlation, would provide better risk prediction, based on family history, than a model based on a highly penetrant mutation alone. To adequately assess the calibration and discriminatory accuracy (Chapter 6) of the various models, one needs cohort data from the target population with baseline measurements of mutation status, family history, and other factors, and with sufficient follow-up to detect several hundred cancers. Although validation studies with small numbers of events have been conducted to assess the calibration of genetically-based models in high risk patients (Bondy et al., 1994; Amir et al., 2003; Quante et al., 2012), there is a need for much larger studies in high risk populations and in the general population. A potential difficulty is the fact that preventive interventions, such as oophorectomy or the use of chemopreventive agents can reduce risks and are usually not included in the risk models.

Although the breast cancer risk models we discussed are widely used, they have modest discriminatory accuracy (Rockhill et al., 2001), with an area under the receiver operating characteristic curve near AUC=0.6. It was hoped that genome-wide association studies (GWAS) that compare SNPs in cases and controls would identify SNPs that would improve discriminatory accuracy. Early studies based on only 7 confirmed SNPs noted that the relative risks were small and indicated that these SNPs would not contribute much to the discriminatory accuracy of models that contain standard risk factors such as family history or age at first live birth (Gail, 2008a, 2009b; Wacholder et al., 2010). Larger GWAS studies identified many more SNPs, but they had even weaker relative risks. Such SNPs can partly account for the polygenic component of risk described at the beginning of Section 9.3. The relative risks from such SNPs seem to act multiplicatively on the relative risks (Antoniou et al., 2008b). The genetic variance in Equation (9.6) from all previously identified SNPs is less than 20% of the polygenic variance required to explain residual familial risk after taking BRCA1 and BRCA2 into account (Ghoussaini and Pharoah, 2009; Michailidou et al., 2013; Park et al., 2012). The explanation for this "missing heritability" may lie in other genetic variants (Ghoussaini and Pharoah, 2009), or in SNPs whose main effects or whose interactions (Zuk et al., 2012) are so small as to be non-detectable by GWAS of practical size (Chatterjee et al., 2013). For predicting risk, it is disappointing that these SNPs contribute only modestly to discriminatory accuracy. Maas et al. (2016) evaluated the potential of 92 such SNPs and numerous epidemiologic risk factors such as family history. A model based on the epidemiologic risk factors had AUC=0.588. A model based only on the 92 SNPs had AUC=0.623. A model with the SNPs and epidemiologic risk factors had AUC=0.648.

Other strong risk factors, such as mammographic density (Chen et al., 2006a; Tice et al., 2008) and detailed histology from biopsies (Hartmann et al., 2005), together with information from SNPs, may lead to improved discriminatory accuracy. Indeed, combining mammographic density, epidemiologic factors and SNPs may lead to an AUC approaching 0.7 for breast cancer (Garcia-Closas et al., 2014; Park et al., 2012). This is still inadequate for applications based on high risk subgroups, however.

This chapter has focused on genetically-based risk models for breast cancer incidence. Risk models, including models like BRCAPRO, are referenced for many other cancers at http://epi.grants.cancer.gov/cancer_risk_prediction/#risk. There is also an exploding literature on SNP-based risk assessment for the incidence of other diseases and on the possible usefulness of SNPs for prognostication following diagnosis.

Chapter 10

Related topics

10.1 Introduction

In this chapter we touch on topics related to absolute risk, including prognosis following disease diagnosis, handling missing data on cause of death, and time-varying covariates or health state. We also discuss applications of absolute risk for individual counseling and for public health prevention strategies. This chapter is not meant to be comprehensive, but to indicate how the ideas in previous chapters are related to other applications and analytical approaches and to provide some key references. Another important related topic, the estimation of residual life in the presence of competing risks, is not discussed here but is treated at length in Jeong (2014).

10.2 Prognosis following disease onset

Although we have emphasized examples and methods for the absolute risk of disease incidence, the concept of absolute risk is also important to guide clinical decisions after disease develops. For example, consider a 65-year-old man just diagnosed with prostate cancer. There is a chance that the man will die of prostate cancer, but he may also die of another competing cause. His absolute risk of dying of prostate cancer is reduced by competing causes of mortality. Albertsen et al. (2005) estimated the chance of dying of prostate cancer as a function of age at diagnosis and pathologic features of the tumor, which are summarized in the Gleason score. The Gleason score indicates the chance that the cancer will spread. Figure 10.1, adapted from Albertsen et al. (2005), depicts the absolute risk of dying of prostate cancer (dark shading) and of dying of other causes (light shading) on the scale of years since diagnosis for men with a favorable Gleason score in the range 0 to 2. The chance that a man diagnosed with Gleason score 0-2 prostate cancer at age 65 years will die within 20 years is 80%, but the chance he will die of prostate cancer is only about 5%. Prostate cancer treatment with radiation or surgery carries a substantial risk of side effects, such as impotence or incontinence. One option for a man with a low risk of dying of prostate cancer is "active surveillance", whereby the patient is monitored with prostate-specific antigen (PSA) testing, but no cancer treatments are given unless subsequent data indicate cancer progression. In contrast, a 65-year-old man diagnosed with Gleason score 9 has a 60% chance of dying of prostate cancer within 10 years without surgical or radiation treatment (Albertsen et al., 2005). Such high absolute risk justifies treatment.

Other examples of the use of absolute risk for prognosis include the probability of dying of breast cancer following diagnosis (Schairer et al., 2004), the absolute risk of a local breast cancer recurrence (Gray, 1988), and the absolute risk of local lung cancer recurrence (with distant metastases and other causes of death as a competing risks) (Consonni et al., 2015). In some settings, competing consequences of treatment are studied. For example, bone marrow transplantation for refractory or relapsed leukemia can result in leukemia recurrence or death from treatment complications (Gaynor et al., 1993; Pepe and Mori, 1993).

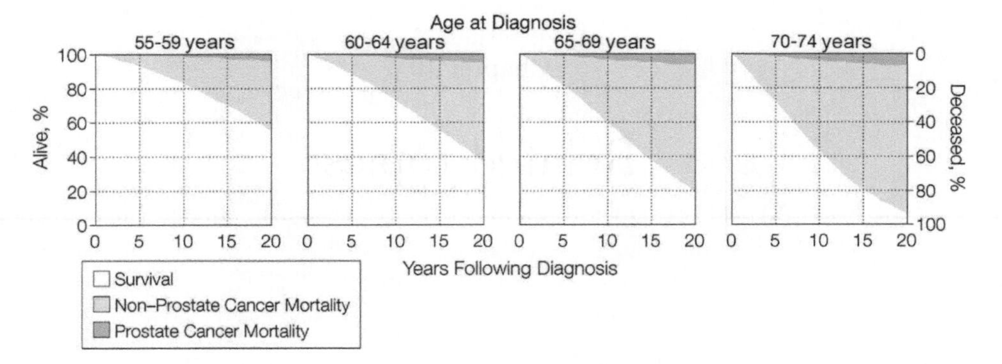

Figure 10.1: Absolute risks of prostate cancer death and non-prostate cancer death, adapted from P. C. Albertsen, J. A. Hanley, and J. Fine. 20-year outcomes following conservative management of clinically localized prostate cancer. *Journal of the American Medical Association*, 293(17):2095–2101, 2005.

Absolute risk estimates often rely on survival analysis methods that were first developed for estimating pure risks following disease diagnosis. Perhaps the first example of covariate modeling in survival analysis concerned the pure risk of death following diagnosis of acute myelogenous leukemia as a function of baseline white cell count (Feigl and Zelen, 1965). Since then, most publications on risk models for prognosis have treated pure risk. The advent of the Cox model (Cox, 1972) facilitated an explosion of papers on prognosis for pure risk. The literature on general features of regression modeling for survival analysis contains valuable lessons that also apply to modeling absolute risk. Such topics include how to code covariates and flexible representations of dose-response for quantitative covariates (e.g., splines), handling missing covariates by imputation or other techniques, such as the expectation-maximization algorithm, model checking by examining residuals and other tests of goodness-of-fit, and re-calibration to adapt a risk model to a new population. There has been less work on the impact of measurement error in predictors, but Khudyakov et al. (2015) found that such measurement error had little impact on the calibration of pure risk in a probit model but could degrade the AUC and mean square error of prediction (Brier criterion). Excellent discussions of these topics are found in classic books on survival and risk modeling, including (Andersen et al., 1993; Harrell, 2001; Kalbfleisch and Prentice, 2002; Steyerberg, 2009; Therneau and Grambsch, 2000; van Houwelingen and Putter, 2012).

10.3 Missing or misclassified information on event type

In previous chapters we ignored the possibility that the type of competing event that occurs may not be recorded. We will refer to causes of death as the competing events, although the competing health outcomes may be other types of events. For example, if the competing events are first cancers of various types and death from other causes, the type of first cancer may not be recorded. Sometimes the cause of death is not captured, and sometimes the cause of death has been misclassified. Although there is some recent work on misclassified outcomes (Ha and Tsodikov, 2015), most publications have dealt with missing cause of death. Simply discarding subjects with missing cause of death ("complete case analysis") can lead to bias, not only in estimates of covariate effects, but also in estimates of the absolute risk itself.

Earlier papers treated unknown cause of death in the absence of covariates (e.g., (Dinse, 1986)). Subsequent literature concerned estimation of covariate effects and cumulative cause-specific baseline hazards, but not absolute risks. Goetghebeur and Ryan (1995) considered the cause-specific hazards model with proportional hazards assumed for covariate effects on each cause-specific hazard. A somewhat restrictive additional assumption was that the cause-specific baseline hazard functions were also proportional. They developed methods to estimate covariate effects and cumulative baseline hazards in the presence of missing data on cause of death, and provided variance estimates for covariate parameter estimates. Dabrowska (1995) avoided the assumption of proportional baseline hazards by employing a parametric model for the probability that a given death was from the cause of interest, given certain covariates and given that a death had occurred at a specific time. Call this probability $\rho(\boldsymbol{W_i}, \boldsymbol{\theta})$, where $\boldsymbol{W_i}$ includes the time the ith subject died as well as covariates $\boldsymbol{Z_i}$ that may affect the cause-specific hazards, and possibly other covariates that predict the type of death but are distinct from $\boldsymbol{Z_i}$. $\boldsymbol{W_i}$ does not include the missing cause of death. Thus, it is assumed that the cause of death information is missing at random, given $\boldsymbol{W_i}$. Lu and Tsiatis (2001) showed how to estimate parameters $\boldsymbol{\theta}$ from subjects with known cause of death and impute the missing cause of death as a Bernoulli variate given $\rho(\boldsymbol{W_i}, \hat{\boldsymbol{\theta}})$. They provide variance estimates for estimates of proportional hazards parameters based on multiple imputation that allow for variability of $\hat{\boldsymbol{\theta}}$, unlike standard variance calculations for multiple imputation (Rubin, 1987).

Gao and Tsiatis (2005) estimated covariate parameters and baseline hazards by using "doubly robust" estimating equations. Let $\Gamma_i = 0, 1, 2$ according as the ith subject was censored or died of causes 1 or 2, respectively. Gao and Tsiatis (2005) defined the probability that a person would be censored or have a known cause of death, $\pi(\boldsymbol{W_i}, I(\Gamma_i > 0), \boldsymbol{\psi})$, where $I(\Gamma_i > 0)$ indicates that the ith subject was not censored, and where $\boldsymbol{\psi}$ represents parameters to be estimated. Assuming that a missing cause of failure Γ_i does not depend on the failure type, conditional on $I(\Gamma_i > 0)$ and $\boldsymbol{W_i}$ (i.e., failure type is missing at random), they used inverse probability weighting of such observations by $\pi(\boldsymbol{W_i}, I(\Gamma_i > 0), \hat{\boldsymbol{\psi}})$ to define estimating equations. To increase efficiency, they added a term to the estimating equations that depended on $\rho(\boldsymbol{W_i}, \hat{\boldsymbol{\theta}})$. These estimating equations have expectation zero if either $\rho(\boldsymbol{W_i}, \boldsymbol{\theta})$ or $\pi(\boldsymbol{W_i}, I(\Gamma_i > 0), \boldsymbol{\psi})$ are correctly specified. Gao and Tsiatis (2005) applied these techniques to a large class of transformation models, including the proportional hazards model and proportional odds model. Lu and Liang (2008) used similar techniques for the additive hazard model.

Although the previous papers provided inference on covariate effects and, in some cases on cumulative baseline hazards, in the presence of missing cause of death, they did not treat absolute risk itself. Lee et al. (2011) used multiple imputation and extended the methods in (Cheng et al., 1998) and (Lu and Tsiatis, 2001) not only for inference on proportional hazards parameters in the cause-specific model but also for absolute risk. Lee et al. (2012) applied these imputation methods to SEER data to estimate the absolute risk of dying from colon cancer as a function of time since diagnosis. In these data, the cause-specific hazards model fit the data better than the Fine-Gray model, but estimates of absolute risk were similar. An advantage of the imputation approach is that it can be used to fit both cause-specific and cumulative incidence models. Nicolaie et al. (2015) partitioned the probability of having the event of interest at time t into the probability of having some event at time t times the conditional probability of having the event of interest given that an event occurred ("vertical modelling"), in a manner similar to (Dabrowska, 1995) and (Lu and Tsiatis, 2001), but used likelihood methods to estimate needed parameters and absolute risk. Moreno-Betancur et al. (2015) used parametric survival models for competing risks that permit likelihood-based estimates of absolute risk in the presence of missing cause of death data. Most of these papers assumed cause-specific hazard models, but Bakoyannis et al. (2010) used multiple imputation as in (Lu and Tsiatis, 2001) to obtain data with imputed complete cause of death information, from which to estimate sub-distribution proportional hazard parameters for the model of Fine and Gray (1999) (see also Lee et al. (2012)).

10.4 Time varying covariates

10.4.1 Fixed versus time-varying covariates and internal versus external time-varying covariates

In previous chapters we have assumed that covariates $\mathbf{Z}$ that affect absolute risk are known at the beginning of the risk projection interval, t_0. Implicitly we assumed that the covariates stayed fixed at their initial values. An exception is deterministic functions of age. For example, in the breast cancer risk model of Gail et al. (1989), there is an interaction between $I(t \geq 50)$ and number of biopsies. For projection intervals $t_0 < t \leq t_0 + \tau$ that include age t =50, the relative hazard for a woman with one or more biopsies decreases at t =50, reducing the absolute risk calculation in Equation (4.1). Suppose the woman is $t_0 = 45$ years old at counseling, and the follow-up duration is τ =10 years. Even before follow-up begins, we know that the indicator $I(t \geq 50)$ will change to 1 at age 50. Thus $I(t \geq 50)$ is an "external" covariate (Kalbfleisch and Prentice, 2002), for which such absolute risk calculations are justified. However, we might want to ask: "What will her absolute risk of breast cancer from age 45 to 55 be if she has a first breast biopsy at age 52?" In order to have a first breast biopsy at age 52, she must not have died or had a diagnosis of breast cancer before age 52, and calculation using Equation (4.1) does not lead to a valid absolute risk calculation. Such a time-dependent covariate is called "internal" by Kalbfleisch and Prentice (2002), who pointed out that a survival calculation like Equation (4.1) that uses covariate values at times after t_0 is not appropriate for internal time-dependent covariates.

Letting $Z(t)$ denote the entire covariate path from time 0 to time t, Kalbfleisch and Prentice (2002) formally defined a time-dependent covariate $Z(t)$ as "external" if for times $0 < u \leq t$, $P(T \in [u, u+du)|Z(u), T \geq u) = P(T \in [u, u+du)|Z(t), T \geq u)$. In other words, the probability of failure at u is not affected by future values of the covariate path beyond time u. An equivalent definition states that the path of $Z(t)$ after time u is not affected by whether or not the subject fails at u. Examples of time-varying external covariates, for which calculations like Equation (4.1) are valid are: interactions of fixed covariates with time, as illustrated in the previous paragraph; any covariate whose path is predetermined irrespective of the status of the individual under study, such as age; and stochastic factors such as air temperature whose probability laws do not depend on parameters of the risk model.

A time-varying covariate that is not external is "internal." Using methods for, e.g., the time-dependent Cox model, one can estimate a quantity such as the cumulative hazard $\int_{t_0}^{u} \lambda_k\{s; \mathbf{z}^k(s)\}ds$. For a given path of the covariate, one can thus get an idea of the time-dependent covariate's impact on the hazard. But, as Kalbfleisch and Prentice (2002) argue, this quantity does not translate into a proper disease risk, because knowing $\mathbf{z}^k(s)$ at a time $s > t_0$ implies survival to s. An additional problem arises with time-varying internal covariates when estimating the Fine-Grey sub-distribution hazard in expression (4.24). Because a person who dies of a competing cause remains in the risk set for estimating the sub-distribution for the cause of interest after the time of death, an internal covariate would not be measurable at the later times, leading to inferential problems, as discussed by several authors (Latouche et al., 2005; Beyersmann and Schumacher, 2008). Andersen and Keiding (2012) also question the interpretation of the sub-distribution hazard defined as the instantaneous risk of failure from cause j at time t among those who are alive or have died of another cause at or before t. Thus, sub-distribution hazard ratios do not have an interpretation as ordinary hazard ratios, regardless of whether the covariate is internal or external.

10.4.2 Joint modeling of covariates and health outcomes, including multistate models

Rather than treating a time-varying-covariate path as a given, as in the usual time-dependent covariate analysis, one can attempt to develop joint stochastic models for the covariate evolution and the competing risk outcomes. Recall the notation $\delta(s) = 0$ if a person is in the initial state 0 (e.g., alive) at time s and $\delta(s) = k$ if a person had transitioned to an absorbing state k (e.g., died of cause k) at or before time s. A joint probability model of the covariate process $\{Z(s) : s \geq 0\}$ and the "state process" $\{\delta(s) : s \geq 0\}$ would allow one to make statements about absolute risk that incorporate the future evolution of time-varying covariates. There is an extensive literature, reviewed by Jewell and Kalbfleisch (1996), Shi et al. (1996), Tsiatis and Davidian (2004), Yu et al. (2004), Rizopoulos (2012) and Proust-Lima et al. (2014), on joint modeling of a longitudinal marker process with a single survival outcome, i.e., $\delta(s) = 0$ or 1. Such joint models lead to predictions that are consistent over time, as defined by Jewell and Nielsen (1993). However, estimation of the joint process parameters often requires numerical integration or simulation techniques, as illustrated by the work of Taylor et al. (2013), who use longitudinal prostate specific antigen (PSA) measurements following radiation treatment for prostate cancer to predict the probability of prostate cancer recurrence. Recent work by Elashoff et al. (2008), Huang et al. (2011) and Andrinopoulou et al. (2014) used joint modeling of a longitudinal marker with competing times to failure. These papers presented results on parameter estimates for cause-specific hazards, but not on absolute risks, whereas Blanche et al. (2015) and Proust-Lima et al. (2016) discussed absolute risk as well. Some limitations of the approach of joint modeling with longitudinal markers include: it is difficult to check model assumptions, which usually involve latent components, with available data; and computations are complex and time-consuming, sometimes implemented via expectation-maximization algorithms or Monte Carlo Markov chain algorithms. Blanche et al. (2015) discussed time-varying estimation of AUC and the Brier statistic for assessing predictions of absolute risk with longitudinal marker data. Ferrer et al. (2016) fitted a joint model for the longitudinal marker (prostate specific antigen) and a general multi-state process, including some non-absorbing states, to describe transitions following diagnosis of prostate cancer.

If the marker covariate $Z(s)$ is discrete, it can be used to define a state in a Markov or semi-Markov process that also includes absorbing states, such as cause-specific death. Such multistate models can be used to compute probabilities like the absolute risk of death from cause k, in the presence of an evolving internal covariate. To illustrate, we consider competing risks of leukemia relapse (k =1) or death without relapse (k =3) following bone marrow transplantation to treat leukemia (Cortese et al., 2013). Here the time scale is time since bone marrow transplantation ($t_0 = 0$), and we might be interested in the absolute risk $r_1(0, \tau; \mathbf{Z} = \mathbf{z})$ of leukemia relapse. If $\mathbf{Z}$ only includes fixed covariates, such as type of leukemia, cause-specific models as in Equation (4.1) or cumulative incidence regression models could be used to estimate $r_1(0, \tau; \mathbf{Z} = \mathbf{z})$ or $r_3(0, \tau; \mathbf{Z} = \mathbf{z})$. A potential complication of bone marrow transplantation is graft versus host disease (GVHD). The first component of $\mathbf{Z}$ might be a discrete time-varying component $Z_1(s) = 1$ if GVHD has developed at or before time s and $Z_1(s) = 0$ otherwise. Figure 10.2, adapted from Cortese et al. (2013), depicts a four state Markov model with two absorbing states, relapse ($k = 1$) or death without relapse ($k = 3$), and with two transient states, in leukemia remission without GVHD ($k = 0$) and in leukemia remission with GVHD ($k = 2$). Cortese et al. (2013) assumed that the transition rates satisfied the proportional hazards form $\alpha_{lk}(t) = \alpha_{lk,0}(t) \exp(\mathbf{Z}'_2\beta_2)$, where $\alpha_{lk,0}(t)$ is a baseline transition rate from state l to state k and baseline covariates $\mathbf{Z}_2$ included age at transplantation and an indicator of whether or not the type of leukemia was acute myelogenous leukemia (AML). Based on methods described in Andersen et al. (1993) (Section VII.2), Andersen and Perme (2008) and Beyersmann et al. (2012) for Markov models, Cortese et al. (2013) estimated the effects of covariates on transition rates and the transition rates themselves. In Markov models, the distribution of sojourn times from the current state to another state depends only on the current state, and not on when a person arrived in the current state. Semi-Markov models also allow dependence on when the person arrived in the current state. Using Markov models, Cortese et al. (2013) found that AML at baseline increased $\alpha_{0,1}(t)$ by 1.75-fold and $\alpha_{2,1}(t)$ by 1.79-fold. Assuming a Markov model, Cortese et al. (2013) considered times $s \in \{0, 1, 3, 6, 12\}$ in months following transplantation and projected the absolute risks of relapse and of death without relapse in the intervals $(s, s + 12]$, separately for those with GVHD at s and those without GVHD at s. At $s = 0$, no patient had GVHD, and the one-year absolute risk of death without relapse ranged from about 0.05 to 0.5, depending on $\mathbf{Z}_2$, whereas risk of relapse ranged from about 0.05 to 0.18. At $s = 3$ months, the absolute risk of death by month 15 ranged from about 0.05 to 0.5 for those with GVHD and from 0.05 to 0.10 for those without GVHD. Thus, onset of GVHD greatly increased the absolute risk of death without relapse.

These calculations assumed a Markov model. If the $\alpha_{21}(t)$ and $\alpha_{23}(t)$ also depend on the time of transition to state 2, then the model would be semi-Markov. Cortese et al. (2013) outlined calculations of absolute risk under a semi-Markov model but presented no methods for estimation nor numerical results. The analyses of Cortese et al. (2013) that begin separately at months 0,1,3,6, and 12 resemble landmark analyses (Section 10.4.3). However, under the Markov model, estimates of the transition rates and relative risk parameters are based on all the follow-up information, not just on the information on covariates (non-absorbing states) up to a given landmark. Moreover, the projections beyond a landmark time in Cortese et al. (2013) use the Markov assumptions, whereas landmark analyses can use more general models, conditional on the covariate history up to the landmark time.

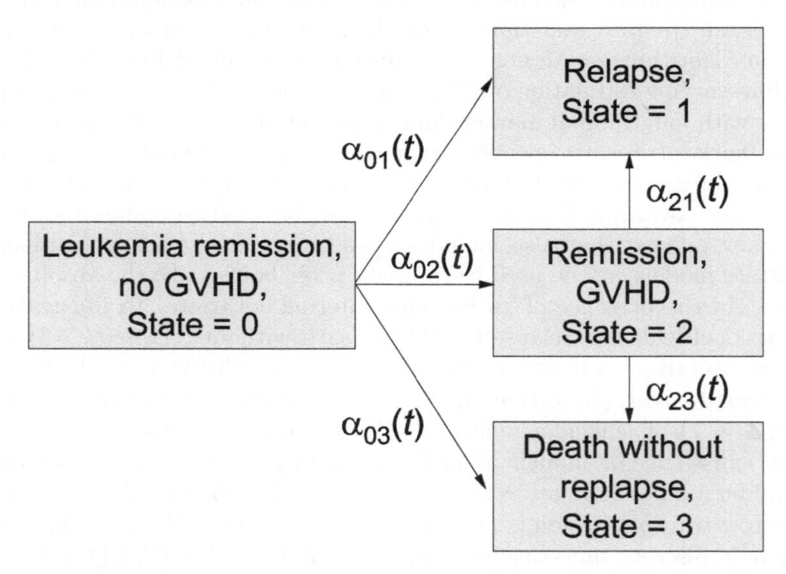

Figure 10.2: Multistate model for patients in leukemia remission following bone marrow transplantation, adapted from G. Cortese, T. A. Gerds, and P. K. Andersen. Comparing predictions among competing risks models with time-dependent covariates. *Statistics in Medicine*, 32(18):3089–3101, 2013.

Cortese et al. (2013) also analyzed the GVHD indicator $Z_1(s)$ as a time-dependent covariate in Cox models for leukemia relapse and for death without relapse. GVHD did not have a statistically significant effect on leukemia relapse but increased the cause-specific hazard of death by 2.85-fold. One could plot the corresponding cumulative hazards, but not interpret them as corresponding to cumulative incidences of relapse and death without relapse, because $Z_1(s)$ is an internal covariate.

We indicate how $r_1(0, \tau; \mathbf{Z})$ can be computed from the model in Figure 10.2, but we suppress the dependence of the transition rates on $\mathbf{Z}$. There are two ways to be in state 1 at time τ. The first is to transit directly from state 0 to state 1, and the second is to transit to state 1 via state 2. The first probability is

$$P_{01}(\tau) = \int_0^\tau \alpha_{01}(t) \exp[-\int_0^t \{\alpha_{01}(u) + \alpha_{02}(u) + \alpha_{03}(u)\}du]dt.$$

To calculate the second probability, we need the probability of being in state 2 at time τ, namely

$$P_{02}(\tau) = \int_0^\tau \alpha_{02}(t) \exp[-\int_0^t \{\alpha_{01}(u) + \alpha_{02}(u) + \alpha_{03}(u)\}du] \exp[-\int_t^\tau \{\alpha_{21}(u) + \alpha_{23}(u)\}du]dt.$$

Then the probability of ending in state 1 by transitioning from state 2 is

$$P_{021}(\tau) = \int_0^\tau P_{02}(t)\Big(\int_t^\tau \alpha_{21}(u) \exp[-\int_t^u \{\alpha_{21}(v) + \alpha_{23}(v)\}dv]du\Big)dt.$$

Finally, $r_1(0, \tau; \mathbf{Z}) = P_{01}(\tau) + P_{021}(\tau)$. By replacing integrated transition rates in these formulas by their empirical estimates and quantities like $\alpha_{01}(t)dt$ by the corresponding increment in the integrated transition rate estimate, one derives estimates of $r_1(0, \tau; \mathbf{Z})$. A general method for estimating such probabilities is given by Equation (7.2.38) in Andersen et al. (1993), who also provide a general variance calculations.

These methods generalize the classical competing risk models in Chapters 3 and 4 by allowing for non-absorbing states in addition to the initial state k=0, and the "state process" $\{\delta(s) : s \geq 0\}$ now takes on values k=2 in addition to the values 1 and 3 for absorbing states. Note that $r_1(0, \tau; \mathbf{Z}) = P(\delta(\tau) = 1)$ can no longer be calculated using the simpler formulas in Chapters 3 and 4.

Klein et al. (1993) used similar methods to study the effects of two time-varying transient conditions following bone marrow transplantation, namely whether or not GVHD had developed by time s and whether or not platelets had recovered to normal levels (PR) by time s. Klein et al. (1993) provided several informative plots for three clinical states, death without leukemia relapse (D), relapse (R), and relapse-free survival (S). The probabilities of each of these states at t =2 years (104 weeks) after transplantation were plotted (figure not shown) as a function of transient state status at various earlier times $0 \leq s \leq 15$ weeks. For example, a patient with PR but no GVHD at week $s = 13$ had a chance of relapse-free survival at two years of about 0.39 compared to only 0.08 for a patient without PR but with GVHD at s =13. Another valuable plot described how the probabilities of D, R, and S changed over time t from $s \leq t \leq 104$ weeks. An example is Figure 10.3, adapted from Klein et al. (1993). This plot depicts the probabilities of R, D and S beyond week $s = 13$ among patients who had experienced PR but not GVHD by week 13. The vertical distance between the top of the plot and the top locus is the probability of R, the distance between the two loci is the probability of D, and the distance from the bottom locus to the bottom of the plot is the probability of S. Klein et al. (1993) presented four separate plots of this type depending on whether or not PR or GVHD had occurred by week $s = 13$.

Simon and Makuch (1984) used a non-homogeneous Markov model to compare the distribution of times to death in patients with an initial tumor response to treatment to the distribution of times to death in patients with without an initial tumor response. Chapters IV and VII in Andersen et al. (1993) describe methods for multistate non-homogeneous Markov models, including covariates, and Andersen and Perme (2008) reviewed this area. de Wreede et al. (2010, 2011) reviewed available software for fitting such models and described the R program, mstate (Putter and Fiocco, 2014), for this purpose. See also Putter et al. (2007) and Cortese and Andersen (2010). Books by Beyersmann et al. (2012), van Houwelingen and Putter (2012) and Geskus (2016) provide a careful discussion of multistate models, including guidance on how to use available software, not only for classical competing risk problems, but also for models with transient states. Geskus (2016) describes computational details and provides programs in SAS and Stata as well as R.

Semi-Markov models allow a sojourn distribution for transition l to k to depend on the time of entry into state l. Weiss and Zelen (1963) gave a general account, but no methods for estimation. Several authors have described non-parametric estimation in the absence of covariates (Lagakos et al., 1978; Meira-Machado et al., 2006; de Una-Alvarez and Meira-Machado, 2015). Wu (1982) described methods for covariates and piecewise constant baseline transition rates. Software in R is available with covariates with certain parametric models (Listwon-Krol and Saint-Pierre, 2015) and with piecewise constant hazards (Jackson, 2011). The R program msm, (Jackson, 2011) also allows for estimation of Markov models from cross-sectional data at several times ("panel data") as well as from continuously observed outcomes. de Wreede et al. (2010) remark that mstate can fit semi-Markov models using a simulation method (Dabrowska, 1995). Datta and Satten (2001) showed that the Aalen-Johansen estimates of transition probabilities and the Nelson-Aalen estimates of cumulative transition rates that were derived for Markov models are also consistent for semi-Markov models, and it is possible that these consistency results also hold with covariates.

10.4.3 Landmark analysis

Multistate models require that the time-varying covariate be discrete. Although it is possible to categorize continuous markers and put them into the multistate framework, this approach may result in loss of information. A more flexible and simpler approach for using accumulating covariate information is "landmark" analysis. Suppose that $\mathbf{Z}(t)$ includes some time-varying internal and external covariates measured at time t, as well as fixed baseline covariates. Suppose a leukemia patient without relapse returns for a consultation at time s and we know the patient's marker history from time $t_0 = 0$ to s, namely $H(s) = \{\mathbf{Z}(t) : 0 \leq t \leq s\}$. The landmark method treats all the information in $H(s)$ at the landmark time s as fixed, and uses standard methods for fixed covariates to estimate absolute risks for times beyond s. One can use any of the methods in Chapter 4 to compute absolute risks $r_k(s, t; H(s))$.

For example, Cortese et al. (2013) used landmark times $s \in \{0, 1, 3, 6, 12\}$ weeks and fit cause-specific hazard models and Fine-Gray models with the "fixed" covariates, age at baseline, AML status, and the GVHD indicator $Z_1(s) = z_1(s)$. The cause-specific models revealed little effect of GVHD on relapse, but GVHD increased the risk of death without relapse, especially for $s = 1$, 3 and 6 weeks. Presence of AML at baseline was a strong risk factor for relapse and for death without relapse. One-year absolute risk projections beyond the landmark time for relapse and for death without relapse from the multistate Markov model (Figure 10.2) agreed well with the landmark projections at the various landmark times, both for the cause-specific hazards landmark model and for the Fine-Gray landmark model. Although the variances of estimates based on the multistate Markov model depend on the Markov assumption, the estimates of transition probabilities and cumulative transition rates are consistent, even when the Markov assumption fails (Datta and Satten, 2001). This may contribute to the good agreement among these various methods.

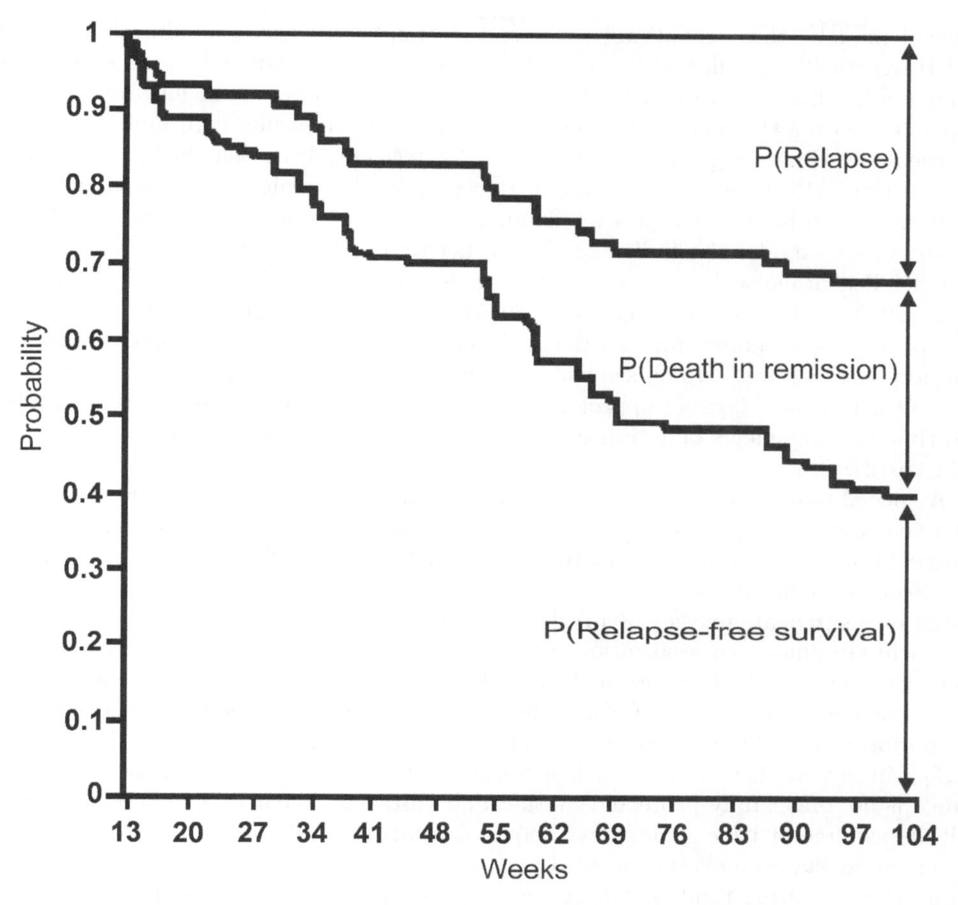

Figure 10.3: Probabilities of leukemia relapse, death without relapse, and relapse-free survival in patients with platelet recovery but no graft versus host reaction in the first 13 weeks following bone marrow transplantation, adapted from J. P. Klein, N. Keiding, and E. A. Copelan. Plotting summary predictions in multistate survival models - probabilities of relapse and death in remission for bone-marrow transplantation patients. *Statistics in Medicine*, 12(24):2315–2332, 1993.

Some advantages of the landmark method include the availability of software for absolute risk modeling with fixed covariates and the extreme flexibility of modeling that is permitted. However, a landmark analysis at time s only includes individuals who survived and remained in follow-up to time s, which is a subset of the original population. This should be kept in mind when projecting risk for members of another target population.

Landmarking has been used in the clinical literature at least since the 1980s. For example, Anderson et al. (1983) recommended a landmark analysis to determine whether cancer patients who survived to time s after treatment and who had a tumor response to treatment by time s had a better prognosis than those who survived to time s without a tumor response. Research on landmarking for risk prediction has been active recently, following the work by Zheng and Heagerty (2005) and van Houwelingen (2007). van Houwelingen (2007) pointed out the practical advantages of landmarking and proposed methods for obtaining smooth landmark projections over a sequence of landmark times. Because each landmark time s induces a different risk model, van Houwelingen (2007) embedded the s-specific covariate parameters and baseline transition rates in a larger flexible parametric class of models, thus smoothing the s-specific quantities across landmark times. Zheng and Heagerty (2005) allowed the model coefficients to vary not only with s but also with times t following the landmark time s, thus relaxing proportional hazards assumptions. Papers extending the method to competing risks and comparing it to multistate modeling followed (van Houwelingen and Putter, 2008; Cortese and Andersen, 2010; van Houwelingen and Putter, 2012; Cortese et al., 2013). Recent work (Nicolaie et al., 2013a) implemented landmark smoothing techniques for competing risks. Another innovation (Nicolaie et al., 2013b) was to model the indicator of whether or not an individual at risk at landmark time s failed of cause k at or before time $s + \tau$ for fixed τ. Following ideas in Andersen et al. (2003) and Klein and Andersen (2005), Nicolaie et al. (2013b) introduced a general class of regression models for this Bernouli outcome and replaced censored observations by "pseudo-observations," which are like jack-knife pseudo-values, to fit models with censored data. Other related flexible approaches for fixed τ are based on time-varying coefficients and time-varying effects of an intermediate outcome during the interval $[0, s]$ (Parast et al., 2011, 2012).

A special issue arises in randomized clinical trials where interest centers on the effect of the fixed covariate Z_2, an indicator of which treatment was randomly assigned. If one uses marker information at subsequent times s beyond the time of randomization, $t_0 = 0$, then the effect of Z_2 can be obscured. Suppose, for example, that the effect of treatment is mediated by a surrogate marker, $Z_1(s)$. If this marker is a perfect surrogate, then conditioning on it will eliminate the association of Z_2 with the clinical outcome, for example survival time (Prentice, 1989). Likewise inclusion of $Z_1(s)$ in a regression model that also includes Z_2 will attenuate the effect of Z_2, if the effect of Z_2 is partly mediated through $Z_1(s)$. If one performs a landmark analysis at time s but ignores mediating marker, $Z_1(s)$, the effect of Z_2 will not be distorted by such mediation effects, but the analysis of times t beyond time s is no longer fully protected by the randomization, because the subset of individuals still disease-free at time s may have acquired treatment imbalances on prognostic factors. For example, suppose overall survival at $t = 10$ years is the same on treatments $Z_2 = 1$ or 0, and that following randomization the distribution of risk factors is the same on the two treatments. Suppose, however, that on treatment 1 only the sickest patients die early, and before time $s = 1$ year, whereas on treatment $Z_2 = 0$ deaths occur in all risk levels before s. Then the population of survivors to the landmark time $s = 1$ year will have a more favorable distribution of risk factors on treatment 1 than on treatment 0. Thus the estimate of treatment effect from year s to year 10 will be biased compared to the estimate of treatment effect from randomization to year 10 that would have been observed without landmarking.

10.5 Risk model applications for counseling individuals and for public health strategies for disease prevention

In earlier chapters we touched on some of the applications of risk models for counseling individuals and for public health strategies for disease prevention. Here we summarize those applications and also introduce new material on two applications: assessing the potential reductions in population absolute risks from interventions to reduce modifiable risk factors; and more efficient allocation of prevention resources.

10.5.1 Use of risk models in counseling individuals

10.5.1.1 Providing realistic risk estimates and perspective

Having a realistic estimate of risk can assist in clinical management for prevention or early disease detection. The perspective gained from a realistic assessment of risk can assist in some decisions, even without a formal risk-benefit analysis. Indeed, one of the motivations for developing BCRAT was that some women seen in clinics for counseling women with a strong family history of breast cancer greatly overestimated their risks. For example, a woman might assume that if her mother had breast cancer she had a 50% chance of getting it, whereas a more realistic lifetime risk might be 18%. On the basis of such misperceptions, she might decide to have a drastic preventive intervention, such as bilateral prophylactic mastectomy.

Another example concerns whether or not a woman in her forties should have annual mammographic screening. There has been continuing debate on this issue. For example, the American Cancer Society recommended annual screening for women beginning at age 45 years, but said that women aged 40-44 should have the opportunity for screening (Oeffinger et al., 2015). The U.S. Preventive Task Force recommended biennial screening for women aged 50–74 years, but not in their forties (USPTF, 2009). However, they said that the choice for women in their forties should be an individual decision, and more recently stressed that such women should weigh the harms and benefits (https://www.uspreventiveservicestaskforce.org/Page/Document/UpdateSummaryFinal/breast-cancer-screening1?ds=1&s=mammography). There is consensus that women aged 50–74 should be screened regularly. It seems reasonable, therefore, that a woman in her forties whose breast cancer risk exceeds that of a 50-year-old woman without risk factors should consider screening, as argued more formally by Gail and Rimer (1998), Gail and Schairer (2010) and Wu et al. (2012). Indeed, Wu et al. (2012) found that 73.6% (11.6 million) of non-Hispanic white women and 30.9% (0.85 million) non-Hispanic black women in their forties in the U.S. had risks above the 50-year old baseline risk and concluded that millions of women in the U.S. in their forties might benefit from mammography screening as much as a low-risk 50-year-old, for whom screening is recommended. van Ravesteyn et al. (2012) reported that women in their forties with twice the average risk had the same harm-benefit ratio as women aged 50–74.

There is increasing use of absolute risk to manage preventive interventions, rather than basing decisions on a single factor, such as age or cholesterol level. Pashayan et al. (2011) compared assigning all women aged 47–79 years to screening mammography (these women have a 10-year risk of invasive breast cancer of 2.5%) to risk-based assignment to screening of women aged 35–79 years whose estimated 10-year risk was at least 2.5%. The estimated risk was based on age and a polygenic risk score derived from 18 SNPs. Pashayan et al. (2011) found with this risk model that one would detect 14% fewer cases but need to give mammograms to 24% fewer women. In addition to the economic advantage to the health care system of screening 24% fewer women, this risk-based screening reduces the inconvenience of mammography and adverse consequences from false positive mammographic screening tests. A model that also included mammographic density and other epidemiologic risk factors would do even better. In Section 10.5.2.3 we consider using risk models to assign women to screening mammography only if their risk is very high, such as in the top 10% of population risk. This approach does not work well unless risk models are very discriminating (i.e., have high AUC), however, because too many cases will arise in women with lower risk. As another example, guidelines for the use of statins to prevent cardiovascular disease rely heavily on 10-year pure risk (Expert Panel on Detection and Evaluation and Treatment of High Blood Cholesterol in Adults, 2001; Stone et al., 2014). Katki et al. (2013) advocated management strategies for women at risk of cervical cancer based on estimated risk of a pre-neoplastic lesion, CIN3, and Kovalchik et al. (2013b) recommended risk-based targeting of low-dose computed tomographic screening for lung cancer. These recommendations are in line with the principle that an intervention is advisable if risk exceeds a particular threshold. This idea is formalized in Equation (6.29) that demonstrates that the choice of threshold reflects the risks and benefits of the intervention. When breast cancer risks are very high, as in women carrying mutations in the breast cancer genes BRCA1 or BRCA2 or in the p53 gene, the risks can exceed high thresholds that reflect substantial adverse effects of intervention, such as prophylactic mastectomy or salpingo-oophorectomy (Chapter 9).

10.5.1.2 More formal risk-benefit analysis for individual counseling

Preventive interventions, such as the use of tamoxifen or raloxifene, can have favorable and unfavorable effects on health outcomes, as described in Sections 6.6.2.2 and 7.4.6. In particular, tamoxifen reduces the risks of breast cancer and hip fractures but increases the risks of endometrial cancer, stroke and pulmonary emboli, which we consider to be severe adverse events. If the patient is willing to associate equal costs (weights) with each of these events, and half those costs with less severe outcomes (*in situ* breast cancer, for which tamoxifen reduces risk, and deep vein thrombosis, for which tamoxifen increases risk), then one can estimate the net benefit (which may be negative) as in Equation (6.40) to assist in the counseling process. It would also be possible to calculate a net benefit using the patient's preferred weights or costs for the various outcomes. When interventions affect multiple outcomes, there is no single risk threshold for e.g breast cancer risk that applies to all women. The net benefit is positive for tamoxifen for a young woman with little baseline risk of endometrial cancer, stroke and pulmonary emboli at a 5-year invasive breast cancer risk threshold of 1.5%. In contrast, a woman in her fifties, whose baseline risks of endometrial cancer, stroke and pulmonary emboli are higher, would need a 5-year breast cancer risk of 4.0% or greater to have a net benefit from tamoxifen (see Table 10 in (Gail et al., 1999a)).

Freedman et al. (2011) compared the net benefit profiles of raloxifene versus tamoxifen for breast cancer prevention in woman aged 50 to 79 with uteri (and therefore at risk of endometrial cancer). We show results from (Freedman et al., 2011) in Table 10.1. Tamoxifen only has a net benefit for women in their fifties with 5-year breast cancer risks $\geq 4.0\%$, and no net benefit in women aged ≥ 60 years. In contrast, raloxifene, which does not increase endometrial cancer risk, has a net benefit for a much broader set of breast cancer risks and ages (Table 10.1). Because raloxifene can be applied beneficially to a larger proportion of the population, it has greater preventive potential. In women who have had a hysterectomy and are therefore not at risk of endometrial cancer, the risk profiles are similar for tamoxifen and raloxifene, and the net benefit is positive for even more women than shown in Table 10.1 (Freedman et al., 2011).

10.5.2 Use of risk models in public health prevention

In addition to their uses in individual counseling, absolute and pure risk models have applications in public health programs to prevent disease (Gail, 2011), as described next.

10.5.2.1 Designing intervention trials to prevent disease

Models of the absolute risk of disease incidence play a key role in designing trials to test preventive interventions. A requirement for such trials is adequate statistical power. Under the proportional hazards assumption (Cox, 1972), the power of such trials depends on the number of incident cases, whose expectation is the sum of the absolute risks of the trial participants. Using BCRAT (model 2 in Costantino et al. (1999)), statisticians at the National Adjuvant Breast and Bowel Project (NSABP) estimated the numbers of women and duration of follow-up needed to observe the required number of incident breast cancers for the Breast Cancer Prevention Trial (P-1 Trial) of tamoxifen (Fisher et al., 1998) and, later, for the NSABP Study of Tamoxifen and Raloxifene (STAR or P-2) trial. The risk model accurately predicted the numbers of incident breast cancers in both these trials.

In addition to power considerations, risk models can play a role in defining eligibility for a trial. For example, in designing the P-1 trial, it was known that tamoxifen had adverse effects. The investigators therefore only wanted to enroll women who had a high enough

Table 10.1: Net benefit indices for tamoxifen and raloxifene chemoprevention by level of 5-year projected risk for invasive breast cancer for white non-Hispanic women with a uterus*

	Tamoxifen			Raloxifene		
5-year) risk (%)	**50–59 years**	**60–69 years**	**70–79 years**	**50–59 years**	**60–69 years**	**70–79 years**
1.5	−133	−310	−325	21	−11	−15
2.0	−105	−283	−298	43	11	7
2.5	−78	−255	−271	65	33	29
3.0	−51	−228	−244	86	55	51
3.5	−25	−202	−217	108	76	71
4.0	3	−175	−190	128	97	93
4.5	29	−148	−164	150	119	115
5.0	56	−121	−137	172	140	136
5.5	83	−95	−111	193	161	157
6.0	109	−69	−84	214	183	179
6.5	135	−42	−58	236	204	199
7.0	162	−15	−32	256	225	221

*Adapted from A. N. Freedman, B. B. Yu, M. H. Gail, J. P. Costantino, B. I. Graubard, V. G. Vogel, G. L. Anderson, and W. McCaskill-Stevens. Benefit/risk assessment for breast cancer chemoprevention with raloxifene or tamoxifen for women age 50 years or older. *Journal of Clinical Oncology*, 29(17):2327–2333, 2011. Freedman et al. (2011) computed life-threatening equivalent events by assigning a weight of 1.0 to life-threatening events (invasive breast cancer, hip fracture, endometrial cancer, stroke, and pulmonary embolism) and a weight of 0.5 to severe events (*in situ* breast cancer and deep vein thrombosis). The net benefit index is the expected number of life-threatening equivalent events in 5 years without chemoprevention in 10,000 such women minus the expected number of life-threatening equivalent events if chemoprevention is used.

risk of breast cancer to have a potential benefit from participation. They chose a 5-year risk of incident invasive breast cancer threshold of 1.66%, which was the risk in an average 60-year-old woman, who they thought might benefit. In order for a woman younger than age 60 to participate, her absolute 5-year risk, calculated from BCRAT had to equal or exceed 1.66%.

10.5.2.2 Assessing absolute risk reduction in a population from interventions on modifiable risk factors

Models of absolute risk with modifiable risk factors afford an opportunity to assess the potential impact on absolute risk in a population of interventions that reduce or eliminate such risk factors. For example, Petracci et al. (2011) developed a breast cancer risk model for Italian women that included age, six non-modifiable risk factors (age at menarche, age at first live birth, education, occupational activity, family history, and biopsy history) and three modifiable risk factors (alcohol consumption, leisure physical activity, and BMI). They calculated average absolute risks of invasive breast cancer in the population in the absence of interventions and in the presence of hypothetical interventions that changed the modifiable risk factors to their lowest risk levels. Pfeiffer and Petracci (2011) devised variance formulas for these criteria based on influence functions.

We now illustrate these criteria with the BC2013 model for breast cancer, that also incorporates information on several modifiable risk factors, including alcohol consumption, hormone replacement therapy use and BMI, in addition to several non-modifiable ones. To assess the impact of changing modifiable risk factors, $\mathbf{Z}_2$, we define the *risk reduction* as

$$d(\mathbf{Z}_1, \mathbf{Z}_2) = \{r(\mathbf{Z}_1, \mathbf{Z}_2) - r(\mathbf{Z}_1, \mathbf{Z}_{20})\}, \tag{10.1}$$

where r denotes the absolute risk estimate, $\mathbf{Z}_1$ the non-modifiable factors, and $\mathbf{Z}_{20}$ the modifiable risk factors set to their lowest risk levels (Petracci et al., 2011; Pfeiffer and Petracci, 2011). The corresponding *fractional risk reduction* is

$$fd(\mathbf{Z}_1, \mathbf{Z}_2) = \{d(\mathbf{Z}_1, \mathbf{Z}_2)/r(\mathbf{Z}_1, \mathbf{Z}_2)\}. \tag{10.2}$$

To evaluate the effects of risk modification at the population level for a given population, the risk reduction and fractional risk reduction are averaged over the entire population or within subgroups. Subgroups can be defined by particular risk factor combinations or by using the Lorenz curve to identify risk factor combinations that confer high risk and account for a given percentage of total population risk. The *mean risk reduction* for a specific subset S is calculated from the formula:

$$\bar{d}(S) = E(d(\mathbf{Z}_1, \mathbf{Z}_2)|(\mathbf{Z}_1, \mathbf{Z}_2) \in S) = \frac{\int_{Z_1,Z_2}\{r(\mathbf{Z}_1, \mathbf{Z}_2) - r(\mathbf{Z}_1, \mathbf{Z}_{20})\}I\{(\mathbf{Z}_1, \mathbf{Z}_2) \in S\}dF(\mathbf{Z}_1, \mathbf{Z}_2)}{\int_{\mathbf{Z}_1,\mathbf{Z}_2} I\{(\mathbf{Z}_1, \mathbf{Z}_2) \in S\}dF(\mathbf{Z}_1, \mathbf{Z}_2)}, \tag{10.3}$$

where $I\{(\mathbf{Z}_1, \mathbf{Z}_2) \in S\} = 1$ if $(\mathbf{Z}_1, \mathbf{Z}_2) \in S$ and 0 otherwise. When S corresponds to the whole population, then (10.3) reduces to

$$\bar{d} = E\{d(\mathbf{Z}_1, \mathbf{Z}_2)\} = \int_{\mathbf{Z}_1,\mathbf{Z}_2} \{r(\mathbf{Z}_1, \mathbf{Z}_2) - r(\mathbf{Z}_1, \mathbf{Z}_{20})\}dF(\mathbf{Z}_1, \mathbf{Z}_2). \tag{10.4}$$

Similarly, the *mean fractional risk reduction in subset* S is

$$mfrr(S) = E\{fd(\mathbf{Z}_1, \mathbf{Z}_2)|(\mathbf{Z}_1, \mathbf{Z}_2) \in S\}. \tag{10.5}$$

A quantity that is more analogous to attributable risk is the *fractional mean risk reduction in subset S*,

$$fmrr(S) = \bar{d}(S)/E\{r(\mathbf{Z}_1, \mathbf{Z}_2)|(\mathbf{Z}_1, \mathbf{Z}_2) \in S\}. \tag{10.6}$$

Table 10.2 shows the effects of the hypothetical interventions that set modifiable risk factors to their lowest risk levels on 20-year average absolute risk of invasive breast cancer in 50-year-old women in the NHS cohort. Calculations are shown separately for all such women, for those with a history of breast cancer in at least one mother, sister or daughter, and for those with risks in the top 10% of risks in the population. Among all such women, the average absolute 20-year risk is 5.86% without intervention. Intervention reduces this risk by 1.09% to 4.77%. The mean fractional risk reduction is 17.3%, close to the fractional mean risk reduction, 18.6%. The absolute risk reduction is 1.51% in women with affected first-degree relatives and 2.50% for women whose risks are in the top 10% of risks. The average risk for women above the 90th decile of risk is 9.20% without intervention and $9.20 - 2.50 = 6.7\%$ with intervention, corresponding to a a mean fractional risk reduction of 26.8% and a fractional mean risk reduction of 27.2%.

The fractional mean risk reduction is analogous to attributable risk and ranges from 18.6% for the entire population to 27.2% for those above the 90th decile of risk, a relative increase of 46%. The average absolute risk reduction is smaller but increases from 1.09% to 2.50%, a relative increase of 129%. The relatively greater absolute risk reduction in women with risks above the 90th decile of risk is a consequence of two features. First such women are in the high risk group partly because they are enriched with modifiable risk factors, that can be reduced by intervention. Second, women at high risk because of non-modifiable risk factors will also experience a larger risk reduction from intervention than women with few non-modifiable risk factors and at lower risk because there are no interactions between modifiable and non-modifiable risk factors in the BC2013 model. Thus the same proportional decrease in risk from intervention will produce a greater absolute reduction in risk among the women at higher risk by virtue of non-modifiable risk factors. Analyses of absolute risk reduction give a different perspective on the public health impact of a hypothetical intervention than does attributable risk or fractional reduction in average absolute risk. Note that even though the absolute risk reduction is greater in the 10% of the women at highest risk, more disease could be prevented by intervening on the entire population because 1.09% is greater than $0.1 \times 2.50\%$.

Table 10.2: Potential reductions in the population risk of invasive breast cancer risk over 20 years from eliminating alcohol consumption, hormone replacement therapy use and BMI>25 kg/m^2 in $N = 2447$ 50-year-old women in the NHS cohort

	Mean absolute risk without intervention (%)	**Reduction in mean absolute risk from intervention (%)**	**Mean fractional risk reduction (%)**	**Fractional mean risk reduction (%)**
Entire population ($N = 2447$)	5.86	1.09	17.3	18.6
Women with at least one affected mother, sister or daughter ($N = 295$)	7.97	1.51	17.7	19.0
Women with risk in the top 10% of risks ($N = 246$)	9.20	2.50	26.8	27.2

It is important to keep in mind the assumptions implicit in such calculations. First, we assumed that there were effective interventions that could reduce exposure to modifiable risks factors. It is difficult to define effective interventions that affect lifestyle factors such as alcohol consumption. Second, we have assumed that the population would accept and adhere to the intervention. Third, we have assumed that the effect of the intervention would be equal to the exposure effects that had previously been estimated from observational data. Unfortunately, interventions that seem to be well justified by observational data are not always beneficial when tested in randomized intervention trials (e.g., (Omenn et al., 1996; Manson et al., 2003)). However, at least these calculations indicate the absolute burden of disease from certain risk factors in the population, whether or not the hypothetical interventions achieve the calculated preventive effects.

10.5.2.3 Implementing a "high risk" intervention strategy for disease prevention

Designing intervention trials and assessing the potential effects on population absolute risk of reducing modifiable risk factors require well calibrated risk models, but not high discriminatory accuracy. Thus models like BCRAT or BC2013 can still be useful in these applications. Higher discriminatory accuracy is needed for the following applications.

In his book, *The Strategy of Preventive Medicine*, Rose (1992) distinguished between the "general population" prevention strategy and the "high risk" prevention strategy. If an intervention is safe enough, one can apply it to the entire population (general population strategy); this approach has the greatest potential for disease prevention. For example, if one could get everyone to lower his or her blood pressure by 2 mmHg by taking a walk each day and eating less salt, one could reduce the incidence of myocardial infarction more than by identifying the members of the population with very high blood pressure and treating them. The general population strategy prevents more disease than the high risk strategy because it applies to many more people and because the risk of myocardial infarction is dispersed throughout the population, and not only in those with very high blood pressure.

Nonetheless, sometimes one is forced to use the high risk strategy of targeting the intervention to a subset of the population at elevated risk. If the intervention has adverse effects, one should only use it on those members of the population whose benefit from reducing the targeted disease outweighs the risks of the adverse effects. This requirement leads to restricting the intervention to a subset of the population with elevated risk of the targeted disease. Resource limitations can also be a reason to use the high risk strategy.

The population impact of the high risk strategy on the targeted disease depends on how much of the total targeted disease burden is concentrated in the high risk subgroup and on the effect of the intervention in reducing the incidence of the targeted disease. If the intervention has few adverse effects, the high risk subgroup can be larger, increasing the proportion of disease that is targeted. If risk models are highly discriminating, they can concentrate those most likely to develop disease in the subgroup, thereby increasing the proportion of the total disease burden that is targeted in the subgroup, called the proportion of cases followed, PCF, in Section 6.5.

To illustrate these points, consider the data on life-threatening events in one year in 100,000 white women aged 50–59 years and with uteri (Table 10.3) (Fisher et al., 1998; Gail et al., 1999a; Gail, 2009b). If none get tamoxifen, 589.6 life-threatening events are expected, including 246.6 invasive breast cancers. If all get tamoxifen, the numbers of breast cancers and hip fractures are cut nearly in half, but the expected numbers of women with endometrial cancer, stroke and pulmonary emboli are increased so much that the expected total number of life-threatening events is 833.5. Thus one cannot employ the general population strategy of giving all women in that age group tamoxifen. The net expected number of life-threatening events prevented by tamoxifen (Gail, 2009b),
$r \times 10^5(1 - .51) + 101.6(1 - .55) + 81.4(1 - 4.01) + 110.0(1 - 1.59) + 50.0(1 - 3.01)$,
depends on the absolute risk of breast cancer, r. For this number to be positive, r needs to exceed the threshold $r^* = 774.3 \times 10^{-5}$. Therefore, in order for a white woman in her fifties to have a net benefit from tamoxifen, her breast cancer risk must be very high. Only about 1% of the population has a risk greater than r^*. Thus the "high-risk" portion of the population is very small, and an intervention that focuses only on high risk women is unlikely to prevent much disease.

As calculated in Gail (2009b), the expected number of life-threatening events is reduced very slightly by giving tamoxifen only to those women with risks above 774.3 per 10^5 (Table 10.4), unless the risk model has very high discriminatory power. For example, giving tamoxifen only to women with BCRAT risk $>r^* = 774.3 \times 10^{-5}$ reduces the expected number of life-threatening events by only 1.4 to 588.2. A model that also includes 7 single nucleotide polymorphisms, BCRAT+7 SNPs, has somewhat higher $AUC = 0.632$. However, giving tamoxifen only to women whose risk with BCRAT+7 SNPs exceeds $r^* = 774.3 \times 10^{-5}$ only reduces the expected number of life-threatening events by 1.6 events, to 587.8. Adding additional SNPs and mammographic density to the model may increase AUC to nearly 0.7 (Garcia-Closas et al., 2014). Even this hard-to-achieve increase in discriminatory accuracy would not reduce the number of life-threatening events by much. A model with perfect discriminatory accuracy, however, would identify the 246 women destined to develop invasive breast cancer (Table 10.3) and target the tamoxifen intervention on them. Because so few women would receive tamoxifen, there would be few life-threatening toxicities, yet

Table 10.3: Numbers of life-threatening events in one year in 100,000 white women aged 50–59 years with uteri, if none get tamoxifen and if all get tamoxifen

Health outcome	**Relative risk**	**Number of events if none get tamoxifen**[a]	**Number of events if all get tamoxifen**
Invasive breast cancer	0.51	246.6	125.8
Hip fracture	0.55	101.6	55.9
Endometrial cancer	4.01	81.4	326.4
Stroke	1.59	110	174.9
Pulmonary embolism	3.01	50	150.5
Total		589.6	833.5

[a] Relative risk compares women given tamoxifen to women given placebo.
From M. H. Gail. Value of adding single-nucleotide polymorphism genotypes to a breast cancer risk model. *Journal of the National Cancer Institute*, 101(13):959–963, 2009. See also Fisher et al. (1998) and Gail et al. (1999a).

the number of breast cancers would be nearly cut in half, resulting in an expected reduction of 119.9 life-threatening events to 469.7 (Table 10.4).

This example illustrates that the high risk prevention strategy may have little public health impact if the high risk subset contains a small proportion of the women who will develop breast cancer, either because the subset is small or because available risk models are not discriminating enough to classify most of the women destined to develop breast cancer as high risk. Of course, the preventive intervention will also have little public health impact if the intervention has a small preventive effect in those who receive it (Janes et al., 2014).

One can think of several approaches to improve the public health impact of the high risk prevention strategy. The most promising is to find safer interventions that can be applied beneficially to a broader high risk subset. For example for women with uteri in their fifties, raloxifene could be used more widely than tamoxifen (Table 10.1). For the example in Table 10.4, 4% of the population would be with treated with raloxifene and would not be at increased endometrial cancer risk, resulting in a reduction of 21 expected life-threatening events, compared to only 1.4 for tamoxifen. For women without uteri, tamoxifen and raloxifene have similar net benefit profiles (Freedman et al., 2011). A second approach is to find interventions with stronger preventive effects on the targeted disease. A third approach is to develop more discriminating risk models to help concentrate those destined to develop the targeted disease in the subset at high risk, but such progress is difficult. Another approach is to build risk models not only for the targeted disease, but for the other endpoints affected by the intervention (Gail, 2012). For example, if one had a model for stroke risk in the absence of intervention, as well as a model for invasive breast cancer risk, one could assess net benefit more accurately and prevent more life-threatening events. In Gail et al. (1999a), one only used age and race to estimate stroke risk, but calculations in Gail (2012) suggest that appreciable improvements can be achieved by modeling both stroke and breast cancer risk. Similarly, a recently developed absolute risk model for endometrial cancer (Pfeiffer et al., 2013) could help identify women who stand to benefit from tamoxifen treatment.

Screening for disease can also be regarded as an intervention, or, at least as the initial part of an intervention that also entails further diagnostic procedures and treatments. Screening for persons at high risk of prevalent disease has risks and benefits, because false positive and false negative screens each have adverse consequences. Risk models usually

Table 10.4: Numbers of life-threatening events expected in one year in 100,000 white women aged 50–59 years with uteri, with tamoxifen given according to risk-based criteria*

Tamoxifen assignment strategy	**Expected number of life-threatening events**	**Reduction in expected life-threatening events**
No tamoxifen	589.6	
BCRAT risk $>r^* = 774.3 \times 10^{-5}$	588.2	1.4
BCRAT+7 SNPs risk $>r^*$	587.8	1.6
Perfect risk model risk $>r^*$	469.7	119.9

*BCRAT is the National Cancer Institute's Breast Cancer Risk Assessment Tool (http://www.cancer.gov/bcrisktool/). The risk model BCRAT+7 SNPs is described in Gail (2008a, 2009b). The perfect risk model assigns all women who are destined to develop breast cancer in one year to the high risk group (risk $>r^*$) and all other women to its complement (risk $\leq r^*$).

need to have high discriminatory accuracy to be useful in deciding who should be screened and who not (Chapter 6). In screening applications, the risk model would ideally predict the probability of screen-detectable prevalent disease, not the absolute risk of disease incidence. However, if prevalence is proportional to the risk of incidence, risk models for incidence can be used to guide screening recommendations.

A key function for evaluating screening is the proportion of cases in the top $p \times 100$ percent of the population at highest risk, called the proportion of cases followed or $PCF(p)$ (Pfeiffer and Gail, 2011) in Section 6.5. Park et al. (2012) studied the potential discriminatory accuracy of a breast cancer risk model that included epidemiologic factors and "foreseeable" SNPs that would be discovered by a genome-wide association study (GWAS) three times as large as the largest GWAS to date. For example, for breast cancer, the largest GWAS had the equivalent of 18,163 cases and controls, and foreseeable SNPs would be based on an hypothetical study of 54,489 cases and controls. They estimated an AUC of 0.67 from such a model. Suppose one assessed the risks of every woman in the population with this model. Using this risk model one could intervene (by giving a screening mammogram) only on the 10% of the population at highest risk. Park et al. (2012) calculated that $PCF(p = 0.1) = 0.255$. Thus, this risk decision rule would give screening mammography to 25.5% of the cases in the entire population, but 74.5% of the cases would not benefit from screening mammography because they are not in this high risk subgroup. The positive predictive value of being in the high risk subgroup is $PPV = \pi PCF(p)/p$, where π is the disease prevalence. This formula highlights the role of $PCF(p)$ in determining a key parameter for screening and high risk prevention strategies, the PPV. For women aged 50–54 years, the prevalence of screen detectable breast cancer was estimated as 0.0031, resulting in $PPV = 0.0031 \times 0.255/0.1 = .0079$. The ratio of women without breast cancer to women with breast cancer in the high risk subgroup is $(1 - PPV)/PPV = 126$. Thus, one needs to give mammographic screens to 127 women to detect one breast cancer in women aged 50–54 years at highest (top 10%) risk. In women aged 40–44, whose prevalence of screen detectable breast cancer is only 0.0016, $(1 - PPV)/PPV = 244$ instead of 126 for women in the top 10% of risk. Clearly, risk-based mammographic screening that focused on women in the top 10% of breast cancer risk would miss many women with cancer, even with the best risk models likely to be available in the foreseeable future, and many of those who would be given mammograms under such a plan would not have breast cancer. More discriminating models are needed for this application.

10.5.2.4 Allocating preventive interventions under cost constraints

Preventive resources are sometimes limited, either because the equipment and personnel are not available or because of cost constraints. In these circumstances, one strategy is to assign the preventive interventions to those at highest risk. For example, magnetic resonance imaging of breast tissue has been recommended only for women whose lifetime risk of breast cancer exceeds 20% (Saslow et al., 2007), partly because the resource is expensive and in short supply. In what follows we consider a setting in which there is only enough money to provide screening mammography to half the population. If one assigns the mammograms at random, one expects to be able to achieve about 50% of the population reduction in breast cancer mortality as could be achieved by giving all women mammograms (which reduces breast cancer mortality by 15% or more (Pace and Keating, 2014)). If one were to first assess breast cancer risk and then allocate mammograms to women in decreasing order of risk until the money ran out, one could hope to achieve a higher proportion of the maximum potential benefit than the 50% from random allocation. This assumes, however, that the cost of risk assessment is small compared to the cost of intervention.

Gail (2009a), using the Lorenz curve of the population risk distribution, showed that the maximum benefit from risk-based allocation of preventive resources could be obtained by maximizing

$$g \times PCF(p) + (1 - g)m \tag{10.7}$$

subject to the cost constraint

$$gk + gp + (1 - g)m \leq h. \tag{10.8}$$

In these expressions, g is the proportion of the population given a risk assessment, k is the ratio of the cost of risk assessment to the cost of the intervention (in our case mammographic screening), p is the proportion of those with risk assessment who have the intervention in descending order from highest to lowest risk, m is the proportion of those not given a risk assessment who were randomly allocated to receive a mammogram, and h is the ratio of the money available to the money required to give mammograms to all women (in our case h =0.5). Choices of g, p, m correspond to various strategies. For example, g =1 implies giving a risk assessment to all. We assumed k =0.02 and used $PCF(p)$ curves corresponding to the risk model BCRAT and to the risk model BCRAT+7SNPs, solved the optimization problems, and calculated the optimal proportions of benefit achieved from Equation (10.7). The optimal strategy assigns g =1, p =0.48, and m =0 for both risk models (Table 10.5). Only 100p =48% of the women get mammograms, because some of the money was used for risk assessment. BCRAT captures 63.2% of the potential benefits of mammography, and BCRAT+7SNPs captures 66.7%. These are both considerable improvements compared to random allocation. Even more of the potential benefit could be captured by more discriminating risk models, but if the cost of risk assessment is too high, it cannot be used for allocation. For models like BCRAT or BC2013, if the cost of risk assessment exceeded about 20% of the cost of the intervention, random allocation would be preferred.

Such calculations indicate that there is a potential public health benefit for risk-based allocation of constrained prevention resources. However, these calculations are based on several assumptions, and sensitivity analyses are needed to gauge the benefit more realistically. In particular, it was assumed that those who come for risk assessment are a random sample of the population, and that those who are offered the intervention will take it.

Table 10.5: Proportion of lives saved with risk-based allocation of mammograms, compared to giving mammograms to all women, if there is only enough money to give mammograms to half the women

Risk model	**Optimal $(g, p, m)^a$**	**Proportion of lives saved compared to giving mammograms to all women**	**Percent improvement versus random allocation**
Random allocation with no risk assessment		0.500	
BCRAT	(1, 0.48, 0)	0.632	26.4%
BCRAT+7SNPs	(1, 0.48, 0)	0.667	33.4%

[a]Abbreviations: g is the proportion of the population given a risk assessment; p is the proportion of those with risk assessment given a mammogram in descending order of risk; m is the proportion of those without a risk assessment who are given a mammogram.

Bibliography

Aalen, O. (1976). Nonparametric inference in connection with multiple decrement models. *Scandinavian Journal of Statistics*, 3:15–27.

Aalen, O., Borgan, O., and Gjessing, H. (2008). *Event History Analysis: A Process Point of View*. Springer-Verlag, New York.

Aalen, O. O. (1978). Nonparametric inference for a family of counting processes. *Annals of Statistics*, 6(4):701–726.

Aalen, O. O. (1989). A linear regression model for the analysis of life times. *Statistics in Medicine*, 8(8):907–925.

Albert, A. (1982). On the use and computation of likelihood ratios in clinical chemistry. *Clinical Chemistry*, 28(5):1113–1119.

Albertsen, P. C., Hanley, J. A., and Fine, J. (2005). 20-year outcomes following conservative management of clinically localized prostate cancer. *Journal of the American Medical Association*, 293(17):2095–2101.

Amir, E., Evans, D. G., Shenton, A., et al. (2003). Evaluation of breast cancer risk assessment packages in the family history evaluation and screening programme. *Journal of Medical Genetics*, 40(11):807–814.

Amir, E., Freedman, O. C., Seruga, B., and Evans, D. G. (2010). Assessing women at high risk of beast cancer: A review of risk asessment models. *Journal of the National Cancer Institute*, 102(10):680–691.

Andersen, P. K., Borgan, O., Gill, R., and Keiding, N. (1993). *Statistical Models Based on Counting Processes*. Springer Series in Statistics. Springer-Verlag, New York.

Andersen, P. K. and Keiding, N. (2012). Interpretability and importance of functionals in competing risks and multistate models. *Statistics in Medicine*, 31(11-12):1074–1088.

Andersen, P. K., Klein, J. P., and Rosthoj, S. (2003). Generalised linear models for correlated pseudo-observations, with applications to multi-state models. *Biometrika*, 90(1):15–27.

Andersen, P. K. and Perme, M. P. (2008). Inference for outcome probabilities in multistate models. *Lifetime Data Analysis*, 14(4):405–431.

Anderson, J. R., Cain, K. C., and Gelber, R. D. (1983). Analysis of survival by tumor response. *Journal of Clinical Oncology*, 1(11):710–719.

Anderson, T. W. (1984). *An Introduction to Multivariate Statistical Analysis, 2nd Edition*. Wiley, New York.

Andrinopoulou, E. R., Rizopoulos, D., Takkenberg, J. J., and Lesaffre, E. (2014). Joint modeling of two longitudinal outcomes and competing risk data. *Statistics in Medicine*, 33(18):3167–78.

Ankerst, D. P., Groskopf, J., Day, J. R., et al. (2008). Predicting prostate cancer risk through incorporation of prostate cancer gene 3. *Journal of Urology*, 180(4):1303–1308.

Ankerst, D. P., Koniarski, T., Liang, Y., et al. (2012). Updating risk prediction tools: A case study in prostate cancer. *Biometrical Journal*, 54(1):127–142.

Antoniou, A., Pharoah, P. D. P., Narod, S., et al. (2003). Average risks of breast and ovarian cancer associated with BRCA1 or BRCA2 mutations detected in case series unselected for family history: A combined analysis of 22 studies. *American Journal of Human Genetics*, 72(5):1117–1130.

Antoniou, A. C., Cunningham, A. P., Peto, J., et al. (2008a). The BOADICEA model of genetic susceptibility to breast and ovarian cancers: updates and extensions. *British Journal of Cancer*, 98(8):1457–1466.

Antoniou, A. C. and Easton, D. F. (2003). Polygenic inheritance of breast cancer: Implications for design of association studies. *Genetic Epidemiology*, 25(3):190–202.

Antoniou, A. C., Hardy, R., Walker, L., et al. (2008b). Predicting the likelihood of carrying a BRCA1 or BRCA2 mutation: validation of BOADICEA, BRCAPRO, IBIS, Myriad and the Manchester scoring system using data from UK genetics clinics. *Journal of Medical Genetics*, 45(7):425–431.

Antoniou, A. C., Pharoah, P. D. P., McMullan, G., et al. (2002). A comprehensive model for familial breast cancer incorporating BRCA1, BRCA2 and other genes. *British Journal of Cancer*, 86(1):76–83.

Antoniou, A. C., Pharoah, P. P. D., Smith, P., and Easton, D. F. (2004). The BOADICEA model of genetic susceptibility to breast and ovarian cancer. *British Journal of Cancer*, 91(8):1580–1590.

Armstrong, G. T. (2010). Long-term survivors of childhood central nervous system malignancies: The experience of the childhood cancer survivor study. *European Journal of Paediatric Neurology*, 14(4):298–303.

Baker, S. G., Cook, N. R., Vickers, A., and Kramer, B. S. (2009). Using relative utility curves to evaluate risk prediction. *Journal of the Royal Statistical Society Series A*, 172(4):729–748.

Bakoyannis, G., Siannis, F., and Touloumi, G. (2010). Modelling competing risks data with missing cause of failure. *Statistics in Medicine*, 29(30):3172–3185.

Begg, C. B. (2002). On the use of familial aggregation in population-based case probands for calculating penetrance. *Journal of the National Cancer Institute*, 94(16):1221–1226.

Benichou, J. and Gail, M. H. (1990a). Estimates of absolute cause-specific risk in cohort studies. *Biometrics*, 46(3):813–826.

Benichou, J. and Gail, M. H. (1990b). Variance calculations and confidence intervals for estimates of the attributable risk based on logistic models. *Biometrics*, 46(4):991–1003.

Benichou, J. and Gail, M. H. (1995). Methods of inference for estimates of absolute risk derived from population-based case-control studies. *Biometrics*, 51(1):182–194.

Berk, R., Brown, L., Buja, A., Zhang, K., and Zhao, L. (2013). Valid post-selection inference. *Annals of Statistics*, 41(2):802–837.

Berry, D. A., Parmigiani, G., Sanchez, J., Schildkraut, J., and Winer, E. (1997). Probability of carrying a mutation of breast-ovarian cancer gene BRCA1 based on family history. *Journal of the National Cancer Institute*, 89(3):227–238.

Beyersmann, J., M., S., and Allignol, A. (2012). *Competing Risks and Multistate Models with R*. Springer, New York.

Beyersmann, J. and Schumacher, M. (2008). Time-dependent covariates in the proportional subdistribution hazards model for competing risks. *Biostatistics*, 9(4):765–776.

Binder, D. A. (1983). On the variances of asymptotically normal estimators from complex surveys. *International Statistical Review*, 51(3):279–292.

Binder, D. A. (1992). Fitting Cox's proportional hazards models from survey data. *Biometrika*, 79(1):139–147.

Binder, N., Gerds, T. A., and Andersen, P. K. (2014). Pseudo-observations for competing risks with covariate dependent censoring. *Lifetime Data Analysis*, 20(2):303–315.

Blanche, P., Proust-Lima, C., Loubere, L., et al. (2015). Quantifying and comparing dynamic predictive accuracy of joint models for longitudinal marker and time-to-event in presence of censoring and competing risks. *Biometrics*, 71(1):102–113.

Bondy, M. L., Lustbader, E. D., Halabi, S., Ross, E., and Vogel, V. G. (1994). Validation of a breast-cancer risk assessment model in women with a positive family history. *Journal of the National Cancer Institute*, 86(8):620–625.

Borgan, O., Goldstein, L., and Langholz, B. (1995). Methods for the analysis of sampled cohort data in the Cox proportional hazards model. *Annals of Statistics*, 23(5):1749–1778.

Brier, G. W. (1950). Verification of forecasts expressed in terms of probability. *Monthly Weather Review*, 78:1–3.

Bruzzi, P., Green, S. B., Byar, D. P., Brinton, L. A., and Schairer, C. (1985). Estimating the population attributable risk for multiple risk-factors using case-control data. *American Journal of Epidemiology*, 122(5):904–913.

Cai, T., Tian, L., Uno, H., Solomon, S. D., and Wei, L. J. (2010). Calibrating parametric subject-specific risk estimation. *Biometrika*, 97(2):389–404.

Chatterjee, N., Chen, Y. H., Maas, P., and Carroll, R. J. (2016). Constrained maximum likelihood estimation for model calibration using summary-level information from external big data sources. *Journal of the American Statistical Association*, 111(513):107–117.

Chatterjee, N., Hartge, P., and Wacholder, S. (2003). Adjustment for competing risk in kin-cohort estimation. *Genetic Epidemiology*, 25(4):303–313.

Chatterjee, N., Kalaylioglu, Z., Shih, J. H., and Gail, M. H. (2006). Case-control and case-only designs with genotype and family history data: Estimating relative risk, residual familial aggregation, and cumulative risk. *Biometrics*, 62(1):36–48.

Chatterjee, N., Kalayliouglu, Z., Shih, J. H., and Gail, M. (2007). Letter to the editor of Biometrics - reply. *Biometrics*, 63(3):965–966.

Chatterjee, N. and Wacholder, S. (2001). A marginal likelihood approach for estimating penetrance from kin-cohort designs. *Biometrics*, 57(1):245–252.

Chatterjee, N., Wheeler, B., Sampson, J., et al. (2013). Projecting the performance of risk prediction based on polygenic analyses of genome-wide association studies. *Nature Genetics*, 45(4):400–405.

Chen, H. Y. and Little, R. J. A. (1999). Proportional hazards regression with missing covariates. *Journal of the American Statistical Association*, 94(447):896–908.

Chen, J. B., Pee, D., Ayyagari, R., et al. (2006a). Projecting absolute invasive breast cancer risk in white women with a model that includes mammographic density. *Journal of the National Cancer Institute*, 98(17):1215–1226.

Chen, S. N. and Parmigiani, G. (2007). Meta-analysis of BRCA1 and BRCA2 penetrance. *Journal of Clinical Oncology*, 25(11):1329–1333.

Chen, Y. Q., Hu, C. C., and Wang, Y. (2006b). Attributable risk function in the proportional hazards model for censored time-to-event. *Biostatistics*, 7(4):515–529.

Cheng, S. C., Fine, J. P., and Wei, L. J. (1998). Prediction of cumulative incidence function under the proportional hazards model. *Biometrics*, 54(1):219–228.

Chiang, C. (1968). *Nonparametric Inference for a Family of Counting Processes.* Wiley, New York.

Claus, E. B., Risch, N., and Thompson, W. D. (1991). Genetic-analysis of breast-cancer in the cancer and steroid-hormone study. *American Journal of Human Genetics*, 48(2):232–242.

Claus, E. B., Risch, N., and Thompson, W. D. (1994). Autosomal-dominant inheritance of early-onset breast-cancer - implications for risk prediction. *Cancer*, 73(3):643–651.

Claus, E. B., Schildkraut, J., Iversen, E. S., Berry, D., and Parmigiani, G. (1998). Effect of BRCA1 and BRCA2 on the association between breast cancer risk and family history. *Journal of the National Cancer Institute*, 90(23):1824–1829.

Colditz, G. A. and Hankinson, S. E. (2005). The Nurses' Health Study: Lifestyle and health among women. *Nature Reviews Cancer*, 5(5):388–396.

Colditz, G. A. and Rosner, B. (2000). Cumulative risk of breast cancer to age 70 years according to risk factor status: data from the Nurses' Health Study. *America Journal of Epidemiology*, 152(10):950–64.

Conjeevaram, H. S., Fried, M. W., Jeffers, L. J., et al. (2006). Peginterferon and ribavirin treatment in African American and Caucasian American patients with hepatitis C genotype 1. *Gastroenterology*, 131(2):470–477.

Consonni, D., Pierobon, M., Gail, M. H., et al. (2015). Lung cancer prognosis before and after recurrence in a population-based setting. *Journal of the National Cancer Institute*, 107(6):djv059.

Cook, N. R. (2007). Use and misuse of the receiver operating characteristic curve in risk prediction. *Circulation*, 115(7):928–935.

Cook, N. R., Buring, J. E., and Ridker, P. M. (2006). The effect of including C-reactive protein in cardiovascular risk prediction models for women. *Annals of Internal Medicine*, 145(1):21–29.

Copas, J. B. (1987). Cross-validation shrinkage of regression predictors. *Journal of the Royal Statistical Society Series B-Methodological*, 49(2):175–183.

Cortese, G. and Andersen, P. K. (2010). Competing risks and time-dependent covariates. *Biometrical Journal*, 52(1):138–158.

Cortese, G., Gerds, T. A., and Andersen, P. K. (2013). Comparing predictions among competing risks models with time-dependent covariates. *Statistics in Medicine*, 32(18):3089–3101.

Costantino, J. P., Gail, M. H., Pee, D., et al. (1999). Validation studies for models projecting the risk of invasive and total breast cancer incidence. *Journal of the National Cancer Institute*, 91(18):1541–1548.

Cox, C. S., Rothwell, S. T., Madans, J. H., et al. (1992). Plan and operation of the NHANES I Epidemiologic Followup Study, 1987. *Vital and Health Statistics Series 1*, 27:1–190.

Cox, D. R. (1958). 2 futher applications of a model for binary regression. *Biometrika*, 45(3-4):562–565.

Cox, D. R. (1959). The analysis of exponentially distributed life-times with two types of failure. *Journal of the Royal Statistical Society. Series B (Methodological)*, 21(2):411–421.

Cox, D. R. (1972). Regression models and life-tables. *Journal of the Royal Statistical*

Society Series B-Statistical Methodology, 34(2):187–202.

Cox, D. R. (1975). Partial likelihood. *Biometrika*, 62(2):269–276.

Cramer, H. (1947). *Mathematical Methods of Statistics.* Princeton University Press, Princeton, NJ.

Dabrowska, D. M. (1995). Estimation of transition probabilities and bootstrap in a semiparametric markov renewal model. *Nonparametric Statistics*, 5:237–259.

D'Agostino, R. B., Grundy, S., Sullivan, L. M., and Wilson, P. (2001). Validation of the Framingham coronary heart disease prediction scores: results of a multiple ethnic groups investigation. *Journal of the American Medical Association*, 286(2):180–7.

Datta, S. and Satten, G. A. (2001). Validity of the Aalen-Johansen estimators of stage occupation probabilities and Nelson-Aalen estimators of integrated transition hazards for non-Markov models. *Statistics and Probability Letters*, 55(4):403–411.

Davison, A. C. and Hinkley, D. V. (1997). *Bootstrap Methods and their Application:.* Cambridge University Press, Cambridge.

de Una-Alvarez, J. and Meira-Machado, L. (2015). Nonparametric estimation of transition probabilities in the non-markov illness-death model: A comparative study. *Biometrics*, 71(2):364–375.

de Wreede, L. C., Fiocco, M., and Putter, H. (2010). The mstate package for estimation and prediction in non- and semi-parametric multi-state and competing risks models. *Computer Methods and Programs in Biomedicine*, 99(3):261–274.

de Wreede, L. C., Fiocco, M., and Putter, H. (2011). mstate: An R package for the analysis of competing risks and multi-state models. *Journal of Statistical Software*, 38(7):1–30.

Delong, E. R., Delong, D. M., and Clarkepearson, D. I. (1988). Comparing the areas under 2 or more correlated receiver operating characteristic curves - a nonparametric approach. *Biometrics*, 44(3):837–845.

Demler, O. V., Pencina, M. J., and D'Agostino, R. B. (2012). Misuse of Delong test to compare AUCs for nested models. *Statistics in Medicine*, 31(23):2577–2587.

Demnati, A. and Rao, J. N. K. (2010). Linearization variance estimators for model parameters from complex survey data. *Survey Methodology*, 36(2):193–201.

Deville, J. C. (1999). Variance estimation for complex statistics and estimators: linearization and residual techniques. *Survey Methodology*, 25(2):193–204.

Dinse, G. E. (1986). Nonparametric prevalence and mortality estimators for animal-experiments with incomplete cause-of-death data. *Journal of the American Statistical Association*, 81(394):328–336.

Dupuy, A. and Simon, R. M. (2007). Critical review of published microarray studies for cancer outcome and guidelines on statistical analysis and reporting. *Journal of the National Cancer Institute*, 99(2):147–157.

Easton, D. F., Ford, D., Bishop, D. T., et al. (1995). Breast and ovarian-cancer incidence in BRCA1-mutation carriers. *American Journal of Human Genetics*, 56(1):265–271.

Efron, B. (1978). Regression and ANOVA with zero-one data - measures of residual variation. *Journal of the American Statistical Association*, 73(361):113–121.

Efron, B. (1986). How biased is the apparent error rate of a prediction rule. *Journal of the American Statistical Association*, 81(394):461–470.

Efron, B. (2014). Estimation and accuracy after model selection. *Journal of the American Statistical Association*, 109(507):991–1007.

Elashoff, R. M., Li, G., and Li, N. (2008). A joint model for longitudinal measurements and survival data in the presence of multiple failure types. *Biometrics*, 64(3):762–71.

Expert Panel on Detection and Evaluation and Treatment of High Blood Cholesterol in Adults (2001). Executive summary of the third report of the national cholesterol education program (NCEP) expert panel on detection, evaluation, and treatment of high blood cholesterol in adults (Adult Treatment Panel III). *Journal of the American Medical Association*, 285(19):2486–2497.

Fan, J. and Li, R. (2001). Variable selection via nonconcave penalized likelihood and its oracle properties. *Journal of the American Statistical Association*, 96(456):1348–1360.

Fan, J. and Li, R. (2002). Variable selection for Cox's proportional hazards model and frailty model. *Annals of Statistics*, 30(1):74–99.

Feigl, P. and Zelen, M. (1965). Estimation of exponential survival probabilities with concomitant information. *Biometrics*, 21(4):826–838.

Ferrer, L., Rondeau, V., Dignam, J., et al. (2016). Joint modelling of longitudinal and multi-state processes: Application to clinical progressions in prostate cancer. *Statistics in Medicine*, 35(22):3933–3948.

Fine, J. P. (1999). Analysing competing risks data with transformation models. *Journal of the Royal Statistical Society. Series B: Statistical Methodology*, 61(4):817–830.

Fine, J. P. (2001). Regression modeling of competing crude failure probabilities. *Biostatistics*, 2(1):85–97.

Fine, J. P. and Gray, R. J. (1999). A proportional hazards model for the subdistribution of a competing risk. *Journal of the American Statistical Association*, 94(446):496–509.

Fisher, B., Costantino, J. P., Wickerham, D. L., et al. (1998). Tamoxifen for prevention of breast cancer: Report of the national surgical adjuvant breast and bowel project P-1 study. *Journal of the National Cancer Institute*, 90(18):1371–1388.

Fisher, R. A. (1918). The correlation between relatives on the supposition of mendelian inheritance. *Transactions of the Royal Society of Edinburgh*, 52:399–433.

Fitzmaurice, G. M., Kenward, M. G., Molenberghs, G., Verbeke, G., and Tsiatis, A. A. (2015). Missing Data: Introduction and Preliminaries, pages 3–22. *Handbooks of Modern Statistical Methods*. CRC Press, Taylor and Francis Group, Chapman and Hall, Boca Raton, FL.

Ford, D., Easton, D. F., Stratton, M., et al. (1998). Genetic heterogeneity and penetrance analysis of the BRCA1 and BRCA2 genes in breast cancer families. *American Journal of Human Genetics*, 62(3):676–689.

Freedman, A. N., Yu, B. B., Gail, M. H., et al. (2011). Benefit/risk assessment for breast cancer chemoprevention with raloxifene or tamoxifen for women age 50 years or older. *Journal of Clinical Oncology*, 29(17):2327–2333.

Friedman, J., Hastie, T., and Tibshirani, R. (2010). Regularization paths for generalized linear models via coordinate descent. *Journal of Statistical Software*, 33(1):1–22.

Friedman, M. (1982). Piecewise exponential models for survival-data with covariates. *Annals of Statistics*, 10(1):101–113.

Gail, M. (1975). Review and critique of some models used in competing risk analysis. *Biometrics*, 31(1):209–222.

Gail, M. and Chatterjee, N. (2004). Some biases that may affect kin-cohort studies for estimating the risks from identified disease genes. In Lin, D. Y. and J., H. P., editors, *Proceedings of the Second Seattle Symposium in Biostatistics: Analysis of Correlated*

Data, pages 175–187, New York. Springer.

Gail, M. and Rimer, B. (1998). Risk-based recommendations for mammographic screening for women in their forties. *Journal of Clinical Oncology*, 16(9):3105–3114.

Gail, M. H. (2008a). Discriminatory accuracy from single-nucleotide polymorphisms in models to predict breast cancer risk. *Journal of the National Cancer Institute*, 100(14):1037–1041.

Gail, M. H. (2008b). Estimation and interpretation of models of absolute risk from epidemiologic data, including family-based studies. *Lifetime Data Analysis*, 14(1):18–36.

Gail, M. H. (2009a). Applying the Lorenz curve to disease risk to optimize health benefits under cost constraints. *Statistics and Its Interface*, 2(2):117–121.

Gail, M. H. (2009b). Value of adding single-nucleotide polymorphism genotypes to a breast cancer risk model. *Journal of the National Cancer Institute*, 101(13):959–963.

Gail, M. H. (2011). Personalized estimates of breast cancer risk in clinical practice and public health. *Statistics in Medicine*, 30(10):1090–1104.

Gail, M. H. (2012). Using multiple risk models with preventive interventions. *Statistics in Medicine*, 31(23):2687–2696.

Gail, M. H., Brinton, L. A., Byar, D. P., et al. (1989). Projecting individualized probabilities of developing breast cancer for white females who are being examined annually. *Journal of the National Cancer Institute*, 81(24):1879–86.

Gail, M. H., Costantino, J. P., Bryant, J., et al. (1999a). Weighing the risks and benefits of tamoxifen treatment for preventing breast cancer. *Journal of the National Cancer Institute*, 91(21):1829–1846.

Gail, M. H., Costantino, J. P., Pee, D., et al. (2007). Projecting individualized absolute invasive breast cancer risk in african american women. *Journal of the National Cancer Institute*, 99:1782–1792.

Gail, M. H. and Mai, P. L. (2010). Comparing breast cancer risk assessment models. *Journal of the National Cancer Institute*, 102(10):665–668.

Gail, M. H., Pee, D., Benichou, J., and Carroll, R. (1999b). Designing studies to estimate the penetrance of an identified autosomal dominant mutation: Cohort, case-control, and genotyped-proband designs. *Genetic Epidemiology*, 16(1):15–39.

Gail, M. H., Pee, D., and Carroll, R. (2001). Effects of violations of assumptions on likelihood methods for estimating the penetrance of an autosomal dominant mutation from kin-cohort studies. *Journal of Statistical Planning and Inference*, 96(1):167–177.

Gail, M. H., Pee, D., and D. Carroll, R. (1999c). Kin-cohort designs for gene characterization. *Journal of the National Cancer Institute Monographs*, 26:55–60.

Gail, M. H. and Pfeiffer, R. M. (2005). On criteria for evaluating models of absolute risk. *Biostatistics*, 6(2):227–39.

Gail, M. H., Pfeiffer, R. M., Wheeler, W., and Pee, D. (2008). Probability of detecting disease-associated single nucleotide polymorphisms in case-control genome-wide association studies. *Biostatistics*, 9(2):201–215.

Gail, M. H. and Schairer, C. (2010). Comments and response on the uspstf recommendation on screening for breast cancer. *Annals of Internal Medicine*, 152(8):540.

Gao, G. Z. and Tsiatis, A. A. (2005). Semiparametric estimators for the regression coefficients in the linear transformation competing risks model with missing cause of failure. *Biometrika*, 92(4):875–891.

Garcia-Closas, M., Gunsoy, N. B., and Chatterjee, N. (2014). Combined associations of genetic and environmental risk factors: implications for prevention of breast cancer. *Journal of the National Cancer Institute*, 106(11). doi: 10.1093/jnci/dju305.

Gaynor, J. J., Feuer, E. J., Tan, C. C., et al. (1993). On the use of cause-specific failure and conditional failure probabilities: Examples from clinical oncology data. *Journal of the American Statistical Association*, 88(422):400–409.

Gerds, T. A., Andersen, P. K., and Kattan, M. W. (2014). Calibration plots for risk prediction models in the presence of competing risks. *Statistics in Medicine*, 33(18):3191–3203.

Gerds, T. A., Cai, T. X., and Schumacher, M. (2008). The performance of risk prediction models. *Biometrical Journal*, 50(4):457–479.

Gerds, T. A., Scheike, T. H., and Andersen, P. K. (2012). Absolute risk regression for competing risks: Interpretation, link functions, and prediction. *Statistics in Medicine*, 31(29):3921–3930.

Gerds, T. A., Scheike, T. H., Blanche, P., and Ozenne, B. (2017). riskregression: Risk regression models and prediction scores for survival analysis with competing risks. *CRAN R Project.*

Geskus, R. B. (2011). Cause-specific cumulative incidence estimation and the Fine and Gray model under both left truncation and right censoring. *Biometrics*, 67(1):39–49.

Geskus, R. B. (2016). *Data Analysis with Competing Risks and Intermediate States.* Chapman and Hall/CRC Biostatistics Series. CRC Press, Taylor and Francis Group.

Ghoussaini, M. and Pharoah, P. D. P. (2009). Polygenic susceptibility to breast cancer: current state-of-the-art. *Future Oncology*, 5(5):689–701.

Gini, C. (1912). Variabilita e mutabilita. *Studi Economico-Giuridici dell'Universita di Cagliari*, 3:1–158.

Giraud, C. (2015). *Introduction to High-Dimensional Statistics*, volume 139 of *Monographs on Statistics and Applied Probability.* CRC Press, Taylor and Francis Group, Chapman and Hall, Boca Raton, FL.

Gneiting, T. and Raftery, A. E. (2007). Strictly proper scoring rules, prediction, and estimation. *Journal of the American Statistical Association*, 102(477):359–378.

Goetghebeur, E. and Ryan, L. (1995). Analysis of competing risks survival data when some failure types are missing. *Biometrika*, 82(4):821–833.

Goldie, C. M. (1977). Convergence theorems for empirical Lorenz curves and their inverses. *Advances in Applied Probability*, 9(4):765–791.

Gong, G., Quante, A. S., Terry, M. B., and Whittemore, A. S. (2014). Assessing the goodness of fit of personal risk models. *Statistics in Medicine*, 33(18):3179–3190.

Graf, E., Schmoor, C., Sauerbrei, W., and Schumacher, M. (1999). Assessment and comparison of prognostic classification schemes for survival data. *Statistics in Medicine*, 18(17-18):2529–2545.

Graubard, B. I. and Fears, T. R. (2005). Standard errors for attributable risk for simple and complex sample designs. *Biometrics*, 61(3):847–855.

Graubard, B. I., Flegal, K. M., Williamson, D. F., and Gail, M. H. (2007). Estimation of attributable number of deaths and standard errors from simple and complex sampled cohorts. *Statistics in Medicine*, 26(13):2639–2649.

Gray, R. J. (1988). A class of k-sample tests for comparing the cumulative incidence of a competing risk. *The Annals of Statistics*, 16(3):1141–1154.

Gray, R. J. (2009). Weighted analyses for cohort sampling designs. *Lifetime Data Analysis*, 15(1):24–40.

Greenland, S. and Drescher, K. (1993). Maximum-likelihood-estimation of the attributable fraction from logistic-models. *Biometrics*, 49(3):865–872.

Greenwood, M. (1926). The natural duration of cancer. *Reports on Public Health and Medical Subjects. London: Her Majesty's Stationery Office*, 33:126.

Grill, S., Ankerst, P. A., Gail, M. H., Chatterjee, N., and Pfeiffer, R. M. (2016). Comparison of approaches for incorporating new information into existing risk prediction models. *Statistics in Medicine*, 99(99):99–999.

Ha, J. and Tsodikov, A. (2015). Semiparametric estimation in the proportional hazard model accounting for a misclassified cause of failure. *Biometrics*, 71(4):941–949.

Hall, J. M., Lee, M. K., Newman, B., et al. (1990). Linkage of early-onset familial breast-cancer to chromosome-17q21. *Science*, 250(4988):1684–1689.

Hampel, F. R. (1974). Influence curve and its role in robust estimation. *Journal of the American Statistical Association*, 69(346):383–393.

Han, P. and Lawless, J. F. (2016). Comment. *Journal of the American Statistical Association*, 111(513):118–121.

Hand, D. J. and Yu, K. (2001). Idiot's Bayes - not so stupid after all? *International Statistical Review*, 69(3):385–398.

Harrell, F. E. J. (2001). *Regression Modeling Strategies. With Applications to Linear Models, Logistic Regression, and Survivial Analysis.* Springer Series in Statistics. Springer-Verlag, New York.

Hartmann, L. C., Sellers, T. A., Frost, M. H., et al. (2005). Benign breast disease and the risk of breast cancer. *New England Journal of Medicine*, 353(3):229–237.

Hastie, T., Tibshirani, R., and Friedman, J. (2009). *The elements of statistical learning, data mining, inference and prediction.* Springer-Verlag, New York.

Heagerty, P. J., Lumley, T., and Pepe, M. S. (2000). Time-dependent ROC curves for censored survival data and a diagnostic marker. *Biometrics*, 56(2):337–344.

Heagerty, P. J. and Zheng, Y. Y. (2005). Survival model predictive accuracy and ROC curves. *Biometrics*, 61(1):92–105.

Henderson, R. and Keiding, N. (2005). Individual survival time prediction using statistical models. *Journal of Medical Ethics*, 31(12):703–706.

Hilden, J. and Gerds, T. A. (2014). A note on the evaluation of novel biomarkers: do not rely on integrated discrimination improvement and net reclassification index. *Statistics in Medicine*, 33(19):3405–3414.

Hopper, J. L., Southey, M. C., Dite, G. S., et al. (1999). Australian breast cancer family study. population-based estimate of the average age-specific cumulative risk of breast cancer for a defined set of protein-truncating mutations in BRCA1 and BRCA2. *Cancer Epidemiology Biomarkers and Prevention*, 8(9):741–747.

Hosmer, D. W. and Lemeshow, S. (1980). Goodness of fit tests for the multiple logistic regression-model. *Communications in Statistics Part A-Theory and Methods*, 9(10):1043–1069.

Huang, X., Li, G., Elashoff, R. M., and Pan, J. (2011). A general joint model for longitudinal measurements and competing risks survival data with heterogeneous random effects. *Lifetime Data Analysis*, 17(1):80–100.

Iversen, E. S. and Chen, S. N. (2005). Population-calibrated gene characterization: Estimating age at onset distributions associated with cancer genes. *Journal of the American Statistical Association*, 100(470):399–409.

Jackson, C. H. (2011). Multi-state models for panel data: The msm package for R.

Journal of Statistical Software, 38(8):1–28.

Janes, H., Pepe, M. S., and Gu, W. (2008). Assessing the value of risk predictions by using risk stratification tables. *Annals of Internal Medicine*, 149(10):751–760.

Janes, H., Pepe, M. S., and Huang, Y. (2014). A framework for evaluating markers used to select patient treatment. *Medical Decision Making*, 34(2):159–167.

Janssens, A. C. J. W., Deng, Y., Borsboom, G. J. J. M., et al. (2005). A new logistic regression approach for the evaluation of diagnostic test results. *Medical Decision Making*, 25(2):168–177.

Jeong, J. H. (2014). *Statistical Inference on Residual Life*. Statistics for Biology and Health. Springer, New York.

Jewell, N. P. and Kalbfleisch, J. D. (1996). Marker processes in survival analysis. *Lifetime Data Analysis*, 2(1):15–29.

Jewell, N. P. and Nielsen, J. P. (1993). A framework for consistent prediction rules based on markers. *Biometrika*, 80(1):153–164.

Kalbfleisch, J. D. and Prentice, R. L. (2002). *The Statistical Analysis of Failure Time Data*. Wiley, Hoboken, NJ.

Kang, S., Cai, J., and Chambless, L. (2013). Marginal additive hazards model for case-cohort studies with multiple disease outcomes: an application to the Atherosclerosis Risk in Communities (ARIC) study. *Biostatistics*, 14(1):28–41.

Kaplan, E. L. and Meier, P. (1958). Nonparametric estimation from incomplete observations. *Journal of the American Statistical Association*, 53(282):457–481.

Katki, H. A., Schiffman, M., Castle, P. E., et al. (2013). Benchmarking CIN3+ risk as the basis for incorporating HPV and Pap cotesting into cervical screening and management guidelines. *Journal of Lower Genital Tract Disease*, 17(supplement):S28–35.

Kenward, M. G. and Carpenter, J. (2007). Multiple imputation: current perspectives. *Statistical Methods in Medical Research*, 16(3):199–218.

Kerr, K. F., Wang, Z., Janes, H., et al. (2014). A critical review. *Epidemiology*, 25(1):114–121.

Khudyakov, P., Gorfine, M., Zucker, D., and Spiegelman, D. (2015). The impact of covariate measurement error on risk prediction. *Statistics in Medicine*, 34(15):2353–2367.

Klein, J. P. and Andersen, P. K. (2005). Regression modeling of competing risks data based on pseudovalues of the cumulative incidence function. *Biometrics*, 61(1):223–229.

Klein, J. P., Keiding, N., and Copelan, E. A. (1993). Plotting summary predictions in multistate survival models - probabilities of relapse and death in remission for bone-marrow transplantation patients. *Statistics in Medicine*, 12(24):2315–2332.

Korn, E. L. and Graubard, B. I. (1999). *Analysis of Health Surveys*. Wiley series in probability and statistics. Wiley, New York.

Korn, E. L. and Simon, R. (1990). Measures of explained variation for survival-data. *Statistics in Medicine*, 9(5):487–503.

Korn, E. L. and Simon, R. (1991). Explained residual variation, explained risk, and goodness of fit. *American Statistician*, 45(3):201–206.

Kovalchik, S. A. and Pfeiffer, R. M. (2013). Population-based absolute risk estimation with survey data. *Lifetime Data Analysis*, 12(459):721–741.

Kovalchik, S. A., Ronckers, C. M., Veiga, L. H. S., et al. (2013a). Absolute risk prediction of second primary thyroid cancer among 5-year survivors of childhood cancer. *Journal of Clinical Oncology*, 31(1):119–127.

Kovalchik, S. A., Tammemagi, M., Berg, C. D., et al. (2013b). Targeting of low-dose CT screening according to the risk of lung-cancer death. *New England Journal of Medicine*, 369(3):245–254.

Kraft, P. and Thomas, D. C. (2000). Bias and efficiency in family-based gene-characterization studies: Conditional, prospective, retrospective, and joint likelihoods. *American Journal of Human Genetics*, 66(3):1119–1131.

Kupper, L. L., McMichael, A. J., and Spirtas, R. (1975). A hybrid epidemiologic study design useful in estimating relative risk. *Journal of the American Statistical Association*, 70(351):524–528.

Lagakos, S. W., Sommer, C. J., and Zelen, M. (1978). Semi-markov models for partially censored data. *Biometrika*, 65(2):311–317.

Langholz, B. and Borgan, O. (1997). Estimation of absolute risk from nested case-control data. *Biometrics*, 53(2):767–774.

Langholz, B. and Thomas, D. C. (1990). Nested case-control and case-cohort methods of sampling from a cohort: A critical comparison. *American Journal of Epidemiology*, 131(1):169–176.

Langholz, B. and Thomas, D. C. (1991). Efficiency of cohort sampling designs: Some surprising results. *Biometrics*, 47(4):1563–1571.

Latouche, A., Porcher, R., and Chevret, S. (2005). A note on including time-dependent covariate in regression model for competing risks data. *Biometrical Journal*, 47(6):807–814.

Lee, M., Cronin, K. A., Gail, M. H., Dignam, J. J., and Feuer, E. J. (2011). Multiple imputation methods for inference on cumulative incidence with missing cause of failure. *Biometrical Journal*, 53(6):974–993.

Lee, M., Cronin, K. A., Gail, M. H., and Feuer, E. J. (2012). Predicting the absolute risk of dying from colorectal cancer and from other causes using population-based cancer registry data. *Statistics in Medicine*, 31(5):489–500.

Leeb, H. (2005). The distribution of a linear predictor after model selection: Conditional finite-sample distributions and asymptotic approximations. *Journal of Statistical Planning and Inference*, 134(1):64–89.

Lemeshow, S. and Hosmer, D. W. (1982). A review of goodness of fit statistics for use in the development of logistic-regression models. *American Journal of Epidemiology*, 115(1):92–106.

Li, Y., Tian, L., and Wei, L. J. (2011). Estimating subject-specific dependent competing risk profile with censored event time observations. *Biometrics*, 67(2):427–435.

Liao, J. G. and McGee, D. (2003). Adjusted coefficients of determination for logistic regression. *American Statistician*, 57(3):161–165.

Liddell, F. D. K., McDonald, J. C., and Thomas, D. C. (1977). Methods of cohort analysis - appraisal by application to asbestos mining. *Journal of the Royal Statistical Society Series A-Statistics in Society*, 140(4):469–491.

Lin, D. Y. (2000). On fitting Cox's proportional hazards models to survey data. *Biometrika*, 87(1):37–47.

Lin, D. Y. and Ying, Z. (1993). Cox regression with incomplete covariate measurements. *Journal of the American Statistical Association*, 88(424):1341–1349.

Lin, D. Y. and Ying, Z. (1994). Semiparametric analysis of the additive risk model. *Biometrika*, 81(1):61–71.

Listwon-Krol, A. and Saint-Pierre, P. (2015). Multi-state semi-Markov models, version 1.4.1.

Liu, D., Zheng, Y., Prentice, R. L., and Hsu, L. (2014). Estimating risk with time-to-event data: An application to the women's health initiative. *Journal of the American Statistical Association*, 109(506):514–524.

Lloyd-Jones, D. M., Leip, E. P., Larson, M. G., et al. (2006). Prediction of lifetime risk for cardiovascular disease by risk factor burden at 50 years of age. *Circulation*, 113(6):791–798.

Lockhart, R., Taylor, J., Tibshirani, R. J., and Tibshirani, R. (2014). A significance test for the lasso. *Annals of Statistics*, 42(5):518–531.

Lorenz, M. O. (1905). Methods of measuring the concentration of wealth. *Publications of the American Statistical Association*, 9(70):209–219.

Lu, K. F. and Tsiatis, A. A. (2001). Multiple imputation methods for estimating regression coefficients in the competing risks model with missing cause of failure. *Biometrics*, 57(4):1191–1197.

Lu, W. B. and Liang, Y. (2008). Analysis of competing risks data with missing cause of failure under additive hazards model. *Statistica Sinica*, 18(1):219–234.

Luo, X. D., Tsai, W. Y., and Xu, Q. (2009). Pseudo-partial likelihood estimators for the Cox regression model with missing covariates. *Biometrika*, 96(3):617–633.

Maas, P., Barrdahl, M., and Joshi, A. D. e. a. (2016). Breast cancer risk from modifiable and nonmodifiable risk factors among white women in the United States. *JAMA Oncology*, 2(10):1295–1302.

Mann, H. B. and Whitney, D. R. (1947). On a test of whether one of two random variables is stochastically larger than the other. *The Annals of Mathematical Statistics*, 18(1):50–60.

Manson, J. E., Hsia, J., Johnson, K. C., et al. (2003). Estrogen plus progestin and the risk of coronary heart disease. *New England Journal of Medicine*, 349(6):523–534.

Mark, S. D. and Katki, H. (2001). Influence function based variance estimation and missing data issues in case-cohort studies. *Lifetime Data Analysis*, 7(4):331–344.

Mark, S. D. and Katki, H. A. (2006). Specifying and implementing nonparametric and semiparametric survival estimators in two-stage (nested) cohort studies with missing case data. *Journal of the American Statistical Association*, 101(474):460–471.

Martinussen, T., Holst, K. K., and Scheike, T. H. (2016). Cox regression with missing covariate data using a modified partial likelihood method. *Lifetime Data Analysis*, 22(4):570–588.

Matsuno, R. K., Costantino, J. P., Ziegler, R. G., et al. (2011). Projecting individualized absolute invasive breast cancer risk in Asian and Pacific Islander American women. *Journal of the National Cancer Institute*, 103(12):951–961.

McClish, D. K. (1989). Analyzing a portion of the ROC curve. *Medical Decision Making*, 9(3):190–195.

McDowell, A., Engel, A., Massey, J. T., and Maurer, K. (1981). Plan and operation of the Second National Health and Nutrition Examination Survey, 1976-1980. *Vital Health Statistics Series 1*, 15:1–114.

McNemar, Q. (1947). Note on the sampling error of the difference between correlated proportions or percentages. *Psychometrika*, 12(2):153–157.

Meinshausen, N., Meier, L., and Buehlmann, P. (2009). p-values for high-dimensional regression. *Journal of the American Statistical Association*, 104(488):1671–1681.

Meira-Machado, L., de Una-Alvarez, J., and Cadarso-Suarez, C. (2006). Nonparametric estimation of transition probabilities in a non-markov illness-death model. *Lifetime Data Analysis*, 12(3):325–344.

Mertens, A. C., Liu, Q., Neglia, J. P., et al. (2008). Cause-specific late mortality among 5-year survivors of childhood cancer: The childhood cancer survivor study. *Journal of the National Cancer Institute*, 100(19):1368–1379.

Metz, C. E. (1978). Basic priniciples of ROC analysis. *Seminars in Nuclear Medicine*, 8(4):283–298.

Michailidou, K., Hall, P., Gonzalez-Neira, A., et al. (2013). Large-scale genotyping identifies 41 new loci associated with breast cancer risk. *Nature Genetics*, 45(4):353–361.

Michaud, D. S., Midthune, D., Hermansen, S., Leitzmann, M., and Harlan, L. S. (2005). Comparison of cancer registry case ascertainment with SEER estimates and self-reporting in a subset of the NIH-AARP diet and health study. *Journal of Registry Management*, 32:70–75.

Miettinen, O. (1976). Estimability and estimation in case-referent studies. *American Journal of Epidemiology*, 103:226–235.

Molenberghs, G., Fitzmaurice, G., Kenward, M. G., Tsiatis, A., and Verbeke, A. G. (2015). *Handbook of Missing Data Methodology*. Handbooks of Modern Statistical Methods. CRC Press, Taylor and Francis Group, Chapman and Hall, Boca Raton, FL.

Molinaro, A. M., Simon, R., and Pfeiffer, R. M. (2005). Prediction error estimation: a comparison of resampling methods. *Bioinformatics*, 21(15):3301–3307.

Moreno-Betancur, M., Rey, G., and Latouche, A. (2015). Direct likelihood inference and sensitivity analysis for competing risks regression with missing causes of failure. *Biometrics*, 71(2):498–507.

Moskowitz, C. S. and Pepe, M. S. (2004). Quantifying and comparing the accuracy of binary biomarkers when predicting a failure time outcome. *Statistics in Medicine*, 23(10):1555–1570.

Nelson, W. (1969). Hazard plotting for incomplete failure data. *Journal of Quality Technology*, 1:27–52.

Nicolaie, M. A., van Houwelingen, H. C., and Putter, H. (2015). Vertical modelling: Analysis of competing risks data with missing causes of failure. *Statistical Methods in Medical Research*, 24(6):891–908.

Nicolaie, M. A., van Houwelingen, J. C., de Witte, T. M., and Putter, H. (2013a). Dynamic prediction by landmarking in competing risks. *Statistics in Medicine*, 32(12):2031–2047.

Nicolaie, M. A., van Houwelingen, J. C., de Witte, T. M., and Putter, H. (2013b). Dynamic pseudo-observations: A robust approach to dynamic prediction in competing risks. *Biometrics*, 69(4):1043–1052.

Oeffinger, K. C., Fontham, E. H., and Etzioni, R. e. a. (2015). Breast cancer screening for women at average risk: 2015 guideline update from the American Cancer Society. *Journal of the American Medical Association*, 314(15):1599–1614.

Olsen, J. H., Moller, T., Anderson, H., et al. (2009). Lifelong cancer incidence in 47 697 patients treated for childhood cancer in the Nordic countries. *Journal of the National Cancer Institute*, 101(11):806–813.

Omenn, G. S., Goodman, G. E., Thornquist, M. D., et al. (1996). Effects of a combination of beta carotene and vitamin A on lung cancer and cardiovascular disease. *New England Journal of Medicine*, 334(18):1150–1155.

Pace, L. E. and Keating, N. L. (2014). Risk and benefits of screening mammography. *JAMA-Journal of the American Medical Association*, 312(6):649–650.

Paik, M. C. and Tsai, W. Y. (1997). On using the Cox proportional hazards model with missing covariates. *Biometrika*, 84(3):579–593.

Parast, L., Cheng, S. C., and Cai, T. X. (2011). Incorporating short-term outcome information to predict long-term survival with discrete markers. *Biometrical Journal*, 53(2):294–307.

Parast, L., Cheng, S. C., and Cai, T. X. (2012). Landmark prediction of long-term survival incorporating short-term event time information. *Journal of the American Statistical Association*, 107(500):1492–1501.

Park, J. H., Gail, M. H., Greene, M. H., and Chatterjee, N. (2012). Potential usefulness of single nucleotide polymorphisms to identify persons at high cancer risk: an evaluation of seven common cancers. *Journal of Clinical Oncology*, 30(17):2157–62.

Pashayan, N., Duffy, S. W., Chowdhury, S., et al. (2011). Polygenic susceptibility to prostate and breast cancer: implications for personalised screening. *British Journal of Cancer*, 104(10):1656–1663.

Patterson, B. H., Dayton, C. M., and Graubard, B. I. (2002). Latent class analysis of complex sample survey data. *Journal of the American Statistical Association*, 97(459):721–741.

Pauker, S. G. and Kassirer, J. P. (1975). Therapeutic decision-making - cost-benefit analysis. *New England Journal of Medicine*, 293(5):229–234.

Pauker, S. G. and Kassirer, J. P. (1980). The threshold approach to clinical decision-making. *New England Journal of Medicine*, 302(20):1109–1117.

Peirce, C. S. (1884). The numerical measure of the success of predictions. *Science*, 4(93):453–454.

Pencina, M. J., D'Agostino, R. B., and Steyerberg, E. W. (2011). Extensions of net reclassification improvement calculations to measure usefulness of new biomarkers. *Statistics in Medicine*, 30(1):11–21.

Pencina, M. J., D'Agostino, R. B., and Vasan, R. S. (2008). Evaluating the added predictive ability of a new marker: From area under the ROC curve to reclassification and beyond. *Statistics in Medicine*, 27(2):157–172.

Pepe, M. S. (2003). *The Statistical Evaluation of Medical Tests for Classification and Prediction*. Oxford University Press, New York.

Pepe, M. S., Fan, J., Feng, Z., Gerds, T., and Hilden, J. (2015). The net reclassification index (NRI): A misleading measure of prediction improvement even with independent test data sets. *Statistics in Biosciences*, 7(2):282–295.

Pepe, M. S., Feng, Z., Huang, Y., et al. (2008). Integrating the predictiveness of a marker with its performance as a classifier. *American Journal of Epidemiology*, 167(3):362–368.

Pepe, M. S. and Janes, H. (2013). *Methods for Evaluating Prediction Performance of Biomarkers and Tests*, pages 107–142. Lecture Notes in Statistics: Proceedings. Springer, New York.

Pepe, M. S., Janes, H., and Li, C. I. (2014). Net risk reclassification p values: Valid or misleading? *Journal of the National Cancer Institute*, 106(4). doi: 10.1093/jnci/dju041.

Pepe, M. S., Kerr, K. F., Longton, G., and Wang, Z. (2013). Testing for improvement in prediction model performance. *Statistics in Medicine*, 32(9):1467–1482.

Pepe, M. S. and Mori, M. (1993). Kaplan-Meier, marginal or conditional-probability curves in summarizing competing risks failure time data. *Statistics in Medicine*, 12(8):737–751.

Petracci, E., Decarli, A., Schairer, C., et al. (2011). Risk factor modification and projections of absolute breast cancer risk. *Journal of the National Cancer Institute*, 103(13):1037–1048.

Pfeiffer, R. M. (2013). Extensions of criteria for evaluating risk prediction models for public health applications. *Biostatistics*, 14(2):366–381.

Pfeiffer, R. M. and Gail, M. H. (2011). Two criteria for evaluating risk prediction models. *Biometrics*, 67(3):1057–1065.

Pfeiffer, R. M., Gail, M. H., and Pee, D. (2001). Inference for covariates that accounts for ascertainment and random genetic effects in family studies. *Biometrika*, 88(4):933–948.

Pfeiffer, R. M., Park, Y., Kreimer, A. R., et al. (2013). Risk prediction for breast, endometrial, and ovarian cancer in white women aged 50 y or older: Derivation and validation from population-based cohort studies. *PLoS Med*, 10(7):e1001492.

Pfeiffer, R. M. and Petracci, E. (2011). Variance computations for functionals of absolute risk estimates. *Statistics & Probability Letters*, 81(7):807–812.

Pharoah, P. D. P., Antoniou, A., Bobrow, M., et al. (2002). Polygenic susceptibility to breast cancer and implications for prevention. *Nature Genetics*, 31(1):33–36.

Pintilie, M. (2006). *Competing Risks : A Practical Perspective*. John Wiley & Sons, Ltd, Chichester, UK.

Pires, A. M. and Branco, J. A. (2002). Partial influence functions. *Journal of Multivariate Analysis*, 83(2):451–468.

Pötscher, B. M. (1991). Effects of model selection on inference. *Econometric Theory*, 7(2):163–185.

Prentice, R. L. (1986). A case-cohort design for epidemiologic cohort studies and disease prevention trials. *Biometrika*, 73(1):1–11.

Prentice, R. L. (1989). Surrogate endpoints in clinical-trials - definition and operational criteria. *Statistics in Medicine*, 8(4):431–440.

Prentice, R. L., Kalbfleisch, J. D., Peterson, A. V., et al. (1978). Analysis of failure times in presence of competing risks. *Biometrics*, 34(4):541–554.

Preston, D. L., Lubin, J. H., Pierce, D. A., and McConney, M. E. (1993). *Epicure User's Guide*. Seattle, WA.

Proust-Lima, C., Dartigues, J. F., and Jacqmin-Gadda, H. (2016). Joint modeling of repeated multivariate cognitive measures and competing risks of dementia and death: a latent process and latent class approach. *Statistics in Medicine*, 35(3):382–398.

Proust-Lima, C., Sene, M., Taylor, J. M. G., and Jacqmin-Gadda, H. (2014). Joint latent class models for longitudinal and time-to-event data: A review. *Statistical Methods in Medical Research*, 23(1):74–90.

Putter, H., Fiocco, M., and Geskus, R. B. (2007). Tutorial in biostatistics: Competing risks and multi-state models. *Statistics in Medicine*, 26(11):2389–2430.

Putter, H.and de Wreede, L. and Fiocco, M. (2014). Package 'mstate' : Data preparation, estimation and prediction in multi-state models. In the CRAN repository for R programs.

Qi, L. H., Wang, C. Y., and Prentice, R. L. (2005). Weighted estimators for proportional hazards regression with missing covariates. *Journal of the American Statistical Association*, 100(472):1250–1263.

Qin, J. (2000). Combining parametric and empirical likelihoods. *Biometrika*, 87(2):484–490.

Quante, A. S., Whittemore, A. S., Shriver, T., Strauch, K., and Terry, M. B. (2012). Breast cancer risk assessment across the risk continuum: genetic and nongenetic risk factors contributing to differential model performance. *Breast Cancer Research*, 14(6). doi: 10.1198/1186/bcr3352.

Rao, J. N. K. and Scott, A. J. (1987). On simple adjustments to chi-square tests with sample survey data. *Annals of Statistics*, 15(1):385–397.

Rebolledo, R. (1980). Central limit theorems for local martingales. *Zeitschrift für Wahrscheinlichkeitstheorie und Verwandte Gebiete*, 51(3):269–286.

Redmond, C. K. and Costantino, J. P. (1996). *Design and current status of the NSABP breast cancer prevention trial*, pages 309–317. Adjuvant Therapy of Breast Cancer V: in series on Recent Results in Cancer Research. Springer-Verlag, Heidelberg.

Reid, N. and Crepeau, H. (1985). Influence functions for proportional hazards regression. *Biometrika*, 72(1):1–9.

Reulen, R. C., Frobisher, C., Winter, D. L., et al. (2011). Long-term risks of subsequent primary neoplasms among survivors of childhood cancer. *Jama - Journal of the American Medical Association*, 305(22):2311–2319.

Risch, N. (1990). Linkage strategies for genetically complext traits. 1. multilocus models. *American Journal of Human Genetics*, 46(2):222–228.

Rizopoulos, D. (2012). *Joint Models for Longitudinal and Time-to-Event Data*. CRC Biostatistics Series. Chapman and Hall, Boca Raton.

Robins, J. M. and Rotnitzky, A. (1992). *Recovery of Information and Adjustment for Dependent Censoring using Surrogate Markers*, pages 297–331. AIDS Epidemiology-Methodological Issues. Birkhäuser, Boston.

Robison, L. L., Armstrong, G. T., Boice, J. D., et al. (2009). The childhood cancer survivor study: A National Cancer Institute-supported resource for outcome and intervention research. *Journal of Clinical Oncology*, 27(14):2308–2318.

Rockhill, B., Spiegelman, D., Byrne, C., Hunter, D. J., and Colditz, G. A. (2001). Validation of the Gail et al. model of breast cancer risk prediction and implications for chemoprevention. *Journal of the National Cancer Institute*, 93(5):358–366.

Rose, G. A. (1992). *The Strategy of Preventive Medicine*. Oxford University Press, Oxford.

Rosthoj, S., Andersen, P. K., and Abildstrom, S. Z. (2004). SAS macros for estimation of the cumulative incidence functions based on a Cox regression model for competing risks survival data. *Computer Methods and Programs in Biomedicine*, 74(1):69–75.

Rubin, D. B. (1976). Inference and missing data. *Biometrika*, 63(3):581–590.

Rubin, D. B. (1987). *Multiple Imputation for Nonresponse in Surveys*. Wiley, New York.

Saha, P. and Heagerty, P. J. (2010). Time-dependent predictive accuracy in the presence of competing risks. *Biometrics*, 66(4):999–1011.

Samuelsen, S. O. and Eide, G. E. (2008). Attributable fractions with survival data. *Statistics in Medicine*, 27(9):1447–1467.

SAS Institute Inc. (2011). *Base SAS 9.3 Procedures Guide*. SAS Institute, Cary, NC.

Saslow, D., Boetes, C., Burke, W., et al. (2007). American cancer society guidelines for breast screening with MRI as an adjunct to mammography. *Ca-a Cancer Journal for Clinicians*, 57(2):75–89.

Schairer, C., Mink, P. J., Carroll, L., and Devesa, S. S. (2004). Probabilities of death from breast cancer and other causes among female breast cancer patients. *Journal of the National Cancer Institute*, 96(17):1311–1321.

Schatzkin, A., Subar, A. F., Thompson, F. E., et al. (2001). Design and serendipity in establishing a large cohort with wide dietary intake distributions: The National Institutes of Health-American Association of Retired Persons diet and health study. *American Journal of Epidemiology*, 154(12):1119–1125.

Schaubel, D. E. and Wei, G. (2007). Fitting semiparametric additive hazards models using standard statistical software. *Biometrical Journal*, 49(5):719–730.

Scheike, T. H. and Zhang, M.-J. (2002). An additive-multiplicative Cox-Aalen regression model. *Scandinavian Journal of Statistics*, 29(1):75–88.

Scheike, T. H. and Zhang, M.-J. (2003). Extensions and applications of the Cox-Aalen survival model. *Biometrics*, 59(4):1036–1045.

Scheike, T. H. and Zhang, M. J. (2011). Analyzing competing risk data using the R timereg package. *Journal of Statistical Software*, 38(2):1–15.

Scheike, T. H., Zhang, M.-J., and Gerds, T. A. (2008). Predicting cumulative incidence probability by direct binomial regression. *Biometrika*, 95(1):205–220.

Schonfeld, S. J., Pee, D., Greenlee, R. T., et al. (2010). Effect of changing breast cancer incidence rates on the calibration of the Gail model. *Journal of Clinical Oncology*, 28(14):2411–2417.

Schoop, R., Graf, E., and Schumacher, M. (2008). Quantifying the predictive performance of prognostic models for censored survival data with time-dependent covariates. *Biometrics*, 64(2):603–610.

Self, S. G. and Prentice, R. L. (1988). Asymptotic distribution theory and efficiency results for case-cohort studies. *The Annals of Statistics*, 16(1):64–81.

Shah, B. V. (2002). Calculus of Taylor deviations. In *Joint Statistical Meetings, ASA*.

Shen, Y. and Cheng, S. C. (1999). Confidence bands for cumulative incidence curves under the risk model. *Biometrics*, 55(4):1093–1100.

Shi, M., Taylor, J. M., and Munoz, A. (1996). Models for residual time to AIDS. *Lifetime Data Analysis*, 2(1):31–49.

Simon, R. and Makuch, R. W. (1984). A non-parametric graphical representation of the relationship between survival and the occurrence of an event - application to responder versus non-responder bias. *Statistics in Medicine*, 3(1):35–44.

Simon, R. M., Paik, S., and Hayes, D. F. (2009). Use of archived specimens in eevaluation of prognostic and predictive biomarkers. *Journal of the National Cancer Institute*, 101(21):1446–1452.

Sorensen, P. and Andersen, P. K. (2000). Competing risks analysis of the case-cohort design. *Biometrika*, 87(1):49–59.

Spiegelhalter, D. J. and Knill-Jones, R. P. (1984). Statistical and knowledge-based approaches to clinical decision-support systems, with an application in gastroenterology. *Journal of the Royal Statistical Society. Series A*, 147(1):35–77.

Spiegelman, D., Colditz, G. A., Hunter, D., and Hertzmark, E. (1994). Validation of the Gail et-al model for predicting individual breast-cancer risk. *Journal of the National Cancer Institute*, 86(8):600–607.

StataCorp. (2015). *Stata Statistical Software: Release 14*. StataCorp L, College Station, TX.

Steliarova-Foucher, E., Stiller, C., Kaatsch, P., et al. (2004). Geographical patterns and time trends of cancer incidence and survival among children and adolescents in Europe since the 1970s (the ACCIS project): An epidemiological study. *Lancet*, 364(9451):2097–2105.

Sterne, J. A. C., White, I. R., Carlin, J. B., et al. (2009). Multiple imputation for missing data in epidemiological and clinical research: potential and pitfalls. *British Medical Journal*, 338:b2393. doi: 10.1136/bmj.b2393.

Steyerberg, E. W. (2009). *Clinical Prediction Models. A Practical Approach to Development, Validation, and Updating.* Springer Series in Statistics for Biology and Health. Springer-Verlag, New York.

Steyerberg, E. W., Borsboom, G., van Houwelingen, H. C., Eijkemans, M. J. C., and Habbema, J. D. F. (2004). Validation and updating of predictive logistic regression models: a study on sample size and shrinkage. *Statistics in Medicine*, 23(16):2567–2586.

Steyerberg, E. W., Eijkemans, M. J. C., Harrell, F. E., and Habbema, J. D. F. (2000). Prognostic modelling with logistic regression analysis: a comparison of selection and estimation methods in small data sets. *Statistics in Medicine*, 19(8):1059–1079.

Stone, N. J., Robinson, J. G., Lichtenstein, A. H., et al. (2014). 2013 ACC/AHA guideline on the treatment of blood cholesterol to reduce atherosclerotic cardiovascular risk in adults. a report of the American College of Cardiology/American Heart Association Task Force on Practice Guidelines. *Journal of the American College of Cardiology*, 63(25):2889–2934.

Struewing, J. P., Hartge, P., Wacholder, S., et al. (1997). The risk of cancer associated with specific mutations of BRCA1 and BRCA2 among Ashkenazi Jews. *New England Journal of Medicine*, 336(20):1401–1408.

Svahn-Tapper, G., Garwicz, S., Anderson, H., et al. (2006). Radiation dose and relapse are predictors for development of second malignant solid tumors after cancer in childhood and adolescence: A population-based case-control study in the five Nordic countries. *Acta Oncologica*, 45(4):438–448.

Taylor, J. M. G., Park, Y., Ankerst, D. P., et al. (2013). Real-time individual predictions of prostate cancer recurrence using joint models. *Biometrics*, 69(1):206–213.

Therneau, T. M. and Grambsch, P. M. (2000). *Modeling Survival Data: Extending the Cox Model.* Statistics for Biology and Health. Springer, New York.

Tibshirani, R. (1996). Regression shrinkage and selection via the Lasso. *Journal of the Royal Statistical Society Series B-Methodological*, 58(1):267–288.

Tice, J. A., Cummings, S. R., Smith-Bindman, R., et al. (2008). Using clinical factors and mammographic breast density to estimate breast cancer risk: development and validation of a new predictive model. *Annals of Internal Medicine*, 148(5):337–47.

Travis, L. B., Hill, D., Dores, G. M., et al. (2005). Cumulative absolute breast cancer risk for young women treated for Hodgkin lymphoma. *Journal of the National Cancer Institute*, 97(19):1428–1437.

Tsiatis, A. (1975). Nonidentifiability aspect of problem of competing risks. *Proceedings of the National Academy of Sciences of the United States of America*, 72(1):20–22.

Tsiatis, A. A. (1980). A note on a goodness-of-fit test for the logistic regression-model. *Biometrika*, 67(1):250–251.

Tsiatis, A. A. (2005). Competing risks. In Armitage, P. and Colton, T., editors, *Encyclopedia of Biostatistics*, volume 2, pages 1025–1035. John Wiley & Sons, Ltd., Chichester.

Tsiatis, A. A. and Davidian, M. (2004). Joint modeling of longitudinal and time-to-event data: An overview. *Statistica Sinica*, 14(3):809–834.

Tucker, M. A., Jones, P. H. M., Boice Jr., J. D., et al. (1991). Therapeutic radiation at a young age is linked to secondary thyroid cancer. *Cancer Research*, 51(11):2885–2888.

Tyrer, J., Duffy, S. W., and Cuzick, J. (2005). A breast cancer prediction model incorporating familial and personal risk factors. *Statistics in Medicine*, 24(1):156–156.

Uno, H., Cai, T., Tian, L., and Wei, L. J. (2007). Evaluating prediction rules for t-year survivors with censored regression models. *Journal of the American Statistical Association*, 102(478):527–537.

USPTF (2009). Screening for breast cancer: U.S. Preventive Services Task Force recommendation statement. *Annals of Internal Medicine*, 151(10):716–26.

Van Calster, B. and Vickers, A. J. (2015). Calibration of risk prediction models: Impact on decision-analytic performance. *Medical Decision Making*, 35(2):162–169.

Van Calster, B., Vickers, A. J., Pencina, M. J., et al. (2013). Evaluation of markers and risk prediction models: Overview of relationships between NRI and decision-analytic measures. *Medical Decision Making*, 33(4):490–501.

van Houwelingen, H. C. (2000). Validation, calibration, revision and combination of prognostic survival models. *Statistics in Medicine*, 19(24):3401–3415.

van Houwelingen, H. C. (2007). Dynamic prediction by landmarking in event history analysis. *Scandinavian Journal of Statistics*, 34(1):70–85.

van Houwelingen, H. C., Bruinsma, T., Hart, A. A. M., van't Veet, L. J., and Wessels, L. F. A. (2006). Cross-validated Cox regression on microarray gene expression data. *Statistics in Medicine*, 25(18):3201–3216.

van Houwelingen, H. C. and Putter, H. (2008). Dynamic predicting by landmarking as an alternative for multi-state modeling: an application to acute lymphoid leukemia data. *Lifetime Data Analysis*, 14(4):447–463.

van Houwelingen, H. C. and Putter, H. (2012). *Dynamic Prediction in Clinical Survival Analysis*. Monographs on Statistics and Applied Probability. CRC Press, Taylor and Francis Group, Boca Raton, FL.

van Houwelingen, J. C. (2001). Shrinkage and penalized likelihood as methods to improve predictive accuracy. *Statistica Neerlandica*, 55(1):17–34.

Van Houwelingen, J. C. and Le Cessie, S. (1990). Predictive value of statistical models. *Statistics in Medicine*, 9(11):1303–25.

van Ravesteyn, N. T., Miglioretti, D. L., Stout, N. K., et al. (2012). Tipping the balance of benefits and harms to favor screening mammography starting at age 40 years: A comparative modeling study of risk. *Annals of Internal Medicine*, 156(9):609–617.

Vecchio, T. J. (1966). Predictive value of a single diagnostic test in unselected populations. *New England Journal of Medicine*, 274(21):1171–1173.

Verweij, P. J. M. and Van Houwelingen, H. C. (1994). Penalized likelihood in Cox regression. *Statistics in Medicine*, 13(23-24):2427–2436.

Viallon, V., Ragusa, S., Clavel-Chapelon, F., and Benichou, J. (2009). How to evaluate the calibration of a disease risk prediction tool. *Statistics in Medicine*, 28(6):901–16.

Vickers, A. J., Cronin, A. M., and Begg, C. B. (2011). One statistical test is sufficient for assessing new predictive markers. *BMC Medical Research Methodology*, 11:13.

Vickers, A. J. and Elkin, E. B. (2006). Decision curve analysis: A novel method for evaluating prediction models. *Medical Decision Making*, 26(6):565–574.

Vickers, A. J., Elkin, E. L., and Steyerberg, E. (2009). Net reclassification improvement and decision theory. *Statistics in Medicine*, 28(3):525–526.

Visvanathan, K., Chlebowski, R. T., Hurley, P., et al. (2009). American Society of

Clinical Oncology clinical practice guideline update on the use of pharmacologic interventions including tamoxifen, raloxifene, and aromatase inhibition for breast cancer risk reduction. *Journal of Clinical Oncology*, 27(19):3235–3258.

Wacholder, S., Hartge, P., Prentice, R., et al. (2010). Performance of common genetic variants in breast-cancer risk models. *New England Journal of Medicine*, 362(11):986–993.

Wacholder, S., Hartge, P., Struewing, J. P., et al. (1998). The kin-cohort study for estimating penetrance. *American Journal of Epidemiology*, 148(7):623–630.

Wang, C. Y. and Chen, H. Y. (2001). Augmented inverse probability weighted estimator for Cox missing covariate regression. *Biometrics*, 57(2):414–419.

Wasserman, L. and Roeder, K. (2009). High-dimensional variable selection. *Annals of Statistics*, 37(5 A):2178–2201.

Weinstein, M. C., Fineberg, H. V., S., E. A., et al. (1980). *Clinical Decision Analysis*. W.B. Saunders, Philadelphia.

Weiss, G. H. and Zelen, M. (1963). A stochastic model for interpretation of clinical trials. *Proceedings of the National Academy of Sciences of the United States of America*, 50(5):988–994.

Whittemore, A. S. (1997). Logistic regression of family data from case-control studies. *Biometrika*, 84(4):989–990.

Wieand, S., Gail, M. H., James, B. R., and James, K. L. (1989). A family of nonparametric statistics for comparing diagnostic markers with paired or unpaired data. *Biometrika*, 76(3):585–592.

Wilson, P. W. F., D'Agostino, R. B., Levy, D., et al. (1998). Prediction of coronary heart disease using risk factor categories. *Circulation*, 97(18):1837–1847.

Woodruff, R. S. (1971). Simple method for approximating variance of a complicated estimate. *Journal of the American Statistical Association*, 66(334):411–414.

Wooster, R., Neuhausen, S. L., Mangion, J., et al. (1994). Localization of a breast-cancer susceptibility gene, BRCA2, to chromosome 13q12-13. *Science*, 265(5181):2088–2090.

Wu, L. C., Grabaud, B. I., and Gail, M. H. (2012). Tipping the balance of benefits and harms to favor screening mammography starting at age 40 years. *Annals of Internal Medicine*, 157(8):597; author reply 597–8.

Wu, S. C. (1982). A semi-Markov model for survival-data with covariates. *Mathematical Biosciences*, 60(2):197–206.

Xu, Q., Paik, M. C., Luo, X. D., and Tsai, W. Y. (2009). Reweighting estimators for Cox regression with missing covariates. *Journal of the American Statistical Association*, 104(487):1155–1167.

Yates, J. F. (1982). External correspondence: Decompositions of the mean probability score. *Organizational Behavior and Human Performance*, 30(1):132–156.

Yu, M. G., Law, N. J., Taylor, J. M. G., and Sandler, H. M. (2004). Joint longitudinal-survival-cure models and their application to prostate cancer. *Statistica Sinica*, 14(3):835–862.

Zhang, D. D., Zhou, X.-H., Freeman Jr., D. H., and Freeman, J. L. (2002). A non-parametric method for the comparison of partial areas under ROC curves and its application to large health care data sets. *Statistics in Medicine*, 21(5):701–715.

Zhang, H. H. and Lu, W. (2007). Adaptive lasso for Cox's proportional hazards model. *Biometrika*, 94(3):691–703.

Zhang, X., Zhang, M.-J., and Fine, J. (2011). A proportional hazards regression model for the subdistribution with right-censored and left-truncated competing risks data. *Statistics in Medicine*, 30(16):1933–1951.

Zheng, Y., Cai, T., Jin, Y., and Feng, Z. (2012). Evaluating prognostic accuracy of biomarkers under competing risk. *Biometrics*, 68(2):388–396.

Zheng, Y. Y. and Heagerty, P. J. (2005). Partly conditional survival models for longitudinal data. *Biometrics*, 61(2):379–391.

Zhou, H. B. and Pepe, M. S. (1995). Auxiliary covariate data in failure time regression. *Biometrika*, 82(1):139–149.

Zöllner, S. and Pritchard, J. K. (2007). Overcoming the winner's curse: Estimating penetrance parameters from case-control data. *American Journal of Human Genetics*, 80(4):605–615.

Zuk, O., Hechter, E., Sunyaev, S. R., and Lander, E. S. (2012). The mystery of missing heritability: Genetic interactions create phantom heritability. *Proceedings of the National Academy of Sciences of the United States of America*, 109(4):1193–1198.

Index

D

J

K

L

M

N

O

P

R

S